Clinical
Veterinary
Language

Clinical Veterinary Language

Joann L. Colville, DVM
Retired, Veterinary Technology Program
North Dakota State University
Fargo, North Dakota

Sharon A. Oien, MT(ASCP)NM
Retired, School of Career and Continuing Education
University of Alaska, Fairbanks
Fairbanks, Alaska

ELSEVIER

3251 Riverport Lane
St. Louis, Missouri 63043

CLINICAL VETERINARY LANGUAGE

ISBN: 978-0-323-09602-7

Notices

Knowledge and best practice in this field are constantly changing. As new research and experience broaden our understanding, changes in research methods, professional practices, or medical treatment may become necessary.

Practitioners and researchers must always rely on their own experience and knowledge in evaluating and using any information, methods, compounds, or experiments described herein. In using such information or methods they should be mindful of their own safety and the safety of others, including parties for whom they have a professional responsibility.

With respect to any drug or pharmaceutical products identified, readers are advised to check the most current information provided (i) on procedures featured or (ii) by the manufacturer of each product to be administered, to verify the recommended dose or formula, the method and duration of administration, and contraindications. It is the responsibility of practitioners, relying on their own experience and knowledge of their patients, to make diagnoses, to determine dosages and the best treatment for each individual patient, and to take all appropriate safety precautions.

To the fullest extent of the law, neither the Publisher nor the authors, contributors, or editors, assume any liability for any injury and/or damage to persons or property as a matter of products liability, negligence or otherwise, or from any use or operation of any methods, products, instructions, or ideas contained in the material herein.

Library of Congress Cataloging-in-Publication Data

Colville, Joann.
   Clinical veterinary language / Joann L. Colville, Sharon A. Oien.
      p. ; cm.
   Includes bibliographical references and index.
   ISBN 978-0-323-09602-7 (pbk.)
   I. Oien, Sharon A.   II. Title.
   [DNLM: 1. Veterinary Medicine—Problems and Exercises.   2. Veterinary Medicine—
Terminology—English.   SF 610]
   SF610
   636.089001'4—dc23

2013010227

Vice President and Publisher: Linda Duncan
Content Strategy Director: Penny Rudolph
Content Manager: Shelly Stringer
Publishing Services Manager: Catherine Jackson
Project Manager: Rhoda Bontrager
Design Direction: Karen Pauls

Printed in China

Last digit is the print number: 9 8 7 6 5 4 3 2

PREFACE

Welcome to *Clinical Veterinary Language*. Our hope is that as you work your way through the book you will become comfortable with the "veterinary speak" that is used every day in veterinary medicine.

Why another medical terminology book? Between the two of us, we have several years of experience in teaching medical terminology to students studying in both the veterinary medical and human medical fields. One thing that struck us as we searched for relevant terminology textbooks was that many of the books currently available rely heavily on anatomy and physiology as their foundation for learning. They are, in effect, anatomy and physiology books in disguise. We wanted something different—a book that emphasizes learning and understanding the veterinary (medical) clinical language, not anatomy and physiology.

Early on we discovered that there is no way to separate anatomy from veterinary clinical language. Many attempts are sitting in virtual and real trashcans. What makes *Clinical Veterinary Language* different is that the emphasis in this book is not on learning individual bone names, how muscle groups work, or the details of digestion. While anatomy is an obvious starting point, we believe learning clinical veterinary language will become more relevant to you if it is associated with clinical applications. We want you to understand and interpret the words you will encounter as you begin a career in veterinary medicine as part of the veterinary team.

ORGANIZATION

Clinical Veterinary Language is divided into two sections. The first section, "Understanding Clinical Veterinary Language," concentrates on word parts, building and deconstructing medical terms, and explaining the importance of having a solid knowledge of clinical veterinary language. This section also introduces animal species, anatomic terms unique to veterinary medicine, directional and positional terms, and the organization of the body as a whole.

The second section, "Building the Clinical Veterinary Language," covers Chapters 4-15 and focuses on specific body systems. You will build a veterinary vocabulary (and a mythical animal) system by system starting from the outside with the skin of the animal, and going inward. In each chapter you will find:

- pronunciation guides to the word parts that are introduced in the chapter
- case studies that emphasize the word parts that are introduced in the chapter, as well as a review of word parts previously introduced
- brief introductions to the system functions by introducing word parts, prefixes, and suffixes
- brief introductions to the anatomy of each system by introducing word parts, prefixes, and suffixes
- tables of the clinical word roots, prefixes, and suffixes that are introduced in the chapter

    Each word part is accompanied by its definition, an example of a medical term that uses it, and a listing of the word parts used to create the term.
- tickets in the outer margins of the pages for each word part being introduced

    This will allow you to quickly find a word part and identify it as a prefix, suffix, or combining word form. These tickets are gold and red.
- numerous exercises throughout the chapters

    Exercises allow you to practice what you have learned so far. They include building words, defining terms, matching, and interpretation. Some of the exercises accompany case studies and others deal with information found in the text and tables. Throughout the exercises there will always be questions to help you review previous chapters' word parts.

- lists of terms that defy word analysis

    These terms are commonly used words, such as *laceration* and *abrasion*, that cannot be broken down into word parts to determine their meanings. They are terms that just have to be learned but with practice will become familiar to you.

- tables of abbreviations

    Many abbreviations are used in veterinary medicine. Rather than present them to you all at once in a separate chapter, we decided to give you a few at a time. The abbreviations are presented in tables in the same way as word parts and are accompanied by blue tickets in the outer margins of the page.

- answers to the exercise questions

    No looking in the back of the book for the answers. They are found at the end of each chapter.

In addition to these features you will also find scattered throughout the chapters "quick tips" to help you remember a word part. Light bulbs, exclamation points, and magnifying glasses are attention grabbers that present an interesting fact, warn of possible confusion, or help clarify a word part or concept.

The Appendices include:
- Combining Forms, Prefixes, and Suffixes Alphabetized According to Word Part
- Combining Forms, Prefixes, and Suffixes Alphabetized According to Definition
- Abbreviations
- Terms That Defy Word Analysis

LEARNING AIDS FOR THIS TEXT

Your goal in learning clinical veterinary language is to be able to divide complex terms into understandable component pieces (i.e., prefixes, combining forms, and suffixes). These pieces can then be shuffled and used in many other combinations to build an even larger clinical veterinary vocabulary.

Pronunciation System

Some clinical veterinary terms are hard to pronounce, especially if you have never heard them spoken. At the beginning of each chapter is a list of the word parts that are discussed in that chapter, along with their pronunciations. These word parts are represented as a prefix, combining form, or suffix. The notation for a prefix is the word part followed by a hyphen (e.g., poly-). The notation for a combining form (the word root and its vowel) is the word root followed by a forward slash (/) and its vowel (e.g., arthr/o). The notation for a suffix is a hyphen followed by the word part (e.g., -pathy).

The pronunciation system that we use is an easy method for mastering the sounds of clinical veterinary language. It is not overloaded with linguistic marks. The following rules apply:

1. Hyphens are used to separate syllables.
2. Any vowel with a dash above it represents the long sound:

ā	as in	sāy
ē	as in	mē
ī	as in	pīe
ō	as in	gō
ū	as in	ūniform

3. Any vowel that is followed by the letter "h" represents the short sound:

ah	as in	about
eh	as in	pet
ih	as in	pit
oh	as in	not
uh	as in	mutt

4. Unique vowel combinations are as follows:

aw	as in	caught
ər	as in	butter
oo	as in	loot
oy	as in	boy

5. Stressed syllables are noted in bold type, as in **class**-room. Terms that use the same word part may emphasize different syllables (e.g., hepatocyte = heh-**paht**-ō-**cīt** vs. hepatitis = **heh**-pah-**tī**-tuhs).

Phonetic spelling has no place in clinical veterinary language. Some word parts are pronounced alike, but they are spelled differently. This is because of their different meanings. For example, "hydr/o" and "hidr/o" have identical pronunciations (**hī**-drō). However, when *hydro* is found in a term, it means water, whereas *hidro* means sweat. In addition, even when terms are spelled correctly, incorrect pronunciation can lead to misunderstanding and possibly a wrong diagnosis. As an example, the tube leading from the urinary bladder to the outside of the body is the urethra (ū-**rē**-thrah), and the tube leading from one kidney to the urinary bladder is the ureter (**ūr**-eh-tər). These two structures are easily confused because their spellings and pronunciations are so similar.

Tickets

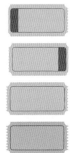

A yellow and red ticket is placed in the outer margin of the page for each word part that is discussed. Besides using hyphens and forward slashes to identify the various word parts, the design for each ticket is an additional clue to the type of word part. Because you would look for a prefix at the beginning (far left) of a word, a ticket with a red band to the left designates a prefix. A suffix is found at the end of a word (far right); thus the ticket with a red band at the right designates a suffix. Word roots and their combining vowels are found in the middle of words; their tickets are plain, with no red bands.

A blue ticket is placed in the outer margin of the page for each abbreviation that is discussed.

Road Signs

Signs are erected at the side of roads to provide information to road users. So it is with the road signs that you will find in the tables of this text. These signs, like any other traffic control devices, command attention and convey a clear and simple meaning.

That's Interesting

When you see the light bulb, you can expect to learn something. Oftentimes it will be a mnemonic that will aid your memory. Other times, the information is merely something interesting on the subject.

Clarify

The magnifying glass is used when information needs to be clarified, i.e., when a single word is not sufficient for a definition.

Watch Out!

The exclamation point on a sign is an indication to take heed, be careful, and think twice. Incorrect usage of clinical veterinary language can lead to misunderstanding and possibly a wrong diagnosis.

EVOLVE WEBSITE

Elsevier has created a website to support *Clinical Veterinary Language* (http://evolve.elsevier.com/Colville/vetlanguage). The website includes both student and instructor resources.

The Student Resources include:

- Interactive games
  - Hangman: guess the letters in a clinical veterinary word
  - Part Puzzler: practice dividing terms appropriately
  - Listen and Spell: hone your spelling skills as you listen to a word and then type it as you think it should appear
  - Word Shop: drag and drop word parts in the order necessary to create the correct term that matches its definition
- Flashcards: study word parts without having to create your own set!
- Audio Glossary: search for and listen to highlighted words from the text and their definitions

The Instructor Resources include:

- Image Collection: contains all of the images from the book
- Test Bank: 500 questions with answers and rationales
- PowerPoint lecture presentations
- Suggestions for classroom activities
- Access to all student resources

ACKNOWLEDGMENTS

Writing a textbook is not like writing a work of fiction. In fiction the author can write whatever comes to mind. In a textbook there must be accuracy, accountability, and completeness. When we set out to create *Clinical Veterinary Language* we knew we wanted to be as complete and accurate as possible. We also knew we couldn't do it all by ourselves. We would need help. And we found the best. These are the people without whose assistance and guidance this book would never have materialized.

- Teri Merchant, Content Manager, Elsevier (retired). Teri was our initial taskmaster, calendar watcher, and go-to answer person. She encouraged, nudged, and cajoled us into getting started with our endeavor. Then she retired from Elsevier.
- Shelly Stringer, Content Manager, Elsevier. Shelly stepped in when Teri retired, and the transition was very smooth. Now she is encouraging, nudging, and cajoling us into completing our project. If you're reading this, she succeeded.
- Burt Oien. If you ever want to test the effectiveness of your textbook, give it to a retired accounting professor and have him go through it as if he were a beginning veterinary student. He was invaluable in finding many things we took for granted or just plain overlooked. We also discovered a great proofreader.
- Tom Colville. He was our accuracy and completeness guy. After more than 40 years in the veterinary profession he provided the "it would make more sense or be more accurate if…" input. His other input included that of proofreader and devil's advocate. He exceled at both.
- Dawn Colville, artist. Dawn used her talent as an artist to create most of the original artwork in *Clinical Veterinary Language*. She took on the challenge of digital drawing and mastered it beautifully.
- Rhoda Bontrager, Project Manager, Elsevier. Rhoda was our deadline master. When *Clinical Veterinary Language* was finally written and submitted, she directed the editing process with efficiency and promptness. Rhoda and all her nameless, faceless assistants took what we thought was a pretty good book and made it better.

Disclaimer: We have tried to be as complete and accurate as possible in presenting terms that defy word analysis and abbreviations. Some regional terms or abbreviations may not be used where you work. Others that you are familiar with may not be included in our lists. The fault is ours alone and we welcome your input.

The Scribble Sisters
Joann Colville and Sharon Oien

CONTENTS

Chapter 1

Getting to Know Your Patients

Animals have their own language of purrs, barks, whinnies, moos, baas, oinks, bleats, hisses, squeaks, and peeps. As smart as we humans are, we have yet to become fluent in their language.

The Scribble Sisters

OUTLINE

ANIMAL SPECIES
- Cats = Feline
- Dogs = Canine
- Horses, Ponies, Donkeys, Mules, and Hinnies = Equine
- Cattle = Bovine
- Sheep = Ovine
- Goats = Caprine
- Pigs = Porcine = Swine
- Birds (commercial/domesticated) = Poultry = Avian
- Birds (companion animals) = Avian
- Rabbits = Lagomorph = Leporine
- Ferrets = Musteline
- Pocket Pets = Guinea Pigs, Hamsters, Gerbils, Mice, and Rats = Rodents

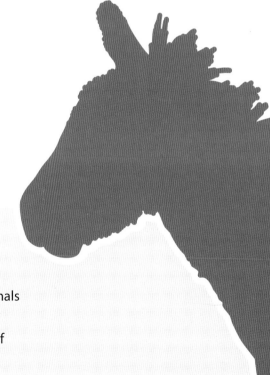

LEARNING OBJECTIVES

When you have completed this chapter, you will be able to:

1. Learn the common terms that have been developed to describe animals at various stages of their lives.

2. Identify the common terms used to indicate birthing and grouping of animals.

"People who work in human medicine have it easy because they have to work with only one species." Have you heard that before? Or how about this one? *"People in human medicine have to learn only one set of normal values for their patients."* Both statements are a bit exaggerated but to some degree true. However, people who work in human medicine do not get to pet their patients on the head; or rub their bellies; or run around with their patients tied on a lead rope/leash; or worry about getting kicked, bitten, run over, or scratched by their patients. When you work in veterinary medicine, you get to do all this and more.

Before you can learn the language of veterinary medicine, you have to know the patients of veterinary medicine. Your patients are real animals—literally.

ANIMAL SPECIES

It is true that you work with a variety of species in veterinary medicine. Any living nonhuman member of the Animal Kingdom is a potential patient. Over the years, one-word terms have been developed to describe animals at various stages of life, groups of animals, breeding capabilities, and the birthing process for different species of animals. These terms have universal meaning. The following lists are not all-inclusive. Many lists that are similar to these contain different or additional terms, especially for groups of animals. The following categories should include terms that appear on all or most of those lists. When you are working in the veterinary field, you should be familiar with these terms for the more common species that you will encounter.

Cats = Feline (fē-līn)

- A **tom** is an intact male. He has not been castrated/neutered and is capable of breeding a female.
- A **sire** is the male parent of his offspring.
- A **queen** is an intact female. She has not been spayed/neutered and can be bred, can go through pregnancy, and can give birth.
- A **dam** is the female parent of her offspring.
- A **kitten** is a young feline.
- **Queening** is the process of giving birth to kittens.
- A **litter** is a group of kittens born of the same pregnancy.
- A group of cats is called a **clowder,** a **cluster,** or a **pounce.**

Dogs = Canine (kā-nīn)

- A **dog/stud** is an intact male. He has not been castrated/neutered and is capable of breeding a female.
- A **sire** is the male parent of his offspring.
- A **bitch** is an intact female. She has not been spayed/neutered and can be bred, can go through pregnancy, and can give birth.
- A **dam** is the female parent of her offspring.
- A **whelp/pup** is a young canine.
- **Whelping** is the process of giving birth to whelps/pups.
- A **litter** is a group of whelps/pups born of the same pregnancy.
- A **pack** is a group of (usually) unrelated dogs. This term is used most commonly with wild adult dogs. A **kennel** is a group of domesticated dogs.

EXERCISE 1-1 *Meet Them!*

Fill in the shaded area as you compare the specific terms related to dogs and cats.

	The Dog	The Cat
1. The animal species		
2. An unrelated group of the species		
3. The female parent of her offspring		
4. The male parent of his offspring		
5. The young of the species (only one)		
6. The young of the species (a group born of the same pregnancy)		
7. A male that has not been neutered/castrated		
8. An intact male, capable of breeding with a female		
9. An intact female, capable of giving birth to young		
10. The process of giving birth to young		

Check your answers at the end of the chapter, Answers to Exercises.

Horses, Ponies, Donkeys, Mules, and Hinnies = Equine (ē-kwīn)

Horses

- A **stallion** is an intact male older than 4 years. He has not been castrated/neutered and is capable of breeding a female.
- A **gelding** is a castrated/neutered male horse.
- A **sire** is the male parent of his offspring.
- A **mare** is an intact female older than 4 years. She has not been spayed/neutered and can be bred, can go through pregnancy, and can give birth.
- A **dam** is the female parent of her offspring.
- A **colt** is an intact male younger than 4 years.
- A **filly** is an intact female younger than 4 years.
- A **foal** is what you call a young equine when you do not know the sex.
- A **weanling** is a young equine that has been weaned from its mother but is younger than 1 year.
- A **yearling** is an equine that is nearly or is just turning 1 year old.
- **Foaling** is the process of giving birth to a colt or filly.
- A group of horses is called a **herd, band, string, team,** or **stable.**

Ponies

- Ponies are adult horses that measure 8.2 to 14.2 hands.
  - **1 hand = 4 inches** at the withers (shoulder).

Donkeys

- Donkeys are long-eared members of the horse family.
- A donkey is also called an **ass** or a **burro.**
- A **jack** is an intact male. He has not been castrated/neutered and is capable of breeding a female.
- A **sire** is the male parent of his offspring.
- A **jenny** is an intact female. She has not been spayed/neutered and can be bred, can go through pregnancy, and can give birth.
- A **dam** is the female parent of her offspring.

Mules and Hinnies

- Mules and hinnies are the sterile (not able to reproduce) offspring of a horse and a donkey.
- A **mule** is the offspring of a jack and a mare.
- A **hinny** (**hih-nē**) is the offspring of a stallion and a jenny.
- A group of mules/hinnies is called a **barren** or a **span.**

EXERCISE 1-2 *Match It!*

The terms *dam* (female parent) and *sire* (male parent) are used to denote the parents for many species. However, when animals are bred, another one-word term may come into use. Match the term related to the sexual status or age of an equine with its definition.

_____ 1. Young equine younger than 1 year but weaned from its mother

_____ 2. Adult horse that measures 8.2 to 14.2 hands at the withers

_____ 3. Intact female horse, older than 4 years

_____ 4. What you call a young equine when you don't know the sex

_____ 5. Long-eared member of the horse family

_____ 6. Intact male horse, younger than 4 years

_____ 7. Sterile offspring of a male horse and a female donkey

_____ 8. Equine that is approximately 1 year old

_____ 9. Intact male donkey

_____ 10. Castrated/neutered male horse

colt

donkey

foal

gelding

hinny

jack

mare

pony

weanling

yearling

Check your answers at the end of the chapter, Answers to Exercises.

Cattle = Bovine (bō-vīn)

- A **bull** is an intact male. He has not been castrated/neutered and is capable of breeding a female.
- A **steer** is a castrated/neutered male bovine.
- A **sire** is the male parent of his offspring.
- A **cow** is an intact female. She has not been spayed/neutered (yes, you can spay a cow) and can be bred, can go through pregnancy, and can give birth.
- A **heifer** (hehf-ər) is a young cow that has not yet had her first calf.
- A **dam** is the female parent of her offspring.
- A **calf** is a young bovine.
- A **freemartin** is a (usually sterile) female calf born twin to a bull calf.
- **Calving** is the process of giving birth to calves.
- **Freshening** is the process of a dairy cow calving. This is when she starts being milked. The term is also used when a dairy goat gives birth to a baby goat.
- A **herd** is a group of cattle.

Sheep = Ovine (ō-vīn)

- A **ram** is an intact male. He has not been castrated/neutered and is capable of breeding a female.
- A **wether** (weh-thər) is a castrated/neutered male ovine.
- A **sire** is the male parent of his offspring.
- A **ewe** (yoo) is an intact female. She has not been spayed/neutered and can be bred, can go through pregnancy, and can give birth.
- A **dam** is the female parent of her offspring.
- A **lamb** is a young ovine.
- **Lambing** is the process of giving birth to lambs.
- A **flock** is a group of sheep.

Goats = Caprine (kah-prīn)

- A **buck** is an intact male. He has not been castrated/neutered and is capable of breeding a female.
- A **wether** is a castrated/neutered male caprine.
- A **sire** is the male parent of his offspring.
- A **doe** is an intact female. She has not been spayed/neutered and can be bred, can go through pregnancy, and can give birth.
- A **dam** is the female parent of her offspring.
- A **kid** is a young caprine.
- **Kidding** is the process of giving birth to kids.
- **Freshening** is the process whereby dairy goats give birth to kids. This is when the dairy goat starts to be milked. The term is also used with dairy cows in the process of calving.
- A **herd** is a group of goats.

Pigs = Porcine (pohr-sīn) = Swine

- A **boar** is an intact male. He has not been castrated/neutered and is capable of breeding a female.
- A **barrow** is a male that was castrated/neutered before sexual maturity.
- A **stag** is a male that was castrated/neutered after sexual maturity.
- A **sire** is the male parent of his offspring.
- A **sow** is an intact female. She has not been spayed/neutered and can be bred, can go through pregnancy, and can give birth.
- A **gilt** is a young female pig that has not yet given birth.
- A **dam** is the female parent of her offspring.
- A **pig** is a young porcine.
- **Farrowing** is the process of giving birth to pigs.
- All the pigs born of one pregnancy form a **litter.**
- A **herd** is a group of swine.

EXERCISE 1-3 *Same or Different?*

Fill in the squares to compare the specific terms related to cats from the left column with corresponding terms for horses, sheep, cows, and pigs.

The Cat	The Horse	The Sheep	The Cow	The Pig
1. feline				
2. queening				
3. neutered male				
4. sire				
5. kitten				
6. dam				
7. queen				
8. clowder				
9. tom				

Check your answers at the end of the chapter, Answers to Exercises.

Birds (commercial/domesticated) = Poultry = Avian (ā-vē-ən)

- Birds can be raised for meat, eggs, and feathers.
- Chickens, ducks, turkeys, and geese are the most important domestic poultry.

Chickens

- A **rooster** is an intact male. He has not been castrated/neutered and is capable of breeding a female. He is also known as a **cock.**
- A **cockerel** is a young male chicken between 10 and 32 weeks old.
- A **capon** is a castrated/neutered male chicken.
- A **hen** is an intact female. She has not been spayed/neutered. She can be bred and can lay viable (living, i.e., capable of developing chicks) eggs.
- A **pullet** is an immature female chicken between 10 and 32 weeks old.
- A **chick** is a very young chicken.
- A **broiler/fryer** is a meat-type chicken sent to market at 6.5 weeks old.
- A **roaster** is a meat-type chicken sent to market between 9 (males) and 11 (females) weeks old.
- A **layer** is an egg-type chicken over 32 weeks old.
- A **flock** is a group of chickens, a **brood** is a group of hens, and a **clutch** or a **peep** is a group of chicks.

Ducks

- A **drake** is an intact male. He has not been castrated/neutered and is capable of breeding a female.
- A **duck** is an intact female. She has not been spayed/neutered. She can be bred and can lay viable eggs. This term is also used to designate both sexes.
- A **duckling** is an immature duck of either sex.
- A group of ducks is called a **flock, bunch, brace, paddling,** or **raft.**

Turkeys

- A **tom** is an intact male. He has not been castrated/neutered and is capable of breeding a female.
- A **hen** is an intact female. She has not been spayed/neutered. She can be bred and can lay viable eggs.
- A **poult** is a young turkey of either sex.
- A group of turkeys is called a **rafter.**

Geese

- A **gander** is an intact male. He has not been castrated/neutered and is capable of breeding a female.
- A **goose** is an intact female. She has not been spayed/neutered. She can be bred and can lay viable eggs. This term is also used to designate both sexes.
- A **gosling** is an immature goose of either sex.
- A group of geese is called a **gaggle** or a **flock.**

Birds (companion animals) = Avian

- This group of birds consists of **Psittaciformes** (**siht**-ah-sih-**fohr**-mēz) and **Passeriformes** (**pahs**-ehr-ih-**fohr**-mēz).
- The Psittaciformes are the parrots, including lovebirds, parakeets (budgies), cockatiels, lories, lorikeets, and cockatoos.
- The Passeriformes are perching birds such as canaries, finches, and mynah birds plus just about all the birds you see at your backyard feeder or in the wild.
- A **cock** is an intact male companion bird. He has not been castrated/ neutered.
- A **hen** is an intact female companion bird. She has not been spayed/ neutered.
- A **chick** or a **hatchling** is a baby companion bird of either sex.
- A **gathering, company,** or **pandemonium** is a group of parrots.
- A group of Passeriformes can be called many things but most commonly will be called a **flock.**

EXERCISE 1-4 *Match It!*

Not all birds are equal. Decide from which group of avians listed on the right each bird in the list on the left belongs to. The first bird is identified as an example.

			Avians
1.	*geese*	gosling	chickens
2.		layer	companion birds
3.		drake	ducks
4.		pullet	geese
5.		capon	turkeys
6.		tom	
7.		cockerel	
8.		hatchling	
9.		poult	
10.		broiler/fryer	
11.		gander	
12.		duckling	

Check your answers at the end of the chapter, Answers to Exercises.

Rabbits = Lagomorph (lāg-ah-mohrf) = Leporine (lehp-ah-rīn)

- A **buck** or a **jack** is an intact male. He has not been castrated/neutered and is capable of breeding a female.
- A **doe** or a **jill** is an intact female. She has not been spayed/neutered. She can be bred, can go through pregnancy, and can give birth.
- A **kit, bunny,** or **kitten** is a young rabbit of either sex.
- A group of rabbits is called a **nest, trace, colony,** or **warren.**

Ferrets = Musteline (muhst-ah-līn)

- A **hob** is an intact male. He has not been castrated/neutered and is capable of breeding a female.
- A **gib** is a castrated/neutered male ferret.
- A **jill** is an intact female. She has not been spayed/neutered. She can be bred, can go through pregnancy, and can give birth.
- A **sprite** is a spayed/neutered female ferret.
- A **kit** is a young ferret of either sex.
- A group of ferrets is called a **business.**

Pocket Pets = Guinea Pigs, Hamsters, Gerbils, Mice, and Rats = Rodents

Guinea Pigs = Cavies (singular = cavy [kā-vē])

- A **boar** is an intact male. He has not been castrated/neutered and is capable of breeding a female.

- A **sow** is an intact female. She has not been spayed/neutered. She can be bred, can go through pregnancy, and can give birth.
- A **pup** is a young guinea pig of either sex.
- Giving birth is called **farrowing.**
- A **herd** is a group of guinea pigs.

Hamsters

- A **buck** is an intact male. He has not been castrated/neutered and is capable of breeding a female.
- A **doe** is an intact female. She has not been spayed/neutered. She can be bred, can go through pregnancy, and can give birth.
- A **pup** is a young hamster of either sex.
- A **horde** is a group of hamsters.

Gerbils

- A **buck** is an intact male. He has not been castrated/neutered and is capable of breeding a female.
- A **doe** is an intact female. She has not been spayed/neutered. She can be bred, can go through pregnancy, and can give birth.
- A **pup** is a young gerbil of either sex.
- A **horde** is a group of gerbils.

Mice and Rats = Murine (myoo-**rēn**)

- A **buck** is an intact male. He has not been castrated/neutered and is capable of breeding a female.
- A **doe** is an intact female. She has not been spayed/neutered. She can be bred, can go through pregnancy, and can give birth.
- A **pinkie, kitten,** or **pup** is a young mouse or rat of either sex.
- A **horde, nest,** or **colony** is a group of mice or rats.

EXERCISE 1-5 *Write It!*

Write a term in each blank to complete the sentence.

1. A _____ is an intact male gerbil.

2. The young mouse, rat, gerbil, guinea pig, and hamster are all called _____.

3. A pinkie is a _____.

4. Cavies are _____.

5. The term *murine* refers to _____.

6. _____ is the process that occurs when pigs and guinea pigs give birth.

7. A group of mice or rats is called a _____.

8. A doe is an _____. This means that she has not been spayed/neutered. She can be bred, can go through pregnancy, and can give birth.

9. Guinea pigs, hamsters, gerbils, mice, and rats all belong to the group called _____.

Check your answers at the end of the chapter, Answers to Exercises.

EXERCISE 1-6 *Who Has the Disease?*

Many animal species are susceptible to the same diseases that affect humans. In some cases, the disease is caused by the same virus or bacteria; in other cases, the disease sounds like a human disease but is completely different. In still other cases, animal diseases just have strange names. In the blank before each disease in the following list, write in the name of the species of animal that is susceptible to that disease. The first disease is done as an example.

1. _____horse_____ equine colic

2. _____ feline chin acne

3. _____ bovine herpesvirus 2

4. _____ canine viral hepatitis

5. _____ feline leprosy

6. _____ caprine herpesvirus 1

7. _____ bovine bonkers (a form of food poisoning)

8. _____ murine leukemia virus

9. _____ porcine hepatitis E virus

10. _____ ovine progressive pneumonia

11. _____ feline leukemia virus

12. _____ avian malaria

13. _____ equine influenza

14. _____ murine typhus

15. _____ porcine poliomyelitis

16. _____ equine infectious anemia

17. _____ porcine stress syndrome

18. _____ avian broodiness

19. _____ canine herpesvirus

20. _____ equine allergic rhinitis

Check your answers at the end of the chapter, Answers to Exercises.

EXERCISE 1-7 *Who Are We?*

Fill in the blank areas to identify the various members of the family. The young cat is done as an example.

Common Name of Offspring	Description	My Mother	My Father	My Species
1. kitten	young cat	queen	tom	feline
2. calf				
3.	young pig			
4.	young dog			
5. filly				
6.	female donkey			
7.			drake	
8.	young ferret			
9. mule				
10.				ovine
11.	immature goose			
12.	young rabbit			
13.		hen		
14. kid				
15.	young female pig			
16.				murine
17. gib				
18.				cavies
19.	young hamster			
20.			tom	
21. heifer				
22.	neutered female ferret			
23. capon				
24.	young gerbil			
25. chick				

Check your answers at the end of the chapter, Answers to Exercises.

ANSWERS TO EXERCISES

Exercise 1-1
1. canine; feline
2. pack/kennel (if domesticated); clowder/cluster/pounce
3. dam; dam
4. sire; sire
5. whelp/pup; kitten
6. litter/litter
7. dog/stud; tom
8. dog/stud; tom
9. bitch; queen
10. whelping; queening

Exercise 1-2
1. weanling
2. pony
3. mare
4. foal
5. donkey
6. colt
7. hinny
8. yearling
9. jack
10. gelding

Exercise 1-3
1. equine; ovine; bovine; porcine
2. foaling; lambing; calving; farrowing
3. gelding; wether; steer; barrow or stag
4. sire; sire; sire; sire
5. foal (if you do not know the sex); lamb; calf; pig
6. dam; dam; dam; dam
7. mare; doe; heifer; sow
8. herd/band/string/team/stable; flock; herd; herd
9. stallion; buck; bull; boar

Exercise 1-4
1. geese
2. chickens
3. ducks
4. chickens
5. chickens
6. turkeys
7. chickens
8. companion birds
9. turkeys
10. chickens
11. geese
12. ducks

Exercise 1-5
1. buck
2. pup
3. young mouse or rat
4. guinea pigs
5. mice and rats
6. farrowing
7. horde, nest, or colony
8. intact female
9. rodents

Exercise 1-6
1. horse
2. cat
3. cow
4. dog
5. cat
6. goat
7. cow
8. mouse or rat
9. pig
10. sheep
11. cat
12. bird
13. horse
14. mouse or rat
15. pig
16. horse
17. pig
18. bird
19. dog
20. horse

Exercise 1-7
1. *kitten, young cat, queen, tom, feline*
2. *calf*, young cow, cow, bull, bovine
3. pig, *young pig*, sow, boar, porcine
4. whelp, *young dog*, bitch, dog/stud, canine
5. *filly*, horse younger than 4 years, mare, stallion, equine
6. jenny, *female donkey*, dam, sire, equine
7. duckling, immature duck of either sex, duck, *drake*, avian
8. kit, *young ferret*, jill, hob, musteline
9. *mule*, offspring of horse and donkey, mare, jack, equine
10. lamb, young sheep, ewe, ram, *ovine*
11. gosling, *immature goose*, goose, gander, avian
12. kit/bunny/kitten, *young rabbit*, doe/jill, buck/jack, leporine
13. chick/hatchling, baby companion bird, *hen*, cock, avian
14. *kid*, young goat, doe, buck, caprine
15. gilt, *young female pig*, sow, boar, porcine
16. pinkie/kitten/pup, young mouse or rat, doe, buck, *murine*
17. *gib*, neutered male ferret, jill, hob, musteline
18. pup, young guinea pig, sow, boar, *cavies*
19. pup, *young hamster*, doe, buck, rodent
20. poult, young turkey, hen, *tom*, avian
21. *heifer*, young cow not yet had first calf, cow, bull, bovine
22. sprite, *neutered female ferret*, jill, hob, musteline
23. *capon*, castrated male chicken, hen, rooster/cock, avian
24. pup, *young gerbil*, doe, buck, rodent
25. *chick*, immature female chicken between 10 and 32 weeks old, hen, rooster, avian

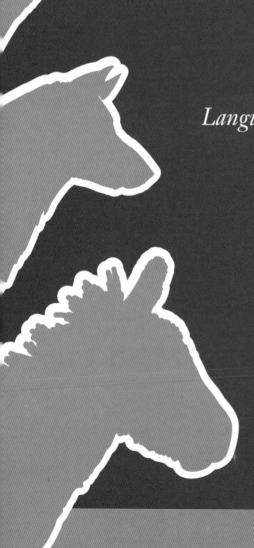

Chapter 2
Assembling a Framework

Language is the means of getting an idea from my brain into yours without surgery.

Mark Amidon

WORD PARTS

-a	ah	-gnosis	**nō**-sihs	-oid	oyd	-plasm	plahzm
-ac	ahck	hyster/o	**hihs**-tehr-ō	-ole	ohl	poly-	**pohl**-ē
-al	ahl	-ia	**ē**-ah	-oma	**ō**-mah	pro-	prō
-ant	ahnt	-ide	īd	oophor/o	ō-**ohff**-ohr-ō	salping/o	sahl-**ping**-ō
-ar	ahr	-ion	shun	-or	ohr	-sarcoma	**sahr-kō**-mah
arthr/o	**arth**-rō	-is	ihs	-ory	**ohr**-ē	-sion	shuhn
-ate	āt	-ism	ihsm	-ose	ōs	-sis	sihs
-ation	**ā**-shun	-ist	ihst	-osis	**ō**-sihs	somat/o	**sō**-mah-tō
chondr/o	**kohn**-drō	-itis	**ī**-tihs	oste/o	**ohs**-tē-ō	-stasis	**stā**-sihs
cost/o	**kohs**-tō	-ium	**ē**-uhm	-ous	uhs	-(t)ic	(t)ihck
dia-	**dī**-ah	-ive	ihv	ovari/o	ō-**vahr**-ē-ō	-tion	shuhn
dys-	dihs	-ize	īz	path/o	**pahth**-ō	-ule	ūhl
-ectomy	**ehck**-tō-mē	log/o	**lō**-gō	-pathy	**pahth**-ē	-um	uhm
eti/o	**ē**-tē-ō	-logy	**lō**-jē	-phyte	fīte	-y	ē
gen/o	**jehn**-ō	neo-	**nē**-ō	plas/o	**plā**-zō		

OUTLINE

LEARNING OBJECTIVES

When you have completed this chapter, you will be able to:

1. Understand the logic of the language of clinical veterinary medicine.

2. Identify and recognize the various parts of medical terms: prefixes, roots, combining forms, and suffixes.

3. Learn a system for analyzing medical terms to determine their meanings.

The Veterinary Healthcare Team

veterinarian
veterinary technician
veterinary assistant
receptionist
support staff

VETERINARY MEDICINE

If you are taking this course, you are probably interested in a career in veterinary medicine, the branch of medicine that deals with the health and welfare of nonhuman animals. That group consists of a lot of animals—everything from blue whales to baby mice. It is the obligation of the veterinary profession to keep animals healthy and to treat them when they are not. It takes an entire team to make this happen; no matter where on the team you sit, your job is vital. And if you are on the team, you have to be able to communicate with your fellow team members and with the public. For this, you need two languages: your native language and clinical veterinary language.

WHY LEARN CLINICAL VETERINARY LANGUAGE?

It is not everyday English, that is for sure. It is not really a foreign language either. So what is clinical veterinary language? It is a fabricated language, very much like its sister language—human medical language, which has evolved over the centuries. However, because veterinary medicine deals with a multitude of animal species, species-specific additions and exclusions are needed in clinical veterinary language. More than 95% of the words that constitute medical language are derived from Greek or Latin words. But do not worry—you do not need to know Greek or Latin to learn clinical veterinary language.

Learning clinical veterinary language at the beginning of your schooling will enable you to build and understand medical terms used in every other veterinary course. To begin with, you will learn how to construct, deconstruct, and analyze words that initially will be unfamiliar to you. When you complete your education, you will be able to read, write, and interpret medical records and laboratory reports; comprehend professional journal articles; and explain all of these to clients if necessary.

Some general words are introduced in Table 2-1 as a preview of things to come. These words are applicable to animal diseases and to veterinary medicine in general.

COMPONENTS OF MEDICAL TERMS

Components of Medical Terms

prefix
combining form (word root and combining vowel or word root alone)
suffix

Reading unfamiliar medical terms can be a daunting experience. If you come across **hysterosalpingo-oophorectomy** in a medical report, you are going to have to know what the word means. The best way to define the word is to deconstruct it, and for this, you have to know the component parts.

Word Root

The word root is the basis for the definition of the word. It tells you what the medical term is about. For example, in the word **arthropathy,** the word root is **arthr,** meaning "joint." When you read, "Dr. Frisbee is concerned that Sparky's limp is being caused by an *arthropathy*," you can identify the word root *arthr* and can determine that Dr. Frisbee thinks something is wrong with one of Sparky's joints.

Some medical terms have more than one word root. For example, if Sparky is exhibiting signs related to both a bone and a joint, Dr. Frisbee might suspect an **osteoarthropathy.** The word root for bone is **oste.** Adding *oste* to *arthr* allows you to identify a condition that involves two structures: a bone and a joint.

Suffix

The suffix is the ending of the word. It can be a syllable (e.g., -*y*), a group of syllables (e.g., -*pathy*), or a word. The suffix modifies the word root and gives it a specific meaning, usually to indicate a procedure, disease, condition, or disorder. In our "limping Sparky" example, the suffix at the end of the word is **-pathy,** which means "disease." Thus Sparky might be suffering from an *arthropathy* (a disease of a joint) or an *osteoarthropathy* (a disease of a bone and a joint).

arthr

oste

-pathy

TABLE 2-1 Words That Are Used with Animal Diseases

Word	Definition	Further Information
zoology	the study of animal life **zoo** *found in words indicates animals.*	Zoology is the branch of biology that relates to the Animal Kingdom, including the structure, embryology, evolution, classification, habits, and distribution of all animals, both living and extinct.
zoonosis (noun) **zoonotic** (adjective)	a disease transmitted from animals to humans	Rabies is a zoonotic disease because it is spread from animals to humans.
enzootic	a disease found in nearly every animal of a species within a limited geographical area; a disease embedded in an area that will occur naturally in unprotected animals	Enzootic pneumonia in dairy calves is found in nearly every calf within a single herd that is housed together, especially if they are indoors.
epizootic (***epidemic*** is the equivalent term in human medicine)	a disease that appears suddenly and spreads rapidly over a large geographical area like a state or country, affecting nearly all unprotected animals	Equine influenza is a viral disease that spreads rapidly throughout the horse population in a large geographical area. Foot and mouth disease in cattle can devastate the cattle industry, as happened in Great Britain in 2001.
morbidity	the number of animals in a population that become sick expressed as a percent of the entire population; also called the *morbidity rate*	The morbidity of enzootic pneumonia in unprotected dairy calves is nearly 100%.
mortality	the number of animals in a population that die from a disease, expressed as a percent of the entire population; also called the *mortality rate*	The mortality of enzootic pneumonia in unprotected dairy calves can be as low as 1%.
acute	sudden onset, and having a short duration	Equine influenza is an acute disease with a high morbidity rate in unprotected animals.
chronic	slow onset, or an abnormal condition that lasts a long time	Cancer can be a chronic disease.

When the suffix **-itis** (meaning "inflammation") is added to word roots, they take on new meanings. **Arthritis** (inflammation of a joint) and **osteoarthritis** (inflammation of a bone and a joint) denote two different diseases. Even though *arthropathy* (involving a joint) and *osteoarthropathy* (involving a bone and a joint) look and sound similar to *arthritis* and *osteoarthritis*, they are different diseases and would have to be recorded in a medical record accurately.

-itis

Combining Vowel

If you look closely at the word *arthropathy*, you will recall that *arthr* was identified as the word root pertaining to a joint, and *-pathy* as the suffix meaning "disease," but a vowel is left over. The **o** between *arthr* and *-pathy* is the combining vowel. A combining vowel is frequently used to link a word root to the suffix or to another word root. The most commonly used combining vowel is the *o*; the **a** is the second most commonly used combining vowel.

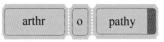

In the word *arthropathy*, the combining vowel *o* is used between the word root and the suffix, but in the term *arthritis* below, no combining vowel is used. There is actually a rule for that. If the suffix begins with a consonant (e.g., *-pathy*) a combining vowel is needed to link the word root to the suffix. If the suffix begins with a vowel (e.g., *-itis*), no combining vowel is needed to link the word root to the suffix.

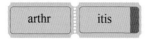

Using Combining Vowels

The *o* vowel is the most commonly used combining vowel.

Use a combining vowel if the suffix begins with a consonant (e.g., arthropathy).

No combining vowel is needed if the suffix begins with a vowel (e.g., arthritis).

A combining vowel is used to link two word roots even if the second word root begins with a vowel (e.g., osteoarthropathy).

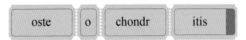

A combining vowel also is used to link two word roots. In the term **osteochondritis** (inflammation of bone and cartilage), the combining vowel *o* is used to link *oste* (bone [the first word root]) and *chondr* (cartilage [the second word root]). The combining vowel *o* is not used to link the word roots to the *-itis* suffix because *-itis* begins with a vowel.

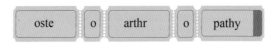

Regardless of whether the second word root begins with a vowel or a consonant, a combining vowel is always used to join the word roots. For example, in the term *osteoarthropathy* (disease of bone and a joint), the *o* combining vowel is used to link *oste* (bone) to *arthr* (joint). The suffix *-pathy* (disease) begins with a consonant, so a combining vowel is needed to link it to the word root.

Combining Form

When medical terms are analyzed and deconstructed into their component parts, the word root and the combining vowel are written together separated by a forward slash (/). This becomes the combining form to which modifiers (e.g., suffixes) are linked. If no combining vowel is needed, the word root becomes the combining form.

The word root for joint is *arthr*; the combining form is **arthr/o.**
The word root for bone is *oste*; the combining form is **oste/o.**
The word root for cartilage is *chondr*; the combining form is **chondr/o.**

When this method is used to deconstruct medical terms, the above examples of terms could be dissected for analysis as follows:

arthr/o/pathy
arthr/itis
oste/o/chondr/itis
oste/o/arthr/o/pathy

Prefix

A prefix is a modifier that can be linked to the front of a combining form or word root to change its meaning. It usually denotes a quantity, location, condition status, or time. Prefixes link directly to a combining form and do not need a combining vowel. If Sparky (Remember him? He was limping.) is exhibiting signs of arthritis in more than one joint, you would have to modify "arthritis" to indicate multiple joint involvement. In this case, **poly-** (meaning "much" or "many") is the appropriate prefix because it indicates that more than one joint is involved. **Polyarthritis** is the term that would be entered into the medical record. Dissected, the term looks like this: **poly/arthr/itis.**

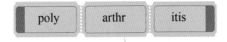

GUIDELINES FOR ANALYZING MEDICAL TERMS

Clinical veterinary language is more easily understood if you treat each medical word as a puzzle that you are attempting to solve. This process also allows for building a greater medical vocabulary when unfamiliar terms can be broken down into recognizable word parts. Just follow these simple guidelines:

1. First, divide the word into its basic component parts: prefix(es), root(s), combining vowel(s), and suffix(es).

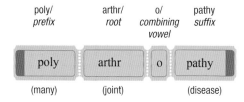

Word to be divided = polyarthropathy = poly/arthr/o/pathy

poly/ prefix	arthr/ root	o/ combining vowel	pathy suffix
poly	arthr	o	pathy
(many)	(joint)		(disease)

2. To define the word, start with the suffix. Next, define the prefix; last, define the root.

(suffix)　(prefix) (root)

Definition = disease of many joints

3. If two or more roots are present, define them from left to right.

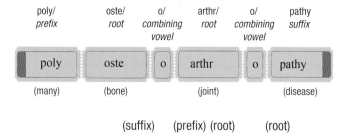

Word to be divided = polyosteoarthropathy = poly/oste/o/arthr/o/pathy

poly/ prefix	oste/ root	o/ combining vowel	arthr/ root	o/ combining vowel	pathy suffix
poly	oste	o	arthr	o	pathy
(many)	(bone)		(joint)		(disease)

(suffix)　(prefix) (root)　　(root)

Definition = disease of many bones and joints

4. Medical words are usually built with roots placed in the order that the organs appear in the body, or in the order in which blood flows through those organs. An exception to this may occur in cases when words are built in the opposite direction of anatomical order (e.g., the order in which an instrument passes through a body part).

   So what about that daunting word *hysterosalpingo-oophorectomy* from the beginning of the chapter? In human medical language, it means "surgical removal of the uterus, oviducts, and ovaries" (a procedure known in clinical veterinary language as a **spay** or **ovariohysterectomy**).

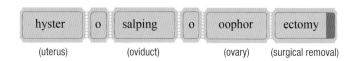

hyster	o	salping	o	oophor	ectomy
(uterus)		(oviduct)		(ovary)	(surgical removal)

    Hyster/o is the combining form for uterus; **salping/o** is the combining form for the oviduct; and **oophor/o** is the human combining form for ovary (in veterinary medicine, we use **ovari/o** as the combining form for ovary). The suffix **-ectomy** means "surgical removal."

Why does veterinary medicine drop the *salping/o?* It is hard to say, but the oviducts are such a small part of what is removed during surgery, someone somewhere must have thought, "Why even bother mentioning them?" And it would be virtually impossible for the ovaries and the uterus to be removed without also taking the oviducts. As for *oophor/o* versus *ovari/o*, *oophor/o* is an outdated term and is seldom used today. You are probably asking yourself, Why even bring up the word if it is so outdated? Well, it is a good word to use to explain how to combine three word roots, and besides it is a fun word to say.

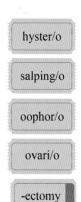

EXERCISE 2-1   *Match It!*

Match word parts from the right column with their descriptions in the left column.

_____ 1. Word part attached at the end of a word

_____ 2. Combination of the root and a vowel

_____ 3. Word part that usually indicates a procedure, disease, condition, or disorder

_____ 4. Word part found at the beginning of a word

_____ 5. Word part that is the basis for the definition of a word

_____ 6. Single vowel (usually an "o") that is added to the end of a root to make the word easier to pronounce

_____ 7. Word part that usually indicates a number, location, status, or time

_____ 8. *arthr/o* is an example of this word part

_____ 9. Every word must have this part

CF = combining form

CV = combining vowel

P = prefix

R = root

S = suffix

Check your answers at the end of the chapter, Answers to Exercises.

EXERCISE 2-2   *Analyze It!*

cost/o

The combining form for the ribs is cost/o. Dissect each term into its basic component parts using forward slashes (/). Then write a short definition for each.

1. costectomy _____

2. costitis _____

3. costochondritis _____

4. polycostopathy _____

5. costoarthritis _____

Check your answers at the end of the chapter, Answers to Exercises.

EXERCISE 2-3 *Build It!*

Write a medical term from each set of word parts, deciding whether you should use the combining vowel or drop it.

1. hyster/o + -pathy _____

2. oste/o + -itis _____

3. poly- + oste/o + -itis _____

4. ovari/o + -ectomy _____

5. poly- + oste/o + chondr/o + -pathy _____

6. chondr/o + -ectomy _____

Check your answers at the end of the chapter, Answers to Exercises.

By mastering this method of analyzing words, you will be able to analyze and build literally thousands of words, spell medical words correctly, and use a medical dictionary intelligently. Clinical veterinary language is going to become understandable, as well as easy—even fun—to learn.

COMMON UNIVERSAL WORD PARTS

Many suffixes used in clinical veterinary language are just as common in ordinary everyday language. Although they have a general meaning, their primary use is to indicate the part of speech. For example, the suffixes **-ac** and **-al** show that the word is an adjective, and **-ation** makes the word a noun. Table 2-2 lists many of the suffixes that you will encounter.

Throughout the following chapters, you will be introduced to word parts that can be used in words that refer to the body as a whole, or in words that refer to a specific system, organ, or tissue. Table 2-3 lists some of the general word parts that are not specific to any one body structure. Note that a few of the word definitions can be used in more than one way: as a suffix or as a word root.

TABLE 2-2	Everyday Suffixes	
Definition	**Suffix**	**Example**
pertaining to	-ac	cardi**ac** arrest
	-al	therm**al** underwear
	-ar	binocul**ar**
	-ia	hypotherm**ia**
	-ide	carbon diox**ide**
	-ive	posit**ive** reaction
	-ory	inflammat**ory** response
	-ous	enorm**ous** quantity
	-(t)ic	microscop**ic** bacteria, asthma**tic**

Continued

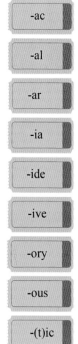

-ac

-al

-ar

-ia

-ide

-ive

-ory

-ous

-(t)ic

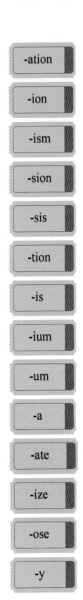

-ation

-ion

-ism

-sion

-sis

-tion

-is

-ium

-um

-a

-ate

-ize

-ose

-y

TABLE 2-2	Everyday Suffixes—cont'd	
Definition	**Suffix**	**Example**
state, condition, action, process, or result	-ation	retard**ation**
	-ion	vis**ion**
	-ism	dwarf**ism**
	-sion	exclu**sion**
	-sis	the**sis**
	-tion	absorp**tion**
structure, thing	-is	analys**is**
	-ium	bacter**ium**
	-um	aquar**ium**
	-a	aquar**ia**

The suffix -a is the plural form of the suffix -um.

to do, to cause, to act upon	-ate	medic**ate**
to engage in a specific activity, to become like, to treat	-ize	crystall**ize**
made up of, characterized by	-ose	cellul**ose**
	-y	fruit**y**

BOX 2-1	Terms That Defy Word Analysis

- benign—does not recur and has a favorable outlook for recovery
- exacerbation—worsening severity of a disease
- idiopathic—a disease of unknown origin
- in vitro—within a glass, a test tube, or another container outside the body
- in vivo—within a living body
- infection—invasion and multiplication of a disease-causing organism in a body tissue
- inflammation—tissue response to injury or destruction, with signs of pain and swelling, redness, and a feeling of warmth; inflammation does not necessarily mean that an infection is involved—only that tissue is injured
- malignant—becoming progressively worse, recurring, leading to death
- remission—improvement in or absence of signs of disease
- signs—objective evidence of disease; observable indicators like body temperature and bleeding
- symptoms—subjective evidence of disease as reported by the patient; what the patient tells you is wrong

WATCH OUT!

Inflammation and *inflammatory* are spelled with a double *m*. *Inflame* and *inflamed* are spelled with a single *m*.

TERMS THAT DEFY WORD ANALYSIS

The words listed in Box 2-1 are words that you will encounter in nearly every system. These words cannot be constructed or deconstructed using traditional word analysis, but they are part of clinical veterinary language. Make yourself some flashcards using these words. The flashcards will come in handy as you learn by practice and experience.

TABLE 2-3   Word Parts Associated with General Body Structure

Word Part	Meaning	Example and Definition	Word Parts
log/o -logy	to study, or to have knowledge of	**chondrology** study of cartilage *The combining form for study or knowledge is log/o; the suffix for study or knowledge is -logy (log/o with a suffix -y).*	chondr/o = cartilage -logy = to study, or to have knowledge of

path/o
-pathy
	disease	**chondropathology**
		the study of disease of the
		   cartilage
			chondr/o = cartilage
			path/o = disease
			-logy = to study, or to
			   have knowledge of

		chondropathy any disease affecting cartilage	chondr/o = cartilage -pathy = disease

-ist
-or
-ant
	a person or a thing
	   that does something
	   specified
		pathologist
		one who studies disease
			path/o = disease
			log/o = to study, or to
			   have knowledge of
			-ist = a person or a
			   thing that does
			   something specified

		injector
		a device for injecting or
		   making an injection
			inject = to introduce a
			   fluid into a living body
			-or = a person or a
			   thing that does
			   something specified

		assistant
		aide, helper, associate,
		   colleague ("The veterinarian's
		   assistant at the clinic always
		   seems to be available to help
		   us whenever we call.")
			assist = give support,
			   aid
			-ant = a person or a
			   thing that does
			   something specified

eti/o	cause	**etiopathology** study of the cause of disease *Often the shortened term **etiology** is used when indicating the cause of a disease or condition.*	eti/o = cause path/o = disease -logy = to study, or to have knowledge of

dia-	through, between,
	   apart, across,
	   complete
		dialog
		an exchange of ideas through
		   conversation
		*The diameter is the
		measurement of a line that
		passes across the circle and
		through its center AND you
		know diarrhea—it goes right
		through your body!*
			dia- = through
			log/o = to study, or to
			   have knowledge of

-gnosis	knowledge	**diagnosis**
		art or act of identifying a
		   disease from its signs and
		   symptoms
		***Signs** = observable indicators
		like body temperature or
		bleeding
		Symptoms = what the patient
		tells you is wrong*
			dia- = through
			-gnosis = knowledge

log/o

-logy

path/o

-pathy

-ist

-or

-ant

eti/o

dia-

-gnosis

Continued

pro-

gen/o

neo-

-oid

-ole

-ule

-osis

-oma

-sarcoma

-phyte

TABLE 2-3 Word Parts Associated with General Body Structure—cont'd

Word Part	Meaning	Example and Definition	Word Parts
pro-	before	**prognosis** the action of prior knowledge; predicting the outcome of an abnormal condition *In veterinary medicine, you will rely just on the signs of a disease to make a diagnosis or a prognosis. The prologue comes in the front of the book, and a promoter starts to work before an event.*	pro- = before -gnosis = knowledge
gen/o	formation or beginning	**pathogenic** pertaining to a substance that causes disease	path/o = disease gen/o = formation or beginning -ic = pertaining to
neo-	new	**neogenic** pertaining to new growth or regeneration	neo- = new gen/o = formation or beginning -ic = pertaining to
-oid	resembling	**osteoid** resembling bone	oste/o = bone -oid = resembling
-ole -ule	indicating something small	**ovariole** a small ovary; one of the tubes of which the ovaries of most insects are composed	ovari/o = ovary -ole = something small
		glandule a small gland or secreting vessel	gland = a group of cells that produce a secretion for use elsewhere in the body -ule = something small
-osis	condition, process, or action; disease or abnormal condition	**osteochondrosis** disease causing severe lesions of the bone and cartilage	oste/o = bone chondr/o = cartilage -osis = disease or abnormal condition
-oma	a tumor or abnormal new growth, a swelling	**osteoma** a tumor composed of bone material *A **tumor** is a localized swelling or protuberance. It does not mean the same as cancer. **Cancer** is an abnormal, uncontrolled growth of cells that does not always produce a tumor.*	oste/o = bone -oma = a tumor
-sarcoma	a malignant new growth arising in bone, cartilage, or muscle that spreads into neighboring tissue or by way of the bloodstream	**chondrosarcoma** a malignant new growth containing cartilage cells	chondr/o = cartilage -sarcoma = malignant new growth arising in bone, cartilage, or muscle
-phyte	abnormal pathological growth	**chondrophyte** an abnormal outgrowth or spur of cartilage	chondr/o = cartilage -phyte = abnormal pathological growth

TABLE 2-3	Word Parts Associated with General Body Structure—cont'd		
Word Part	**Meaning**	**Example and Definition**	**Word Parts**
plas/o	growth, development, or formation	**osteochondroplasia** pertaining to bone and cartilage that are forming or developing	oste/o = bone chondr/o = cartilage plas/o = growth, development, or formation -ia = pertaining to
-plasm	formed material (as of a cell or tissue)	**neoplasm** any new and abnormal growth, specifically one in which cell multiplication is uncontrolled	neo- = new -plasm = formed material
dys-	bad, defective, painful, or difficult	**dysplasia** the process of abnormal or difficult growth	dys- = bad, defective, painful, or difficult -plasia = growth or development
somat/o	body	**somatology** knowledge of the body *Watch out! The word for mouth is* **stoma** (plural, *stomata*).	somat/o = body -logy = to study, or to have knowledge of
-stasis	stopping, slowing, or a stable state	**diastasis** the resting phase of a heartbeat that occurs between filling of the lower chambers of the heart and the start of contraction; also known as **diastole**	dia- = through, between, apart, across, complete -stasis = stopping, slowing, or a stable condition

plas/o

-plasm

dys-

somat/o

-stasis

EXERCISE 2-4 *Build It!*

Start with the word part chondr/o, and then finish writing the terms for these definitions by placing a letter in each blank.

1. disease of the cartilage

   chondro __ __ __ __ __

2. disease affecting several areas of cartilage

   __ __ __ __ *chondro* __ __ __ __ __

3. abnormal growth of cartilage

   __ __ __ *chondro* __ __ __ __ __ __

4. study of cartilage

   chondro __ __ __ __

5. tumor composed of cartilage cells

   chondr __ __ __

6. forming new cartilage growth

   __ __ __ *chondro* __ __ __ __ __

7. malignant growth arising in the cartilage

   chondro __ __ __ __ __ __ __ __

8. cartilage that is forming or growing

   chondro __ __ __ __ __

9. inflammation of the cartilage of a joint

   __ __ __ __ __ *chondr* __ __ __ __

10. pertaining to bone and cartilage

    __ __ __ __ __ *chondr* __ __

11. person who studies cartilage

chondro __ __ __ __ __

12. resembling cartilage

chondr __ __ __

13. abnormal condition of cartilage

chondr __ __ __ __

14. tumor composed of bone and cartilage cells

__ __ __ __ __ chondr __ __ __

15. pathological outgrowth or spur of cartilage

chondro __ __ __ __ __

16. surgical removal of cartilage

chondr __ __ __ __ __ __

Check your answers at the end of the chapter, Answers to Exercises.

COMMON ABBREVIATIONS

Before the advent of computer use to "cut and paste" long words and phrases that are repeated several times, these words and phrases had to be written by hand. This tedious task was alleviated somewhat by the creation of abbreviations that are commonly used throughout veterinary medicine. Starting with this chapter, a few abbreviations will be introduced at the end of each chapter (Table 2-4). The abbreviations introduced will not necessarily be related to the specific chapter system.

| F |
| M |
| C |
| N |
| S |
| DLH |
| DSH |
| K-9 |
| LA |
| SA |

TABLE 2-4 Abbreviations

Abbreviation	Meaning	Example
F	female	Rosie is a F.
	Fahrenheit	Rosie has a normal temperature of 101° F.
M	male	Sparky is a M.
C	castrated	Sparky is a 4-year-old M/C (or M(C) or M/N) Rat Terrier dog.
N	neutered	
S	spayed	Rosie is a F/S Golden Retriever.
DLH	domestic longhair (cat)	Dweezle is a M(C) DLH.
DSH	domestic shorthair (cat)	Rocky is a M/C DSH.
K-9	canine (dog)	Sparky is a K-9 Rat Terrier terror.
LA	large animal	The Frisbee Animal Hospital is both a LA and a SA facility.
SA	small animal	

EXERCISE 2-5 *Recall It!*

Decide whether each of the following statements is True or False. Rewrite to correct the false statements on the lines below.

T F   1. A condition that tends to become progressively worse and leads to death is malignant.

T F   2. Remission is the state of absence of disease activity in patients with a chronic illness.

T F   3. The prefix is the basis for the definition of a word.

T F   4. Cancer is the tissue response to injury or destruction.

T F   5. All medical words require a suffix.

T F   6. Prognosis is the art or act of identifying a disease from its signs and symptoms.

T F   7. For some medical conditions, the cause may not be readily apparent or characterized; these conditions are idiopathic.

T F   8. A yearling is a bovine that is nearly or is just turning 1 year old.

T F   9. A study done <u>in vivo</u> looks at how the body responds to a particular substance, in contrast to <u>in vitro</u> studies, which are done in a test tube or a laboratory dish.

T F   10. Queening is the process of giving birth to kittens.

_____

_____

_____

_____

_____

Check your answers at the end of the chapter, Answers to Exercises.

ANSWERS TO EXERCISES

Exercise 2-1
1. S
2. CF
3. S
4. P
5. R
6. CV
7. P
8. CF
9. R

Exercise 2-2
1. cost/ectomy = surgical removal of ribs
2. cost/itis = inflammation of ribs
3. cost/o/chondr/itis = inflammation of rib cartilage
4. poly/cost/o/pathy = disease affecting many ribs
5. cost/o/arthr/itis = inflammation of the rib joints

Exercise 2-3
1. hysteropathy
2. osteitis
3. polyosteitis
4. ovariectomy
5. polyosteochondropathy
6. chondrectomy

Exercise 2-4
1. *chondro*pathy
2. poly*chondro*pathy
3. dys*chondro*plasia
4. *chondro*logy
5. *chondr*oma
6. neo*chondro*genic
7. *chondro*sarcoma
8. *chondro*genic
9. arthro*chondr*itis
10. osteo*chondr*al
11. *chondro*logist
12. *chondr*oid
13. *chondr*osis
14. osteo*chondr*oma
15. *chondro*phyte
16. *chondr*ectomy

Exercise 2-5
1. T
2. T
3. F—The word root is the basis for the definition of a word.
4. F—Inflammation is the tissue response to injury or destruction.
5. F—All medical words require a word root.
6. F—Diagnosis is the art or act of identifying a disease from its signs and symptoms.
7. T
8. F—A yearling is an equine that is nearly or is just turning 1 year old.
9. T
10. T

Chapter 3

Looking at the Entire Body

The body is the only machine for which there are no spare parts.

Hermann M. Briggs

WORD PARTS

abdomin/o	ahb-**dah**-mehn-ō	end-	ehnd	later/o	**laht**-ər-ō	rostr/o	**rohs**-trō
adip/o	**ahd**-ih-pō	endo-	**ehn**-dō	lip/o	**lī**-pō	sinistr/o	sihn-**ihs**-trō
anter/o	ahn-**tər**-ō	epi-	**ehp**-ih	medi/o	**mē**-dē-ō	spin/o	**spī**-nō
caud/o	**kahw**-dō	ex-	ehcks	mes/o	**mēs**-ō	sub-	suhb
cellul/o	**sehl**-yoo-lō	exo-	**ehcks**-ō	mesi/o	**mēs**-ē-ō	super-	**soo**-pər
chondr/o	**kohn**-drō	extra-	**ehcks**-trah	meta-	**meht**-ah	supra-	**soo**-prah
crani/o	**krā**-nē-ō	hem/o	**hē**-mō	my/o	**mī**-ō	system/o	sihs-**tehm**-ō
cyt/o	**sī**-tō	hemat/o	hē-**mah**-tō	neur/o	**nər**-ō	ten/o	**tehn**-ō
-cyte	sīt	hist/o	**hihs**-tō	organ/o	ohr-**gahn**-ō	tendin/o	**tehn**-dihn-ō
derm/o	**dər**-mō	histi/o	**hihs**-tē-ō	oste/o	**ohs**-tē-ō	tendon/o	**tehn**-dohn-ō
dermat/o	**dər**-mah-tō	hyper-	**hī**-pər	palm/o	**pahl**-mō	tenont/o	**tehn**-ohnt-ō
dextr/o	**dehcks**-trō	hypo-	**hī**-pō	palmar/o	pahl-**mahr**-ō	thorac/o	**thōr**-ah-cō
dia-	**dī**-ah	in-	ihn	peri-	**pehr**-ih	trans-	trahnz
dist/o	**dihs**-tō	infra-	**ihn**-frah	plant/o	**plahn**-tō	ultra-	**uhl**-trah
dors/o	**dohr**-sō	inter-	**ihn**-tər	plantar/o	plahn-**tahr**-ō	ventr/o	**vehn**-trō
ect-	ehct	intra-	**ihn**-trah	poster/o	pō-**stēr**-ō	viscer/o	**vihs**-ər-ō
ecto-	**ehct**-tō	kary/o	**kehr**-ē-ō	proxim/o	**prohck**-sih-mō		

OUTLINE

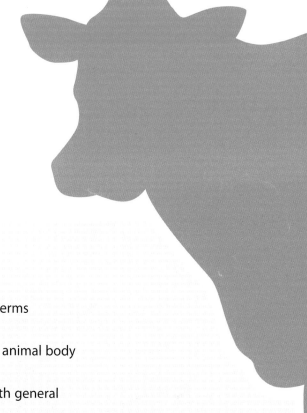

LEARNING OBJECTIVES

When you have completed this chapter, you will be able to:

1. Learn and recognize directional and positional terms, and terms specifically related to animal body areas.

2. Understand terms used to describe the organization of the animal body as a whole.

3. Become familiar with the word parts that are associated with general body structure.

In this chapter you are going to explore some of the similarities and differences between clinical veterinary language and clinical human language when it comes to describing your patients. Not all of the words that are being introduced are medical *terms* per se but are part of clinical veterinary *language*. You will not be able to analyze some of these terms using the methods learned in Chapter 2; you just have to learn them. Your flashcards will help. What may seem daunting at first will become second nature the more you use the terms.

DIRECTIONAL AND POSITIONAL TERMS

Humans walk on two feet; your patients walk on four feet (or their ancestors had four limbs as is the case with snakes and whales). Walking on four feet changes the perspective of the body; therefore, you have to use different terms to denote direction and position. For example, in humans when you point straight up on a standing body, you say the direction is **superior** or toward the head. In a standing cat if you point straight up, you are pointing to the cat's backbone, and you say the direction is **dorsal** or toward the back or top surface. In a standing human body if you pointed to the back, you would be pointing in a **posterior** direction; and in a standing dog if you pointed to the back end of the body toward the tail, you would be pointing in a **caudal** direction. Humans do not have a dorsal direction and four-legged animals do not have a superior direction. Humans do not have a caudal direction and four-legged animals do not have a posterior direction. Table 3-1 describes the common directional terms used to describe a direction or location on a four-legged body. The comparable human terms are included to indicate common terms and when the terms are different. Table 3-2 provides the word parts that are used to create combining forms and prefixes that pertain to direction.

TABLE 3-1	Common Directional Terms		
Veterinary Position or Direction	**Definition**	**Example**	**Comparable Human Term**
right and left	the animal's right side and left side	R L	right and left
median plane	an imaginary plane that runs down the center of the body lengthwise and divides it into equal left and right halves		median plane
medial	toward the median plane		medial

TABLE 3-1	Common Directional Terms—cont'd		
Veterinary Position or Direction	**Definition**	**Example**	**Comparable Human Term**
lateral	away from the median plane		lateral
rostral	toward the tip of the nose when referring to the head		nasal
cranial	toward the head end of the body or in a direction toward the head		superior
	AND		
	on the front of the forelegs above the carpus (the joint corresponding to the human wrist) and on the front of the back legs above the tarsus (the joint corresponding to the human ankle)		anterior
caudal	toward the tail end of the body or in a direction toward the tail		inferior
	AND		
	on the back of the forelegs above the carpus (the joint corresponding to the human wrist) and on the back of the rear legs above the tarsus (the joint corresponding to the human ankle)		posterior

Continued

TABLE 3-1	Common Directional Terms—cont'd		
Veterinary Position or Direction	**Definition**	**Example**	**Comparable Human Term**
transverse plane	divides the body into cranial (front) and caudal (rear) parts		transverse plane
proximal	a position on a limb that is closer to the point of attachment to the body		proximal
distal	a position on a limb that is farther away from the point of attachment to the body		distal
dorsal	toward the animal's back		posterior
	AND		
	the top/front surface of the forelimb distal to the carpus (the joint corresponding to the human wrist) and the top/front surface of the rear legs distal to the tarsus (the joint corresponding to the human ankle)		anterior or the top of the foot
ventral	toward the animal's belly		anterior
dorsal plane	runs lengthwise down the body and divides it into dorsal and ventral portions		frontal plane

TABLE 3-1	Common Directional Terms—cont'd		
Veterinary Position or Direction	**Definition**	**Example**	**Comparable Human Term**
palmar	the back of the forefeet distal to the carpus (the joint corresponding to the human wrist)		palmar, or the palm of the hand
plantar	the back of the rear feet distal to the tarsus (the joint corresponding to the human ankle)		plantar, or the bottom of the foot
superficial or external	toward the surface of the body or body part		superficial or external
deep or internal	toward the center of the body or body part		deep or internal
recumbency	lying down		lying down, reclining

EXERCISE 3-1 *Point to Me!*

You will need to be familiar with several anatomical terms to describe directions. Write a term in each blank to complete the following sentences. Then label these terms on the diagram.

1. What species of animal is this? _____ .

2. The _____ cuts across the body, dividing it into caudal and cranial portions.

3. The front of the forefeet below the carpus or the front of the rear feet below the tarsus is the _____ surface.

4. A direction within the head that is toward the tail is _____ .

5. _____ is within the head and toward the muzzle.

6. The area of the belly is _____.

7. The direction _____ is toward the tail.

8. The term used to describe a location nearer to the point of origin, or closer to the body, is _____.

9. The hoof is located on the _____ end of the leg.

10. The back side of the animal is its _____ side.

11. The _____ is a section through the side of the body that divides the body into dorsal and ventral portions.

12. The back of the rear foot below the tarsus is the _____ surface.

13. The back of the forefoot below the carpus is the _____ surface.

14. The direction toward the head is _____.

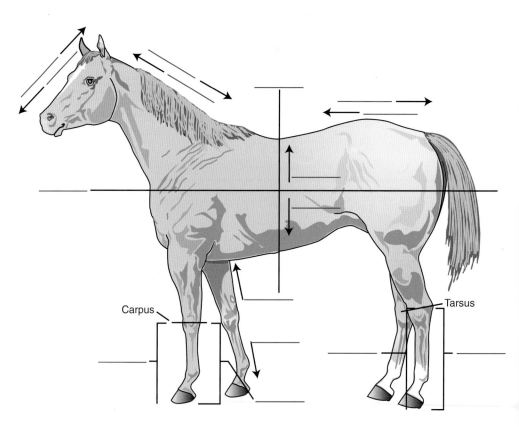

Check your answers at the end of the chapter, Answers to Exercises.

EXERCISE 3-2 *Define Me!*

Each of the descriptions listed below refers to a specific animal, or a location on a specific animal. Place the corresponding number for each description on its silhouette body.

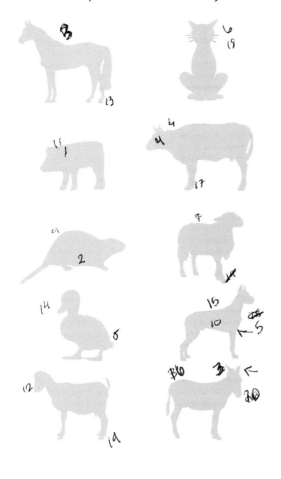

1. the lateral surface of a porcine
2. ventral surface of a rodent
3. a parent of a hinny
4. the cranial end of a bovine
5. the proximal end of a dog's foreleg
6. queening is a process for this species
7. the dorsal surface on an ovine
8. the caudal end of the avian
9. a member of the rodent family
10. the ventral surface on a canine
11. farrowing is a process for this species
12. the rostral area of a caprine
13. the plantar surface on an equine
14. the intact male is a drake
15. whelping is a process for this species
16. jack and jenny are members of this family
17. the palmar surface of a cow
18. the tom is a member of this family
19. the distal end of a goat's rear leg
20. the left ear of the donkey

Check your answers at the end of the chapter, Answers to Exercises.

crani/o

rostr/o

caud/o

poster/o

dors/o

anter/o

TABLE 3-2	Word Parts Associated with Directional Terms		
Word Part	**Meaning**	**Example and Definition**	**Word Parts**
crani/o	head	**cranial** toward the head	crani/o = head -al = pertaining to
		cranium the skull, specifically, the bony case for the brain	crani/o = head -um = structure, thing
		craniectomy surgical removal of part of the skull	crani/o = head -ectomy = surgical removal
rostr/o	nose	**rostral** toward the front of the head; on the head and toward the upper jaw and nose bones *A rostrum is another name for a lectern, the piece of furniture suitable for holding papers used by a person who is standing in front of, and is addressing, a group.*	rostr/o = nose -al = pertaining to
caud/o	tail	**caudal** toward the tail; also the direction specifically in the head toward the tail (the opposite of rostral)	caud/o = tail -al = pertaining to
		caudectomy surgical removal of the tail	caud/o = tail -ectomy = surgical removal
poster/o	rear, behind, after	**posterior** situated toward the rear *In humans, posterior is synonymous with dorsal. In animals, posterior should correctly be limited to use within the head, but posterior is commonly used to mean caudal (e.g., the posterior chamber of the eye).*	poster/o = rear or behind -ior = pertaining to
dors/o	back or top	**dorsal** the back or top of an animal	dors/o = back or top -al = pertaining to
		dorsum the entire dorsal surface of an animal or the upper surface of a body part (as of the nose, tongue, or foot) *When you endorse a check, you sign on the back.*	dors/o = back or top -um = structure or thing
anter/o	front or before	**anterior** situated at the front *In humans, anterior is commonly used to mean "ventral." In animals, anterior is synonymous with cranial. In animals, anterior should correctly be limited to use within the head, but anterior is commonly used to mean "cranial" (e.g., the anterior chamber of the eye).*	anter/o = front or before -ior = pertaining to

TABLE 3-2 Word Parts Associated with Directional Terms—cont'd

Word Part	Meaning	Example and Definition	Word Parts
ventr/o	belly	**ventral** pertaining to the belly	ventr/o = belly -al = pertaining to
		dorsoventral extending from the back toward the belly	dors/o = back or top ventr/o = belly -al = pertaining to
		ventrodorsal extending from the belly toward the back	ventr/o = belly dors/o = back or top -al = pertaining to
later/o	side	**lateral** toward the side, or farther from the midline *In radiography (X-rays), a lateral chest picture is one taken of the side of the chest. The animal is in lateral recumbency.*	later/o = side -al = pertaining to
medi/o mes/o mesi/o	middle	**mediolateral** pertaining to the middle and to one side	medi/o = middle later/o = side -al = pertaining to
		mesoappendix the middle of the appendix	mes/o = middle appendix = appendix
		mesial near to the middle or center	mesi/o = middle -al = pertaining to
palm/o palmar/o	back of forefeet of animals below the carpus	**palmar** pertaining to back of the forefeet below the carpus (the joint corresponding to the human wrist)	palm/o = back of forefeet below the carpus -ar = pertaining to
		palmarodorsal pertaining to the back of the forefeet below the carpus and to the dorsum (the front of the forefeet below the carpus)	palmar/o = back of forefeet below the carpus dors/o = back or top -al = pertaining to
plant/o plantar/o	back of rear feet of animals below the tarsus	**plantar** pertaining to the back of the rear feet below the tarsus	plantar/o = back of rear feet below the tarsus -ar = pertaining to
		plantarodorsal pertaining to the back of the rear feet below the tarsus and to the dorsum (the front of the rear feet below the tarsus)	plantar/o = back of the rear feet below the tarsus dors/o = back or top -al = pertaining to
dist/o	remote, farther away from any point of reference	**distal** the part that is farther away from the point of attachment to the body (e.g., the paw is distal to the knee) *If you go a great distance, you go farther away.*	dist/o = remote, farther away -al = pertaining to
proxim/o	nearest	**proximal** the part that is closer to the point of attachment to the body (e.g., the hip is proximal to the knee) *Something in your proximity is nearest to you.*	proxim/o = nearest -al = pertaining to

ventr/o

later/o

medi/o

mes/o

mesi/o

palm/o

palmar/o

plant/o

plantar/o

dist/o

proxim/o

Continued

TABLE 3-2	Word Parts Associated with Directional Terms—cont'd		
Word Part	**Meaning**	**Example and Definition**	**Word Parts**
trans-	across, through	**transillumination** the passage of a strong beam of light through tissues of the body to enable medical inspection *The trans-Alaska pipeline was built across Alaska.*	trans- = across, through illumination = the use of light sources
endo- end-	within, inner	**endoarthritis** inflammation within a joint *A hyphen is often used between duplicated vowels (e.g., that big word* hysterosalpingo- oophorectomy*); however, when* endo- *is followed by a word part that begins with an* o, *the* o *is dropped, and it is the prefix* end- *that will be used.*	endo- = within arthr/o = joint -itis = inflammation
		endosteitis inflammation within bone	end- = within oste/o = bone -itis = inflammation
ecto- ect-	outside, external	**ectodermatosis** disease or abnormal condition affecting the outer layer of skin *When* ecto- *is followed by a word part that begins with an* o, *the* o *is dropped, and it is the prefix* ect- *that will be used.*	ecto- = outside, external dermat/o = skin -osis = disease or abnormal condition
		ectosteal pertaining to the outside surface of a bone	ect- = outside, external oste/o = bone -al = pertaining to
exo- ex-	out, outside, outer, away from	**exogenous** pertaining to something originating outside, or caused by factors outside the animal *When* exo- *is followed by a word part that begins with an* o, *the* o *is dropped, and it is the prefix* ex- *that will be used.*	exo- = outside gen/o = substance that causes or produces something -ous = pertaining to
		exostosis a bony growth projecting outward from the surface of a bone	ex- = outside ost(e)/o = bone -osis = abnormal condition
in-	in, within, inward, into	**inside** inner side or surface of a thing	in- = in, within, inward, into side = the surface of a body
	not	**inbreeding** deliberately chosen system of breeding to preserve and fix desirable characters *Prefix* in- *also means "not," as in* inactive *(not active) and* inapt *(not appropriate).*	in- = not breeding = the physical act of mating

trans-

endo-

end-

ecto-

ect-

exo-

ex-

in-

TABLE 3-2	Word Parts Associated with Directional Terms—cont'd			
Word Part	**Meaning**	**Example and Definition**	**Word Parts**	
dextr/o	right, or toward the right	**dextroposition** displacement to the right (i.e., a body part normally found on the left side is displaced to the right side) *In Latin, the word for "right" is* dexter, *from which has come the English* dextrous, *meaning "skillful." A person who uses his right hand is expected to be dextrous.*	dextr/o = right or toward the right position = a relative place	dextr/o
sinistr/o	left	**sinistral** left-handed *The Latin* sinister *is the left hand (i.e., the wrong hand). Left-handers were thought to be unlucky.*	sinistr/o = left -al = pertaining to	sinistr/o
		sinistrodextral capable of using both hands with equal ease *Ambidextrous is a more commonly used term for "one who can use both hands with equal ease."* **(ambi- = both)**	sinistr/o = left dextr/o = right -al = pertaining to	

EXERCISE 3-3 *Position It!*

Here you will see numbers located at various places on the dog's head. Describe exactly where the number is placed, and build a term to denote that body position. The first number is given as an example.

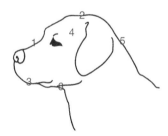

1. _the top of the nose_　　　= _rostrodorsal_

2. _____　　　= _____

3. _____　　　= _____

4. _____　　　= _____

5. _____　　　= _____

6. _____　　　= _____

Check your answers at the end of the chapter, Answers to Exercises.

Recumbency

If an animal is lying down (recumbent), recumbency is modified by adding a beginning term that describes which side of the animal is touching the ground, table, or cage floor. Table 3-3 lists the common positions used in various veterinary practice settings and some of the procedures during which they might be used.

TABLE 3-3	Recumbency Positions		
Position	**Definition**	**Example**	**Used in These Procedures**
dorsal recumbency	lying on the back		many surgical procedures, some radiography (X-ray) procedures
sternal (ventral) recumbency	lying on the belly or sternum (breast bone)		drawing blood samples, intravenous injections (companion animals)
right lateral recumbency	lying on the right side of the body		physical examinations, restraint, radiography procedures
left lateral recumbency	lying on the left side of the body		physical examination, restraint, radiography procedures
oblique recumbency	lying in a tilted position between dorsal or sternal recumbency and lateral recumbency		radiography procedures

VETERINARY REGIONAL ANATOMICAL TERMS

Body Areas

When you are reading, writing, or talking about an animal's body, you can use shortcut anatomical terms to describe a region of the body rather than using a long, wordy description. Some of these terms are used universally for all animals. For example, the withers is the withers on all animals. It is easier to say or write **withers** than to say or write "the area dorsal to the scapula." Other terms are used only for specific species. For example, **pastern** is a term that is used mainly for hoofed animals. This is the area where the leg angles forward, or the area right above the hoof. Table 3-4 lists the commonly used terms that you will have to know to correctly define the regions of an animal's body.

TABLE 3-4	Animal Body Regions	
Area	**Definition**	**Example**
withers	area dorsal (above) to the shoulder blade (scapula) *Cattle and sheep people use some very interesting phrases. One of them is* cast her withers. *It means that while giving birth, the uterus prolapsed and came out with the calf or lamb. The origin of the phrase is a mystery.*	
barrel	trunk of the body formed by the rib cage and the abdomen	
flank	lateral (side) surface of the abdomen between the last rib and the rear legs	
brisket	area at the base of the neck between the front legs that covers the cranial end of the breastbone (sternum)	
poll	top of the head between the bases of the ears	
muzzle	rostral part of the face formed mainly by the upper jaw and nose bones	
tailhead	dorsal part of the base of the tail	

Continued

TABLE 3-4	Animal Body Regions—cont'd	
Area	**Definition**	**Example**
brachium	area on the front leg in animals between the shoulder joint and the elbow joint	
knee	the carpus; area of the joint on the front leg in animals that corresponds to the human wrist *In humans, the knee joints are on the legs. In four-legged animals, the knee joints are on the front legs and the stifle joints are on the rear legs.*	
stifle	area of the joint on the rear leg that corresponds to the human knee	
shin	area of the dorsal surface of the tibia between the stifle joint and the hock	
hock	the tarsus; area of the joint on the rear leg that corresponds to the human ankle (between the shin and foot bones); term used most often in large domestic animals, especially the horse	
cannon	the area over the large bones in the lower legs of hoofed animals that corresponds to the bones of the human hand or foot; located between the knee and the fetlock on the front legs, and between the hock and the fetlock on the rear legs	
fetlock	area of a joint on the lower part of the leg marked by a projection above and behind the hoof; term used most often in hoofed animals although sometimes used in companion animals	

TABLE 3-4	Animal Body Regions—cont'd	
Area	**Definition**	**Example**
pastern	area where the leg angles forward; located between the fetlock and the hoof; term used most often in hoofed animals, although sometimes used in companion animals	
axillary region	armpit; a space medial to the proximal portion of the front leg and lateral to the cranial portion of the thorax	
inguinal region	groin; the fold or hollow where the thigh joins the abdomen	

EXERCISE **3-4** *Name It!*

Define the following anatomical terms, and then label the corresponding areas on the animal.

1. barrel _____

2. brisket _____

3. cannon _____

4. fetlock joint _____

5. flank _____

6. hock _____

7. knee _____

8. muzzle _____

9. pastern _____

10. poll _____

11. stifle joint _____

12. tailhead _____

13. withers _____

Continued

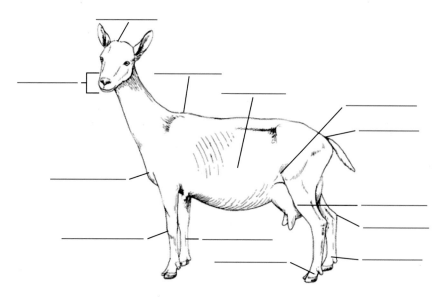

14. What species of animal is this? _____

Check your answers at the end of the chapter, Answers to Exercises.

EXERCISE 3-5 *Position It!*

You have positioned your next patient for examination. For each recumbency position, decide (yes or no) if the body part is touching the table.

	Left Lateral Recumbency	Right Lateral Recumbency	Ventral Recumbency	Dorsal Recumbency
1. barrel				
2. brisket				
3. cannon				
4. fetlock				
5. flank				
6. hock				
7. knee				
8. muzzle				
9. pastern				
10. poll				
11. stifle				
12. tailhead				
13. withers				

Check your answers at the end of the chapter, Answers to Exercises.

Body Cavities

Outside of a dog, a book is man's best friend. Inside of a dog, it's too dark to read.
Groucho Marx

An animal's body is not a solid mass. If you think about it abstractly, the body is composed of two cavities and a hollow tube surrounded by various structures. The two cavities are called the **dorsal cavity** and the **ventral cavity.** The hollow tube is the **gastrointestinal tract.** By now you should be able to deduce that the dorsal cavity is located somewhere above the ventral cavity in a standing four-legged animal (Figure 3-1; Table 3-5).

The dorsal cavity houses the brain and the spinal cord. It runs from inside the skull (where it is called the **cranium** that encloses the brain in the cranial cavity) and continues along the spine (or backbone) as a narrow **spinal cavity** that houses the spinal cord. The dorsal cavity is one continuous cavity.

The ventral cavity is the larger of the two cavities and sits below the dorsal cavity. It is divided into two parts by the **diaphragm,** a thin muscle that stretches across the cavity near the area of the last rib. The two parts of the ventral cavity are (1) the **thoracic cavity, thorax,** or **chest cavity** (located toward the front) and (2) the **abdominal cavity** or **abdomen** (located toward the back). *Thorax* and *abdomen* are the terms commonly used to indicate the two sections of the ventral cavity.

The thorax contains the heart, lungs, and esophagus, and many blood vessels. The abdomen contains the organs of the digestive, urinary, and reproductive systems. You will learn more about these structures in upcoming chapters.

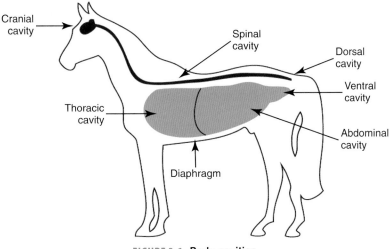

FIGURE 3-1 **Body cavities.**

TABLE 3-5	Word Parts Associated with Body Cavities		
Word Part	**Meaning**	**Example and Definition**	**Word Parts**
crani/o	head, skull	**craniology** study of skulls	crani/o = head, skull -logy = to study, or to have knowledge of
spin/o	spine	**spinous** pertaining to the spine	spin/o = spine -ous = pertaining to
abdomin/o	abdomen	**abdominohysteric** pertaining to the abdomen and the uterus	abdomin/o = abdomen hyster/o = uterus -ic = pertaining to
thorac/o	thorax	**thoracopathy** any disease of the organs or tissues in the thorax	thorac/o = thorax -pathy = disease

crani/o

spin/o

abdomin/o

thorac/o

EXERCISE 3-6 *Position It!*

All of the descriptions below denote a specific location. Define each position or direction. Then place the corresponding number for each location on the body of the dog.

What species of animal is this? _____

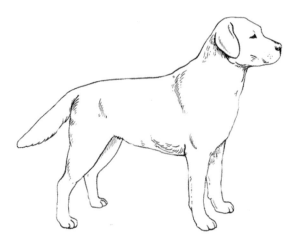

1. lateral surface of the barrel = _____

2. caudal-most point on the body of the dog = _____

3. ventral surface of the thorax = _____

4. cranial half of the transverse plane = _____

5. palmarodorsal surfaces = _____

6. external = _____

7. plantar surfaces = _____

8. rostral = _____

9. dorsointercostal = _____

10. proximal to the hock on the rear leg = _____

Check your answers at the end of the chapter, Answers to Exercises.

ORGANIZATION OF THE BODY AS A WHOLE

In *Clinical Anatomy and Physiology for Veterinary Technicians*, Dr. Tom Colville states, "The animal body is an amazing machine." He is right. It is a complex, well-organized machine with all its parts working together to keep an animal alive and healthy. It is your job as veterinary professionals to help the animal maintain this state of **homeostasis,** or physiological equilibrium. To do this, you must understand the body parts, what they are made of, and how they function. That is the purpose of anatomy and physiology courses. In this section, you are going to explore the language that you need to understand the body as a whole and how to communicate that knowledge to your supervisors and peers and to the lay public.

But first a quick review of the body's anatomy, starting small and working toward large.

Organization of the Body

cells
tissues
organs
systems

Cells

The **cell** is the smallest basic unit of the body. It is made up of a nucleus and cytoplasm surrounded by a cell wall. Cells come in different sizes. Bacterial cells are among the smallest (50,000 bacteria of a certain species could line up in 1 inch). The largest cells are the yolks of bird eggs, and the largest cell of all is the yolk of the ostrich egg (it is the size of a baseball).

Every living thing is made of one or more cells. The horse is a giant compared with a mosquito only because the horse has millions more cells, not because the cells are larger.

Tissues

Many types of cells in the body vary by content and function. If a group of identical cells together perform a specific function, they form a **tissue.** Four types of tissue can be found in the body: **epithelial** (provides physical barriers and glands), **muscle** (contracts to provide movement), **nerve** (analyzes and conducts information), and **connective** (fills spaces, provides support and framework, transports, aids in immunity, and stores energy). Connective tissue can be tendon, cartilage, bone, blood, or fat.

Organs

When two or more tissues work together to perform a unified and specific function, they are collectively called an **organ.** The liver, kidney, lungs, spleen, and brain are just some of the more than 20 organs in an animal's body.

Systems

Sometimes organs work together to perform even more involved tasks. This creates a **system.** Ten systems are present in the body (integumentary, skeletal, muscular, cardiovascular, respiratory, digestive, nervous, endocrine, urinary, and reproductive), and each of the chapters in the next section will explore the language of a specific system. Although you will study these systems individually, remember that the animal body itself is one unit. Its many parts are interrelated and are dependent on each other to make the body a whole.

Table 3-6 lists new word parts that are associated with body structure in general.

cellul/o

cyt/o

-cyte

chondr/o

dermat/o

derm/o

hemat/o

hem/o

histi/o

hist/o

kary/o

lip/o

adip/o

TABLE 3-6 **Word Parts Associated with General Body Structure**

Word Part	Meaning	Example and Definition	Word Parts
cellul/o cyt/o -cyte	cell	**cellulitis** inflammation of cells	cellul/o = cell -itis = inflammation
		chondrocytosis a condition in which there is more than the usual number of cartilage cells	chondr/o = cartilage cyt/o = cell -osis = disease or abnormal condition
		chondrocyte cartilage cell *The combining form for cell is* cyt/o *without an* e. *The suffix for cell is* -cyte *with an* e.	chondr/o = cartilage -cyte = cell
chondr/o	cartilage	**chondrectomy** surgical removal of cartilage	chondr/o = cartilage -ectomy = surgical removal
dermat/o derm/o	skin	**dermatitis** inflammation of skin	dermat/o = skin -itis = inflammation
		dermopathy any disease of the skin	derm/o = skin -pathy = disease
hemat/o hem/o	blood	**hematothorax** collection of blood in the cranial portion of the ventral cavity	hemat/o = blood thorax = thorax
		hemostasis interruption of blood flow to a part of the body; stopping the flow of blood either naturally (e.g., by the formation of a clot) or artificially (e.g., by compression or the use of a tourniquet)	hem/o = blood -stasis = stopping, slowing, or a stable state
histi/o hist/o	tissue	**histiocytosis** abnormal presence of tissue cells (in the blood)	histi/o = tissue cyt/o = cell -osis = disease or abnormal condition
		histology the study of tissues	hist/o = tissue -logy = to study, or to have knowledge of
kary/o	nucleus	**karyogenic** producing a nucleus	kary/o = nucleus gen/o = formation or beginning -ic = pertaining to
lip/o adip/o	fat	**lipectomy** surgical removal of fat	lip/o = fat -ectomy = surgical removal
		adipocyte a cell specialized for the storage of fat *There does not seem to be any rule as to when to use* lip/o *and when to use* adip/o *when referring to fat. Mostly, you will go by common usage.*	adip/o = fat -cyte = cell

TABLE 3-6		Word Parts Associated with General Body Structure—cont'd	
Word Part	**Meaning**	**Example and Definition**	**Word Parts**
my/o	muscle	**myodysplasia** abnormal development of muscles *The Greek word for mouse is* mys; *the Latin word for mouse is* mus. *Muscle movements reminded these Ancients of a mouse crawling around under a blanket.*	my/o = muscle dys- = defective plas/o = growth, development, or formation -ia = pertaining to
neur/o	nerve	**neuritis** inflammation of nerves	neur/o = nerve -itis = inflammation
organ/o	organ	**organectomy** surgical removal of an organ	organ/o = organ -ectomy = surgical removal
oste/o	bone	**osteoliposarcoma** malignant growth containing bony and fatty elements	oste/o = bone lip/o = fat -sarcoma = malignant new growth arising in bone, cartilage, or muscle
system/o	system	**systemic** referring to a specific system or to the body as a whole	system/o = system -ic = pertaining to
tendon/o tendin/o ten/o tenont/o	tendon	**tendonectomy** surgical removal of a tendon	tendon/o = tendon -ectomy = surgical removal
		tendinitis inflammation of a tendon	tendin/o = tendon -itis = inflammation
		tenophyte an abnormal growth in a tendon	ten/o = tendon -phyte = abnormal pathological growth
		tenontology branch of science that studies and specializes in knowledge regarding the tendons Tendon *is spelled with the letter* o, *but the combining form can also be* tendin/o, *spelled with the letter* i. *And to make matters worse, sometimes the word contains just* ten/o.	tenont/o = tendon -logy = to study, or to have knowledge of
viscer/o	viscera (internal organs)	**viscerate** (the modern term for *eviscerate*): to remove an organ from a patient or to remove the contents of an organ	viscer/o = internal organs -ate = to do, to cause, to act upon

my/o

neur/o

organ/o

oste/o

system/o

tendon/o

tendin/o

ten/o

tenont/o

viscer/o

EXERCISE 3-7 *Study It!*

It is only Chapter 3, and you are already becoming a *-logist,* one who is involved with study. For each "specialist" word, write your area of expertise.

1. tenologist _____

2. craniologist _____

3. cytologist _____

4. hematologist _____

5. osteologist _____

6. lipologist _____

7. histologist _____

8. thoracologist _____

9. myologist _____

10. organologist _____

11. abdominologist _____

12. dermatologist _____

13. neurologist _____

14. arthrologist _____

15. hysterologist _____

16. pathologist _____

17. etiologist _____

18. tendinologist _____

19. palmarologist _____

20. viscerologist _____

Check your answers at the end of the chapter, Answers to Exercises.

PREFIXES THAT DESCRIBE POSITION

Prefixes are added to the beginnings of words to modify their meanings. Just as regional terms are used to describe areas of the body, prefixes are used to describe position. The prefixes in Table 3-7 are used in all systems to describe a location.

TABLE 3-7	Prefixes That Describe Position		
Prefix	**Meaning**	**Example and Definition**	**Word Parts**
dia-	through, between, apart, across, complete	**diadermal** acting through the skin (e.g., diadermal ointment)	dia- = through derm/o = skin -al = pertaining to
epi-	on or upon	**epidermis** the layer of skin on top of the dermis	epi- = on or upon derm/o = skin -is = structure, thing
extra-	outside	**extracellular** outside a cell *Extracurricular activities happen outside of school.*	extra- = outside cellul/o = cell -ar = pertaining to
hyper-	above, over, or excess	**hyperplasia** an abnormal growth in normal tissue *A hyper person has excess energy.*	hyper- = excess plas/o = growth, development, or formation -ia = pertaining to
hypo-	under, beneath, below	**hypodermic** below the skin *The hypodermic needle is used to give an injection under the skin.*	hypo- = under, beneath, below derm/o = skin -ic = pertaining to
infra-	below, beneath	**infraspinous** lying below the spine	infra- = below, beneath spin/o = spine -ous = pertaining to
inter-	between, among	**interchondral** between, or connecting, cartilages *Intermural games are played between teams from different schools.*	inter- = between, among chondr/o = cartilage -al = pertaining to
intra-	within	**intracellular** within a cell *Intramural games are played by teams within the same school.*	intra- = within cellul/o = cell -ar = pertaining to
meta-	beyond, after, next	**metastasis** the transfer of disease from one organ to another organ not directly connected to it	meta- = beyond, after, next -stasis = stopping, or slowing, or a stable state
peri-	around, surrounding	**endoperiarthritis** inflammation in and around a joint	endo- = within, inner peri- = around, surrounding arthr/o = joint -itis = inflammation
sub-	below, decrease, under	**subdorsal** pertaining to the area immediately below the dorsal surface	sub- = below, decrease, under dors/o = back or top -al = pertaining to

Continued

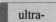

ultra-

TABLE 3-7	Prefixes That Describe Position—cont'd		
Prefix	Meaning	Example and Definition	Word Parts
super-	above, over, exceeding the norm, implying excess	**superman** a man who exceeds the norm	super- = above, over, exceeding the norm, implying excess man = man
supra-	above, over, on top of	**supracranial** on the upper surface of the cranium	supra- = above, over, on top of crani/o = head, skull -al = pertaining to
ultra-	beyond, excess, on the other side of	**ultrasound** sound with a frequency range beyond the upper limit of perception by the human ear	ultra- = beyond, on the other side of sound = sensation perceived by the sense of hearing

EXERCISE 3-8 *Prefix It!*

In the case of many prefixes, there is another prefix whose meaning is opposite. Fill in the following table with the prefix definitions. Then decide whether each pair has the same meaning, or if the meanings are different.

	Prefix	Definition	Prefix	Definition	Same or Different?
1.	epi-		sub-		
2.	extra-		intra-		
3.	super-		supra-		
4.	sub-		hypo-		
5.	hypo-		hyper-		
6.	infra-		hypo-		
7.	inter-		meta-		
8.	dia-		peri-		
9.	hyper-		ultra-		
10.	endo-		exo-		

Check your answers at the end of the chapter, Answers to Exercises.

ANSWERS TO EXERCISES

Exercise 3-1
1. equine
2. transverse plane
3. dorsal
4. caudal
5. rostral
6. ventral
7. caudal
8. proximal
9. distal
10. dorsal
11. dorsal plane
12. plantar
13. palmar
14. cranial

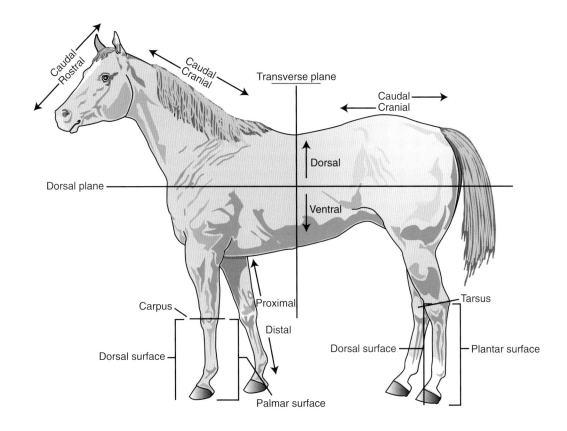

Exercise 3-2

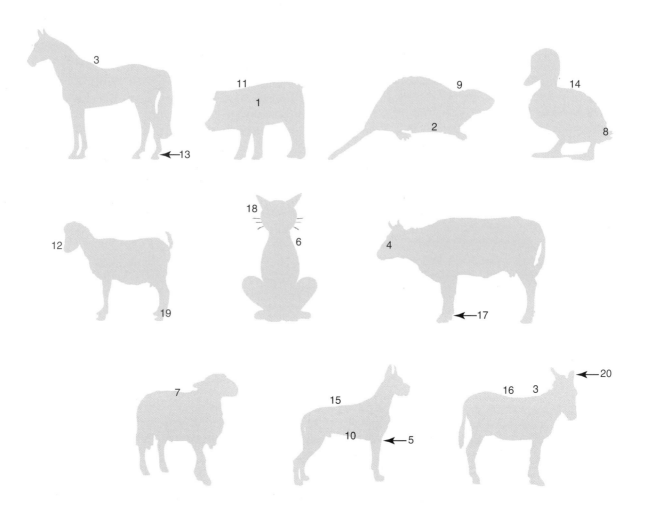

Exercise 3-3

1. top of the nose = rostrodorsal
2. top of the head = craniodorsal
3. under the lower jaw, toward the nose = rostroventral
4. on the left side of the head, in the upper portion = left dorsolateral
5. the back of the head = caudodorsal
6. toward the rear and the underside of the lower jaw = caudoventral

Exercise 3-4

1. barrel—trunk of the body formed by the rib cage and the abdomen
2. brisket—area at the base of the neck between the front legs that covers the cranial end of the breastbone
3. cannon—large bones in the lower legs of hoofed animals; area corresponds to the bones of the human hand or foot
4. fetlock joint—area of the joint on the lower part of leg marked by a projection above and behind the hoof
5. flank—lateral surface of the abdomen between the last rib and the rear legs
6. hock—area of the joint on the rear leg that corresponds to the human ankle (between the shin and the foot bones)
7. knee—area of the joint on the front leg that corresponds to the human wrist in hoofed animals
8. muzzle—rostral part of the face formed mainly by the upper jaw and the nose bones
9. pastern—area where the leg angles forward; located between the fetlock and the hoof
10. poll—top of the head between the bases of the ears
11. stifle joint—area of the joint on the rear leg that corresponds to the human knee
12. tailhead—dorsal part of the base of the tail
13. withers—area dorsal to the shoulder blade
14. This is a caprine.

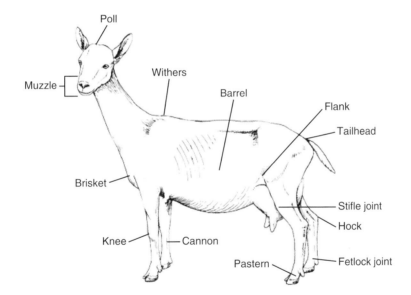

Exercise 3-5

1. barrel: yes, yes, yes, yes
2. brisket: no, no, yes *OR* no (if legs are tucked under), no
3. cannon: yes, yes, yes, no
4. fetlock: yes, yes, yes, no
5. flank: yes, yes, no, no
6. hock: yes, yes, yes, no
7. knee: yes, yes, yes, no
8. muzzle: yes, yes, yes, no
9. pastern: yes, yes, yes, no
10. poll: no, no, no, no
11. stifle: yes, yes, yes, no
12. tailhead: no, no, no, yes
13. withers: yes, yes, no, yes

Exercise 3-6

(The species is canine.)

1. pertaining to the side of the dog in the area of the trunk
2. the tail end of the dog or in a direction toward the tail
3. pertaining to the belly (the underside of the body) in the area of the chest
4. the head end of the front end of the body
5. pertaining to the back of the forefeet and the dorsum (the front of the forefeet)
6. on the outside of the body
7. across the back of the rear foot below the tarsus
8. pertaining to the nose end of the head or the body
9. in the back, between the ribs
10. nearer to the center of the body than the hock (the tarsus, which corresponds to the human ankle)

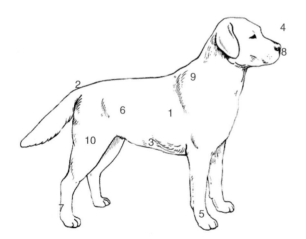

Exercise 3-7

1. tendons
2. head
3. cells
4. blood
5. bone
6. fat
7. tissue
8. thorax
9. muscle
10. organs
11. abdomen
12. skin
13. nerves
14. joints
15. uterus
16. disease
17. cause of things
18. tendons
19. the back of the front feet below the tarsus
20. internal organs

Exercise 3-8

1. on or upon; below or under; Different
2. outside; within; Different
3. above or over; above or over or on top of; Same
4. below or decreased or under; under or beneath or below; Same
5. under or beneath or below; above or over or excess; Different
6. below or beneath; under or beneath or below; Same
7. between or among; beyond or after or next; Different
8. through; around or surrounding; Different
9. above or over or excess; above or over or exceeding the norm; Same
10. within or inner; out or outside; Different

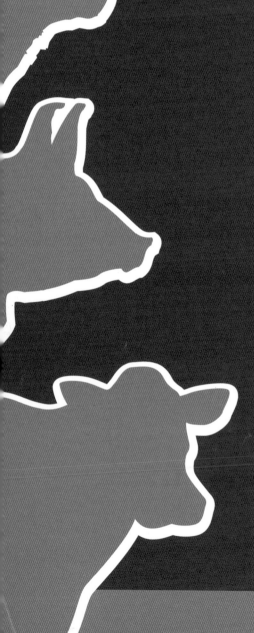

Chapter 4

The Integumentary System

Skin keeps the outside out and the inside in.

Tom Colville

WORD PARTS

a-	ah *or* ā	derm/o	dər-mō	necr/o	neh-krō	-rrhaphy	raff
adip/o	**ahd**-ih-pō	dermat/o	dər-mah-tō	nod/o	**nohd**-ō	scop/o	**skō**-pō
an-	ahn	-ectomy	**ehck**-tō-mē	onych/o	**ohn**-ih-kō	-scope	skōp
aut/o	**ahw**-tō	follicul/o	fohl-**lihck**-kuhl-ō	pachy-	**pahck**-ē	seb/o	**seh**-bō
bi-	bī	-gram	grahm	papul/o	**pahp**-yool-ō	sebac/o	seh-**bā**-shō
bi/o	**bī**-ō	-graph	grahf	para-	**pahr**-ah	-stomy	**stō**-mē
-centesis	sehn-**tē**-sihs	-graphy	**grahf**-ē	-pexy	**pehck**-sē	sudor/o	**soo**-dohr-ō
circum-	**sehr**-kuhm	hidr/o	**hī**-drō	-phyte	fīte	-tomy	**tō**-mē
cor/o	**kohr**-ō	hydr/o	**hī**-drō	pil/o	**pī**-lō	trich/o	**trī**-kō
cornu/o	**kohr**-nū-ō	kerat/o	**kehr**-ah-tō	-plasty	**plahs**-tē	vesicul/o	veh-**sihk**-ū-lō
cutane/o	**kyoo-tā**-nē-ō	lip/o	**lī**-pō	purpur/o	**pər**-pər-ō	xer/o	**zē**-rō
cyst/o	**sihs**-tō	melan/o	**mehl**-ah-nō	py/o	**pī**-ō		

OUTLINE

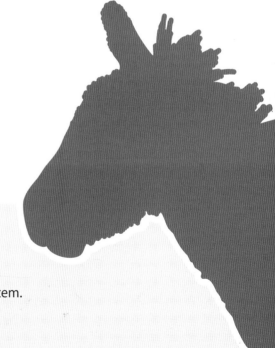

LEARNING OBJECTIVES

When you have completed this chapter, you will be able to:

1 Understand the components and functions of the integumentary system.

2 Identify and recognize the meanings of word parts related to the integumentary system, using them to build or analyze terms.

3 Apply your new knowledge of understanding clinical veterinary language in the context of medical reports.

CASE STUDY 4-1 #2001-923 ALLOVER

Signalment and History: Allover is a 7-year-old M(C) Golden Retriever who was brought to the Frisbee Small Animal Clinic because he had been sluggish and gaining weight, even though he was eating the same amount of food. He sought out warm spots more often than usual, and his skin and hair coat did not look good.

Physical Examination: Upon physical examination, Jess Nelson, the veterinary technician, found that Allover was slightly depressed for a Golden Retriever. His BW was 95 pounds, about 10 pounds over his ideal weight. Allover's TPR was within the expected reference ranges. Jess found **bilateral areas of alopecia** on Allover's body. In other areas, the hair was just thinning. Allover's skin was crusty and scaly all over his body, and there were even some **areas of pyoderma.** Based on Allover's history and clinical signs, Dr. Frisbee suspected that Allover was suffering from **hypothyroidism.** Jess drew blood samples from Allover to submit to the lab to check his level of thyroid hormone.

Diagnosis and Treatment: The results of the lab work confirmed the **diagnosis** of hypothyroidism with secondary **pyoderma,** Dr. Frisbee prescribed oral antibiotics for the **dermatitis, topical** treatment with medicated shampoo for the other **dermatoses,** and a thyroid hormone supplement that probably will have to be given for the rest of Allover's life.

Outcome: At a recheck 1 month later, Allover's skin already looked better. His sores had healed, he was beginning to re-grow his missing hair, and his owners reported that he had more energy than they had seen in a long time. With a controlled diet and more activity, Allover was starting to lose his extra weight.

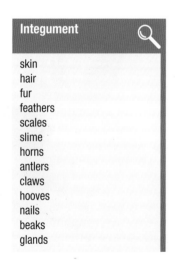

Integument
skin
hair
fur
feathers
scales
slime
horns
antlers
claws
hooves
nails
beaks
glands

INTEGUMENTARY SYSTEM

The integumentary system, or **integument,** is the largest organ of the body; it is the first thing you see when you meet a patient. Think about a goldfish, an iguana, a cat, a frog, a sheep, a parakeet, an elephant, and a giraffe. You will quickly realize that there are big differences in the skin of these animals. Scales, fur, slime, wool, feathers, and hair are all parts of the integumentary system of animals, even though the animals may look very different. The integument of all animals has the same basic structure. It consists of skin and all of its accessory structures, including horns, claws, hooves, nails, beaks, sweat glands, oil glands, mammary glands, scales, feathers, hair, fur, and slime.

You are going to build a prototype animal, system by system. You will discover how each system has its own structures and functions but still plays a vital role for the animal as a whole. The most obvious way to start building your animal is to use a container to hold all of its parts together in one place—skin!

Functions of the Skin

The most important function of the skin is to provide protection by creating a physical barrier. Together, the skin and its accessory structures act to:

- protect internal body structures against injury
- protect the body against bacterial invasion
- protect the body against ultraviolet light damage
- prevent water loss from the body
- aid in camouflage and sexual displays through variations in pigmentation
- detect pain, touch, pressure, and temperature through the nerve endings
- maintain and regulate body temperature
- dispose of waste products
- emit odors (pheromones) that are crucial to the social structure of animal societies

- produce milk in mammary glands for young offspring
- play a part in inflammatory and immune responses, and in wound healing

Table 4-1 lists combining forms for the major structures of the integument. You will note that there are no combining forms for some of the anatomical parts of the integument. A hoof is a hoof, a feather is a feather, and slime is slime. You will also note that more than one combining form is listed for skin and for some other parts of the integumentary system. Do not get too concerned yet about which combining forms should be used for terms like skin or hair. The more you study and use clinical veterinary language, the more you will become familiar with the accepted usage of each word part.

TABLE 4-1	Combining Forms for Integumentary Anatomy		
Word Part	**Meaning**	**Example and Definition**	**Word Parts**
dermat/o derm/o cor/o cutane/o	skin	**dermatologist** specialist in the study of skin	dermat/o = skin log/o = to study, or to have knowledge of -ist = a person who does something specific
		hypodermic a dermatologist uses a hypodermic needle to inject a material under the skin	hypo- = under, beneath, below derm/o = skin -ic = pertaining to
		corium the dermis layer of skin *There are numerous places in the body where the corium is given special recognition. The equine hoof contains a laminar corium in the hoof wall, a solear corium in the sole of the foot, and a cuneal corium in the frog of the hoof.*	cor/o = skin -ium = structure, thing
		subcutaneous something situated or located below or beneath the skin *Many skin diseases have the word* cutaneous *associated with them.* Cutaneous habronemiasis *is a condition of horses caused by fly larvae in a skin wound.* *You probably have noticed that* **hypodermic** *and* subcutaneous *have virtually the same meaning. There is no hard and fast rule as to when you use one or the other term. Again, the more you study and use veterinary medical terms, the more familiar you will become with their accepted usage. For example, you will use hypodermic needles to administer subcutaneous injections.*	sub- = below, decrease, under cutane/o = skin -ous = pertaining to
melan/o	black, dark	**melanoma** tumor arising from melanocytes, the cells that produce the black pigment melanin	melan/o = black, dark -oma = a tumor or abnormal growth
kerat/o	hard, horn-like tissue	**keratodermia** excessive development of the horny layer of skin *Keratin is sometimes used to coat pills when drugs need to pass through the stomach without being digested.*	kerat/o = hard, horn-like tissue derm/o = skin -ia = pertaining to

Continued

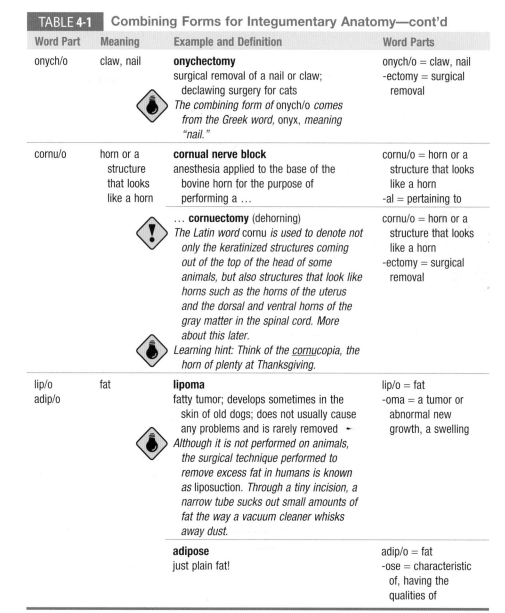

TABLE 4-1		Combining Forms for Integumentary Anatomy—cont'd	
Word Part	**Meaning**	**Example and Definition**	**Word Parts**
onych/o	claw, nail	**onychectomy** surgical removal of a nail or claw; declawing surgery for cats *The combining form of* onych/o *comes from the Greek word,* onyx, *meaning "nail."*	onych/o = claw, nail -ectomy = surgical removal
cornu/o	horn or a structure that looks like a horn	**cornual nerve block** anesthesia applied to the base of the bovine horn for the purpose of performing a …	cornu/o = horn or a structure that looks like a horn -al = pertaining to
		… cornuectomy (dehorning) *The Latin word* cornu *is used to denote not only the keratinized structures coming out of the top of the head of some animals, but also structures that look like horns such as the horns of the uterus and the dorsal and ventral horns of the gray matter in the spinal cord. More about this later.* Learning hint: *Think of the* cornucopia, *the horn of plenty at Thanksgiving.*	cornu/o = horn or a structure that looks like a horn -ectomy = surgical removal
lip/o adip/o	fat	**lipoma** fatty tumor; develops sometimes in the skin of old dogs; does not usually cause any problems and is rarely removed *Although it is not performed on animals, the surgical technique performed to remove excess fat in humans is known as* liposuction. *Through a tiny incision, a narrow tube sucks out small amounts of fat the way a vacuum cleaner whisks away dust.*	lip/o = fat -oma = a tumor or abnormal new growth, a swelling
		adipose just plain fat!	adip/o = fat -ose = characteristic of, having the qualities of

onych/o

cornu/o

lip/o

adip/o

Skin Layers 🔍

epidermis
  melanocytes
  melanin
  keratin
  keratinocytes
dermis
  collagen
  hair follicles
  blood vessels
  glands
  nerves
hypodermis
  collagen
  fat

ANATOMY OF THE INTEGUMENTARY SYSTEM

Skin

Skin is made up of three layers: the **epidermis,** or the most superficial outer layer; the **dermis,** or the deeper middle layer; and the **hypodermis,** or the deepest layer (Figure 4-1).

Epidermis

The epidermis is many cell layers thick over most of the body and is made up of about 95% epithelial cells, most of which are **keratinocytes,** and 5% pigment-producing cells called **melanocytes.** This layer does not contain any blood cells or nerve endings.

    Melanocytes are produced by the bottom layer of the epidermis and stay anchored there, but through long tentacles can reach out and inject pigment into many epidermal cells. The pigment **melanin** produced by the melanocytes is what determines skin

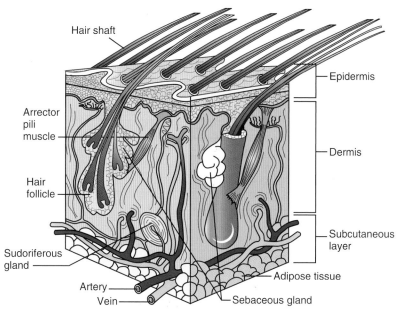

FIGURE 4-1 **Anatomy of skin.** The three layers of skin and the structures located in each. (Adapted from Colville TP: *Clinical Anatomy and Physiology for Veterinary Technicians,* ed 2, St Louis, 2007, Mosby.)

and hair/fur color. The distribution of melanocytes is what gives animals variations in hair coat patterns such as spots, swirls, and stripes, which help animals to camouflage themselves or to show themselves off during sexual displays. Melanin also provides protection against damaging ultraviolet light.

Most **epidermal** cells start out as new keratinocytes in the bottom layer of the epidermis and are gradually pushed upward or more superficially as new cells are produced. As the keratinocytes are pushed upward away from their blood supply in the dermis, they age and eventually die. Thus the outermost layer of the epidermis is made up of dead, dried-up, tough cells that are collectively called **keratin.** Keratin is a protein that provides protection and waterproofing and helps prevent water loss. The thicker the cell layer of dead keratinocytes, the more physical is the protection that it provides. Thick layers of specialized keratin form hair, fur, horns, nails, claws, feathers, and beaks. The outer layer of the epidermis on the footpads is the toughest in the body. It allows animals to safely walk on rough, hot, or cold surfaces.

Dermis

The dermis, the thickest layer of the skin, is made up of tough fibrous tissue called **collagen.** This layer is where hair follicles, glands, nerves, and blood vessels are located. Hair follicles are the site of hair production where the root of a hair is attached. The glands in the dermal layer include **sudoriferous** (sweat) glands, which are involved in body temperature regulation, and **sebaceous** (oil) glands, which provide lubrication for hair and skin. Sebaceous glands also help prevent bacterial growth on the skin. Also located in the **dermal** layer are numerous cell types that are involved in inflammatory and immune responses, as well as in wound healing.

Hypodermis

The hypodermis is a layer of mostly collagen and fatty tissue below the dermis. It is also called the **subcutaneous** layer. This is the layer that attaches the skin to the deeper structures so it does not just fall off the body. The fat in the hypodermis provides insulation, serves as an energy reserve, and helps form the contours of the body. On the footpads, the hypodermis is thicker to provide some shock absorption.

CISE 4-1 *Define Me!*

at you are able to recognize and identify many word parts, complete these sentences by writing in the blank the definitions correspond to the underlined word parts.

1. A <u>hypo</u>dermic needle is placed _____*under*_____ a layer of skin.

2. A <u>melano</u>derm is a person who belongs to one of the _____*Black*_____ races.

3. <u>Epi</u>dermatitis is the term for an inflammation of the _____*outer*_____ layer of skin.

4. A <u>meta</u>-arthritic condition pertains to the _____*after*_____ effects of arthritis.

5. Dermato<u>pathy</u> is a _____*disease*_____ of the skin.

6. Poly<u>onych</u>ia is the presence of too many _____*nails*_____.

7. <u>Lipo</u>sarcoma is a malignant growth arising from _____*fat*_____ cells.

8. <u>Dermatoneuro</u>logy is the study of _____*skin*_____ and _____*nerves*_____.

9. An <u>adipo</u>cyte is a cell composed of _____*fat cell*_____.

10. <u>TRANSDERM</u>® is a sticky patch that can be embedded with various drugs. Its name tells you that the drugs work by being absorbed _____*across*_____ the skin.

11. <u>Kerato</u>derma is a _____*horn like*_____ condition of the skin.

12. Sub<u>cutaneous</u> refers to something under the _____*skin*_____.

13. Hyper<u>plasia</u> is an abnormal or unusual increase in _____*tissue growth*_____.

14. <u>Myo</u>melanosis is a condition in which there is an area of black pigment in _____*muscle*_____.

15. The term <u>cornu</u>ate pertains to the _____*horns*_____ of a bovine, ovine, or caprine.

Check your answers at the end of the chapter, Answers to Exercises.

ANATOMY OF THE ACCESSORY INTEGUMENTARY STRUCTURES

Hair

Hairs are formed in hair follicles. The follicles are located at the level of the dermis but are actually deep indentations of the epidermis. Each hair follicle contains a hair bulb, which is the enlarged inner end of the hair shaft. Associated with each follicle are one or two sebaceous glands and an **arrector pili** muscle. The glands secrete an oily substance called **sebum** that lubricates the hair. When the arrector pili muscle contracts, it pulls the hair more upright or vertical. Think of hair standing on end. It makes the animal look fluffier and bigger, and sometimes more dangerous. This is the arrector pili muscles at work. The arrector pili muscles also cause "goose bumps" or "goose flesh."

The hairs themselves are made up of specialized, keratinized epithelial cells that grow and are lost in cycles that correlate to seasonal changes in the amount of daylight. Most animals shed hair in the spring and grow thick coats in the fall.

Glands

Two types of glands are found all over the body: sebaceous (oil) glands and sudoriferous (sweat) glands. Sebaceous glands are located in the dermal layer. Their ducts may empty into a hair follicle or directly onto the surface of the skin. The substance released by sebaceous glands is **sebum,** an oily substance that lubricates the skin and hair to provide waterproofing. Excess sebum can plug the gland's ducts, forming whiteheads or pimples. As the sebum ages, it turns black and blackheads form.

Sudoriferous glands are sweat glands. Their secretions act to cool the body. These glands are found all over the body in some animals and only at specific locations in others. Only the horse produces enough sweat to become obviously sweaty over its entire body. Two types of sweat glands are known. One type empties directly onto the skin's surface; the other type empties into hair follicles. Sweat glands of the dog that empty onto the skin are located around the nose and between the footpads.

Anal glands in cats, dogs, and other small mammals are specialized glands with which you will become familiar if you work with these animals. These glands are related to the musk glands of skunks and produce a foul-smelling secretion. The glands are located at 4 and 8 o'clock positions to the anus and normally empty each time the animal has a bowel movement. Even though the odor is offensive to us humans, dogs and cats use it to mark their territory or attract a mate. The anal glands may become impacted (obstructed) and infected. When this occurs, they will have to be manually expressed (squeezed) or surgically repaired if they have ruptured. *Caution:* The secretions of the anal glands smell very bad. Table 4-2 provides the word parts that are used to create combining forms for the accessory integumentary structures.

TABLE 4-2	Combining Forms for Accessory Integumentary Anatomy		
Word Part	**Meaning**	**Example and Definition**	**Word Parts**
pil/o trich/o	hair	**piloerection** hair stands "up on end"	pil/o = hair erection = condition of being stiff or elevated
		melanotrichia abnormally increased black color of hair *Are you familiar with* trichinosis, *a parasitic disease caused by eating undercooked* Trichinella-*infected meat, usually pork? The* Trichinella *parasites are very small and slender and are so named because they look like small hairs.*	melan/o = black trich/o = hair -ia = pertaining to
follicul/o	follicle	**folliculitis** inflammation of a follicle, usually a hair follicle *The* **follicle** *is a small bag or sack, kind of like a "cul de sac" of cells. Each body hair sits within a hair follicle.*	follicul/o = follicle -itis = inflammation
sebac/o seb/o	oil, sebum	**pilosebaceous** pertaining to hair follicles and their sebaceous glands	pil/o = hair sebac/o = oil, sebum -(e)ous = pertaining to
		sebum thick oily substance secreted by the sebaceous glands	seb/o = oil, sebum -um = structure, thing
sudor/o hidr/o	sweat	**sudoral** pertaining to sweating	sudor/o = sweat -al = pertaining to
		hidrosis excessive sweating hidr/o *sounds the same, but it does not mean the same as* **hydr/o,** *which means "water" (e.g., water from the fire hydrant).*	hidr/o = sweat -osis = abnormal condition

pil/o

trich/o

follicul/o

sebac/o

seb/o

sudor/o

hidr/o

hydr/o

EXERCISE 4-2 *Label It!*

Write in each blank the name of the structure in the integumentary system that matches its description. Use Figure 4-1 to refresh your memory about the various structures of the integumentary system.

1. _Epidermis_ melanocytes are located here

2. _Sudoriferous_ this is a sweat gland

3. _Dermis_ thickest layer of skin

4. _Dermis_ wound healing and immune responses occur here

5. _Adipose_ this is fat!

6. _Epidermis_ made up of dead, dried-up cells

7. _Follicules_ the sac where hair is formed

8. _Sebum_ secretes an oily substance that lubricates and provides waterproofing

9. _Epidermis_ keratinocytes make up 95% of this layer

10. _Hypodermis_ ~~Arrector muscles~~ also called the subcutaneous layer

11. _Arrector muscles_ this pulls the hair more upright or vertical, and gives goose bumps

12. _Sudoriferous gland_ its secretions cool the body

13. _Epidermis_ the color of the skin is determined here

14. _Epidermis_ no blood cells or nerve endings are found in this layer

15. _Follicules_ where the root of the hair is attached

16. _Hypodermis_ skin does not fall off the body because of this

17. _hair_ one combining form for this structure is *trich/o*

18. _Adipose_ this is an energy reserve

19. _Sebaceous g_ its secretions help prevent bacterial growth on the skin

20. _Sudoriferous g_ this is overactive in hidrosis

Check your answers at the end of the chapter, Answers to Exercises.

TERMS THAT DEFY WORD ANALYSIS

The terms listed in Box 4-1 are similar to words that you will encounter in every system. These words cannot be constructed or deconstructed using traditional word analysis. So what is the best way to learn these terms? Practice, experience, and flash cards. Ask yourself questions like, "What is the difference between an abrasion and a laceration?" or "What is the difference between a keloid and proud flesh?"

BOX 4-1   Terms That Defy Word Analysis

- abrasion—a skin scrape
- abscess—a localized collection of pus
- alopecia—loss of hair, wool, or feathers
- carbuncle—a group of furuncles in adjacent hairs
- cicatrix (*plural* = cicatrices)—a scar
- ecchymosis—blood leaking from a ruptured blood vessel into subcutaneous tissue; a bruise
- epithelium—the cells that cover the internal and external body surfaces and also form many glands
- eschar—dried serum, blood, pus; a scab; the charred surface of a burn
- excoriate—scratch the skin
- fissure—a crack-like lesion in the skin
- furuncle—a boil or skin abscess, usually around follicles
- granulation tissue—new tissue that grows to fill in a wound defect
- infection—the invasion of body tissues by disease-causing microorganisms (e.g., bacteria, viruses, fungi, and parasites) and the reaction of the host tissues to these organisms and the toxins that they produce; not the same as inflammation
- keloid—an overgrowth of scar tissue at the site of injury
- laceration—a rough or jagged skin tear
- palliative—treating the symptoms, but not curing the cause
- papule—a small, solid, usually somewhat pointed elevation of the skin; does not contain pus but is inflamed
- petechia (*plural* = petechiae)—tiny ecchymosis within the dermal layer
- plaque—a raised, flat papule greater than 1 cm
- proud flesh—overgrowth of granulation tissue at the site of injury; also known as *exuberant granulation tissue* (horses)
- pruritus—itching
- purulent—containing or consisting of pus
- sepsis—the systemic inflammatory response induced by an infection
- signalment—a detailed description, including distinctive features, of an animal
- suppurate—to produce or discharge pus
- topical—applied to, designed for, or an action on the surface of the body
- tumor—any mass or swelling; a nodule greater than 2 cm
- ulcer—a circumscribed crater-like lesion of the skin or mucous membrane
- wheal (hives, urticaria)—a circumscribed, elevated papule (pimple) caused by localized edema (collection of fluid between cells)

EXERCISE **4-3** *Ask Yourself!*

Describe in your own words the meanings of the following words.

1. abrasion Skin scrape

2. laceration a rough or jagged skin tear

3. excoriate Scratch the skin

4. fissure Crack like lession in skin

5. incision Cut or wound

6. keloid an overgrowth of scar tissue

7. scar a mark remaining after healing of wound

8. proud flesh overgrowth of graduation tissue

9. granulation tissue New tissue formed in repair of wounds of soft tissue

10. cicatrix a scar

11. papule Solid elevation of skin no puss

12. plaque Solid elevation of skin greater than 1cm in diameter.

13. wheal elevated papule that is redder or paler

14. pus Cells and cellular debris in a thin fluid

15. abscess localized collection of pus in a cavity

16. purulent Containing or forming pus

17. suppurate to produce or discharge pus

18. furuncle boil skin abscess

19. carbuncle a cluster of furuncles in adjacent hairs

20. boil a furuncle

21. eschar Dried serum, blood, pus, a scab

22. ecchymosis a bruise

23. petechia tiny ecchymosis In the dermal layer

24. signalment Animals history deals with age, sex

25. signs Indicators like body temperature.

26. symptoms what the patient says is wrong

27. palliative ___treating symptoms___
28. tumor ___Any mass swelling, new growth___
29. ulcer ___Open sore___
30. inflammation ___tissue is injured, redness swelling___

Check your answers at the end of the chapter, Answers to Exercises.

CASE STUDY 4-2 #2010-443 HOLSTEIN

Signalment and History: An M(C) white adult cat with black patches, named Holstein, was brought to the Frisbee Small Animal Clinic by a local animal rescue organization. He had been living outdoors on his own for a while so his age was indeterminate, although he appeared to be a middle-aged adult. Holstein had been rescued from an abandoned barn, so no history was available.

Physical Examination: Jess performed an initial physical exam. Although Holstein was thin, he was bright, alert, responsive (BAR), and quite happy to be handled. His TPR values were within expected reference ranges. Jess drew blood samples for lab testing. Apparently Holstein was a fighter, not a lover, because he had several skin problems indicating altercations with other cats.

Scattered over his body were small, circular areas of **alopecia.** It appeared that the hairs had been broken off and the **skin was thickened** and crusty. In other areas, the circular areas of alopecia were red in the middle. Dr. Frisbee suspected that these patches could have been due to a **dermatophyte infection,** and cautioned everyone to wash their hands well and change lab coats after handling Holstein. A dermatophyte infection can be a **zoonotic** disease. Many small **superficial and deep abrasions** and **lacerations** were also evident, particularly around Holstein's head and neck. Some seemed to involve only the **epidermis;** others also involved the **dermis,** A few of the wounds extended down to the **hypodermis.** On the left **lateral** side of his neck, Holstein had an **abscess** about the size of a flattened ping pong ball. A small amount of **purulent material** came from an opening at the bottom of the lump when Dr. Frisbee gently pressed it.

Diagnosis: Dr. Frisbee shined an ultraviolet light over Holstein's areas of alopecia. Some of these areas glowed fluorescent green when the light hit them. This confirmed Dr. Frisbee's tentative diagnosis of dermatophytosis. She also diagnosed secondary superficial wounds and an abscess.

Treatment: Once the **diagnosis** of dermatophyte infection was confirmed, Holstein was placed on a treatment schedule of **oral** medications and twice-weekly **topical** application of lime-sulfur dip solution. The hair from around the deeper wounds was clipped so they could be cleaned. The skin and hairs of the white areas contain little or no pigment, but the skin and hairs of the black areas contain a lot of **melanin.**

After microscopically examining the purulent fluid, Dr. Frisbee diagnosed the abscess as probably resulting from a deep bite wound that became **infected.** She anesthetized Holstein, enlarged the opening from which the **purulent material** was draining, and flushed out the lump's cavity so it could heal more rapidly. Holstein was also given a lime-sulfur dip to begin ringworm treatment. Dr. Frisbee cautioned the owner about the zoonotic potential of the disease and that it could also spread to other animals.

Outcome: The rescue organization placed Holstein in a foster home with no other animals. After 2 weeks of treatment for his skin problems, Holstein had gained a little weight and his skin was looking better. The abscess was nearly healed, and purulent material was no longer draining from the opening. His scattered wounds and **abrasions** were nearly healed. The **dermatophyte infection,** however, was going to take longer to heal. Overall, Holstein's **prognosis** for a complete recovery was very good. Three months later, Holstein was back in the clinic with his new owner for his vaccinations. The only evidence of his previous injuries included some areas of **alopecia** and a few **eschars.** The abscess had completely healed.

EXERCISE 4-4   *Case It!*

Read Case Study 4-2, and decide whether each of the following statements is True or False. Rewrite to correct the false statements on the lines below.

T **(F)**   1. A zoonotic disease is one that can be spread from humans to animals.

T **(F)**   2. The diagnosis is a prediction of the outcome of Holstein's disorder.

(T) F   3. Melanin gives Holstein's skin and hair their dark colors.

(T) F   4. A discharge is a substance that is secreted or excreted.

T **(F)**   5. A laceration that is superficial is in the hypodermis.

(T) F   6. Dermatophytosis is a medical term for the cause of Holstein's alopecia.

(T) F   7. A topical medication is rubbed directly onto the skin.

T **(F)**   8. Holstein is a bovine tom.

(T) F   9. Holstein's abscess contained some pus.

(T) F   10. The term *dermatosis* could describe Holstein's problems.

1) Animals to humans

2) Prognosis

5) Deep laceration is the epidermis

8) Feline tom

Check your answers at the end of the chapter, Answers to Exercises.

CASE STUDY 4-3   #1998-459 SUNDANCE

Signalment and History: Sundance, a 10-year-old Appaloosa **gelding** who stands **15 hands high,** was brought to the Frisbee Large Animal Clinic because of wire cuts on his front legs and chest. He was startled in his pasture this morning by a low-flying airplane, and took off at a gallop right into the wire fence that surrounds his pasture.

Physical Examination: Sam Ting, a veterinary technician, performed Sundance's initial physical examination and drew blood samples for laboratory testing. The results of the exam were unremarkable; the TPR was within expected reference ranges. Lab results were all within expected reference ranges. Some of Sundance's wounds were minor **lacerations** and **abrasions** that involved only the **epidermis,** but others extended down to the **dermis,** and some even reached down to the **hypodermis.** One particularly deep laceration on the **lateral** surface of his right front leg was just **proximal** to the **coronary band.**

Treatment: Dr. Murdoch decided that the minor wounds involving only the epidermis could be left to heal on their own. He instructed the owner to clean the wounds every day. Four of the larger and deeper wounds needed to be sutured closed. Sundance was given a sedative. An **intradermal local** anesthetic drug was injected around the wounds, and suture material was used to close the wounds. The needle with the suture material attached was passed through the **epidermis and dermis** on each side of each wound, and the suture material was tied in a square knot to hold the wound closed until it healed. The kind of suture material used would not be absorbed by Sundance's body, so the sutures would have to be cut and removed in 10 days.

The wound down by Sundance's **coronary band** was of particular concern for Dr. Murdoch because a piece of skin was missing, and Dr. Murdoch could not suture the wound closed. He was concerned that as the wound healed, the **granulation tissue** would become **proud flesh.** This is a fairly common complication with deep wounds in the **distal** areas of horses' legs. If this proud flesh forms, it can be removed under local anesthesia, but it tends to grow back.

Outcome: Sundance was brought back to the clinic 10 days later for suture removal. Dr. Murdoch found that the wounds were healing nicely and removed the sutures without the need to sedate Sundance. The wound by the **coronary band** showed no sign of proud flesh. Dr. Murdoch instructed the owner to continue topical treatment of the wound until it had healed. Three months later, Dr. Murdoch visited Sundance's ranch and found only a nickel-sized wound that was nearly healed. Six months after that, Dr. Murdoch was again at the ranch and found only a small **cicatrix** in the area above the coronary band.

EXERCISE 4-5 *Case It!*

Read Case Study 4-3, and circle the best answer in each statement.

1. Sundance is (a neonate), (a castrated male), or (an intact adult male) horse.

2. The soft skin that a horse's hooves grow from is (a laceration), (a coronary band), or (the epidermis).

3. The local anesthetic will induce the absence of sensation in (a small part of the body such as a tooth or an area of skin), (a larger part of the body such as a leg), or (the whole body).

4. Laceration wounds are (jagged tears), (infected), or (burned).

5. Excess healing tissue is called (cicatrix), (proud flesh), or (alopecia).

6. The anesthetic drug was injected (under the skin), (within a vein), or (within the skin).

7. The lateral surface of Sundance's leg is (in the front), (on the back), or (at the side).

8. The distal part of Sundance's leg is (near the hoof), (at the knee), or (on the surface).

9. Absorbable suture material (dissolves in body fluids and disappears), (consists of sharp-pointed pins that are pushed through the tissue and secured by knobs on each end), or (consists of stainless steel wire or staples).

10. An abrasion is (a cut), (a scrape), or (an infected wound).

Check your answers at the end of the chapter, Answers to Exercises.

MORE WORD PARTS

The prefixes, combining forms, and suffixes presented in Table 4-3 can be used to describe more thoroughly conditions or situations involving the integument. Like the word parts you learned in previous chapters, these word parts will be used with many other systems, so you will be seeing them again in upcoming chapters.

a-

an-

aut/o

bi/o

bi-

circum-

cyst/o

necr/o

nod/o

pachy-

papul/o

para-

TABLE 4-3		Word Parts Associated with the Integumentary System	
Word Parts	**Meaning**	**Example and Definition**	**Word Parts**
a- an-	without, no, not	**acellular** no cells are present	a- = without, no, not cellul/o = cell -ar = pertaining to
		anhidrosis the inability to sweat	an- = without, no, not hidr/o = sweat -osis = disease or abnormal condition
aut/o	self	**autodermic** pertaining to a patient's own skin; term is applied to skin grafts using the patient's own skin	aut/o = self derm/o = skin -ic = pertaining to
bi/o	life	**endobiosis** condition of an organism that lives within another (a parasite) *Do not confuse* bi/o *with the prefix* **bi-** *meaning two (as in* bicycle *with its two wheels).*	endo- = within bi/o = life -osis = disease or abnormal condition
circum-	around	**circumflex** describes a structure that is bent around like a bow *The distance around a circle is its circumference.*	circum- = around flex = capable of being bent; pliable
cyst/o	sac containing fluid, a bladder	**pilocystic** sometimes used to describe dermoid (resembling skin) tumors, which are hollow and contain hair *Be careful!* cyst/o *may refer to one of several sacs or bladders that contain a fluid: the keratin cyst of skin, the fluid-filled gall bladder, or the bladder which collects urine formed by the kidneys.*	pil/o = hair cyst/o = a sac containing fluid -ic = pertaining to
necr/o	death	**necrobiosis** abnormal condition of the death of living tissue; another word for gangrene	necr/o = death bi/o = life -osis = disease or abnormal condition
nod/o	knot	**nodule** a small knot; a small solid lesion measuring <2 cm	nod/o = knot -ule = small
pachy-	thick	**pachyderma** a condition of thick skin *Elephants and rhinoceroses are sometimes referred to as pachyderms.*	pachy- = thick derm/o = skin -a = structure, thing
papul/o	pimple, solid lesion <1 cm	**papular** pertaining to a pimple	papul/o = pimple -ar = pertaining to
para-	near, beside, abnormal, apart from	**parabiosis** the union of two individual animals, as twins joined together *A veterinary* para*professional such as a veterinary technician or a veterinary assistant works alongside a veterinarian.*	para- = near, beside, abnormal, apart from bi/o = life -osis = disease or abnormal condition

TABLE 4-3	Word Parts Associated with the Integumentary System—cont'd		
Word Parts	**Meaning**	**Example and Definition**	**Word Parts**
-phyte	abnormal pathological growth	**dermatophyte** a diseased growth on the skin *The term* dermatophyte *is used to describe a fungal growth of the skin = ringworm.*	dermat/o = skin -phyte = abnormal pathological growth
purpur/o	purple	**purpura** a condition of purple *Purpura is a purplish coloration, visible through the epidermis and caused by blood leaking into the tissue—the "black and blue" bruise.*	purpur/o = purple -a = structure, thing
py/o	pus	**pyoarthrosis** abnormal condition of pus in a joint	py/o = pus arthr/o = joint -osis = disease or abnormal condition
vesicul/o	blister, small sac	**vesiculectomy** surgical removal of a blister	vesicul/o = blister, small sac -ectomy = surgical removal
xer/o	dry	**xeroderma** a condition of dry skin *Frustrated with the slow mimeograph machines and the cost of photography, in 1937 an American law student invented a "dry" way of copying—the Xerox machine.*	xer/o = dry derm/o = skin -a = structure, thing

-phyte

purpur/o

py/o

vesicul/o

xer/o

EXERCISE 4-6 *Case It!*

Read again Case Study 4-1. Then write the words from the right column in the blanks to match their definitions in the left column.

CASE STUDY 4-1 #2001-923 ALLOVER

Signalment and History: Allover is a 7-year-old M(C) Golden Retriever who was brought to the Frisbee Small Animal Clinic because he had been sluggish and gaining weight, even though he was eating the same amount of food. He sought out warm spots more often than usual, and his skin and hair coat did not look good.

Physical Examination: Upon physical examination, Jess Nelson, the veterinary technician, found that Allover was slightly depressed for a Golden Retriever. His BW was 95 pounds, about 10 pounds over his ideal weight. Allover's TPR was within the expected reference ranges. Jess found bilateral areas of alopecia on Allover's body. In other areas, the hair was just thinning. Allover's skin was crusty and scaly all over his body, and there were even some areas of pyoderma. Based on Allover's history and clinical signs, Dr. Frisbee suspected that Allover was suffering from hypothyroidism. Jess drew blood samples from Allover to submit to the lab to check his level of thyroid hormone.

Diagnosis and Treatment: The results of the lab work confirmed the diagnosis of hypothyroidism with secondary pyoderma. Dr. Frisbee prescribed oral antibiotics for the dermatitis, topical treatment with medicated shampoo for the other dermatoses, and a thyroid hormone supplement that probably will have to be given for the rest of Allover's life.

Outcome: At a recheck 1 month later, Allover's skin already looked better. His sores had healed, he was beginning to re-grow his missing hair, and his owners reported that he had more energy than they had seen in a long time. With a controlled diet and more activity, Allover was starting to lose his extra weight.

Dermatitis 1. inflammation of the skin

hypothyroid 2. underactive thyroid gland

Diagnosis 3. knowledge of a disease gained by studying through its symptoms

alopecia 4. loss of hair from the body

Dermatosis 5. any nonspecific skin problem

pyoderma 6. moist patches on skin with a creamy material covering them

Bilateral Symmetry 7. the right half of an animal is the mirror image of the left half

Topical 8. medication applied to body surfaces such as skin

alopecia

bilateral symmetry

dermatitis

dermatosis

diagnosis

hypothyroid

pyoderma

topical treatment

Check your answers at the end of the chapter, Answers to Exercises.

TESTING AND TREATMENT PROCEDURES

In addition to describing the integument and conditions involving the integument, you will have to be able to describe testing and treatment procedures performed on the structures of the integument. Table 4-4 provides the word parts that are used to create combining forms and suffixes pertaining to testing and treatment procedures.

TABLE 4-4	Word Parts Associated with Diagnosis and Treatment		
Word Part	**Meaning**	**Example and Definition**	**Word Parts**
-tomy	surgical incision	**craniotomy** surgical incision into the skull, sometimes done to remove contents to decrease the size of the head of a dead fetus and facilitate delivery *A* **tome** *is an instrument for cutting. Think of Tom as doing the cutting and it will be easier to remember three of the suffixes about surgical procedures: -tomy, -stomy, and -ectomy. Look—Tom is there every time!*	crani/o = head, skull -tomy = surgical incision
-stomy	surgical creation of a new permanent opening	**hysterosalpingostomy** surgical creation of an opening between the uterus and the oviduct **Stoma** *is the name sometimes given to the opening created by -stomy surgery.*	hyster/o = uterus salping/o = oviduct -stomy = surgical creation of a new permanent opening
-ectomy	surgical removal	**onychectomy** removal of a claw; a declaw procedure	onych/o = claw -ectomy = surgical removal
-plasty	surgical repair	**epidermatoplasty** surgical repair of the outer layer of skin *This term is used in describing skin grafts.*	epi- = on or upon dermat/o = skin -plasty = surgical repair
-rrhaphy	suture	**dermorrhaphy** suture of the skin	derm/o = skin -rrhaphy = suture
-pexy	surgical fixation, stabilization, firmly attached	**hysteropexy** surgical fixation of a displaced uterus	hyster/o = uterus -pexy = surgical fixation, stabilization
-centesis	surgical puncture	**abdominocentesis** procedure done to drain off fluid that accumulated in the abdomen	abdomin/o = abdomen -centesis = surgical puncture
-graphy	method of recording	**myography** a technique in which muscle activity is recorded; may be referred to as an *EMG (electromyography)*, which tests for nerve damage or inflammation	my/o = muscle -graphy = method of recording
-graph	instrument used to write or record	**myograph** the instrument for recording muscle activity	my/o = muscle -graph = instrument used to write or record
-gram	written record produced; something recorded or written	**myogram** a written record produced by the myograph instrument *Compare these suffixes and their use in the* telegram *(the written message), which is made by the* telegraph *machine through a process known as* telegraphy.	my/o = muscle -gram = written record produced; something recorded or written

-tomy

-stomy

-ectomy

-plasty

-rrhaphy

-pexy

-centesis

-graphy

-graph

-gram

Continued

-scope

scop/o

TABLE 4-4	Word Parts Associated with Diagnosis and Treatment—cont'd		
Word Part	**Meaning**	**Example and Definition**	**Word Parts**
-scope	instrument for examining or viewing	**endoarthroscope** instrument for examining the interior of a joint *You are familiar with many "scopes": microscope, stethoscope, telescope, oscilloscope, and periscope.*	endo- = within, inner arthr/o = joint -scope = instrument for examining or viewing
scop/o	examine, view	**necroscopy** process of examination of a body after death; word is sometimes shortened to **necropsy**	necr/o = death scop/o = examine, view -y = made up of, characterized by

EXERCISE 4-7 *Write It!*

Remember—when you define a word, you start with the suffix. Next, you define the prefix, and last, you define the word root. Using the following word parts, construct the medical word and define it. Some terms will not have all the word parts. Some terms will have more than one word root. The first medical term is done as an example.

Suffix	Prefix	Combining Form	The Word!	Definition
-osis	hypo-	hidr/o	hypohidrosis	an abnormal diminished secretion of sweat
1. -ous	pachy-	hemat/o	Pachy ~~Poly~~hematous	pertaining thicken blood
2. -ium	epi-	crani/o	epicranium	scalp musle cover head
3. -itis	poly-	chondr/o	polychondytis	inflam of cartilages
4. thorax	—	py/o hem/o	hemothorax	pus blood in thorax
5. -osis	hyper-	lip/o	hyperlipasis	abnormal con of excess fat.
6. -plasty	—	neur/o	Neuroplasty	surgical repair of nerves
7. -ia	—	hist/o hydr/o	histohydria	excess water in tissue
8. -logy	—	onych/o path/o	pathology	study of diseases.
9. -al	supra-	spin/o	supraspinal	something above the spine
10. -osis	a-	trich/o	atrichosis	No hair

Check your answers at the end of the chapter, Answers to Exercises.

ABBREVIATIONS

At the end of this chapter and the others that follow you will find tables that do not provide word parts but do provide abbreviations that are commonly used in clinical veterinary language, especially in medical records and professional communications (Table 4-5).

TABLE 4-5	Abbreviations	
Abbreviation	**Meaning**	**Example**
pt	patient	In veterinary medicine, the animal is the pt and the owner is the client.
PE	physical exam	A PE should be performed at the start of every veterinary visit.
hx	history	Sparky has a hx of vomiting.
YOB	year of birth	Oscar's YOB is 1999.
wt	weight	A growing problem in SA medicine is the wt of many pt. Like many people, many pets are becoming obese.
R/O	rule out	Sometimes diagnostic tests are performed to R/O conditions or diseases.
®	right	Take a ® lateral X-ray of Rosie's thorax.
Ⓛ	left	The medial surface of the Ⓛ metatarsal joint was oozing a mucopurulent fluid.
CC	chief complaint	The CC for Roxie is a Ⓛ rear leg myalgia.
BAR	bright, alert, responsive	Physical examination: Sparky was BAR and was limping on his left hind leg.
DDN	dull, depressed, nonresponsive	Physical examination: Bruiser was DDN with numerous facial and cervical lacerations.
T P R	temperature pulse respiration	Physical examination: Dweezle's TPR was within the reference range.
FUO	fever of unknown origin	Physical examination: Bruiser was displaying a 105° F FUO.
BW	body weight	Sparky has a hx of a loss of 5 lbs BW between January and March.
BD/LD	big dog/little dog (used when describing a specific type of dogfight wound)	History: Sparky had been in a BD/LD fight that resulted in a laceration on his left hind leg.
dx	diagnosis	Dx: BD/LD laceration on ® foreleg proximal to the carpus and distal to the elbow
ddx	differential diagnosis	The ddx for the wounds could be animal abuse or self-trauma.
DOA	dead on arrival	Neither Sparky nor Bruiser was DOA, even though Bruiser was DDN.
GSW	gunshot wound	Physical examination: Rosie has a GSW on her thorax, just caudal to the point of the left elbow.
HBC	hit by car	History: Initially, we thought this was an HBC, but upon physical examination, we discovered a GSW.
Stat	immediately (if not sooner)	Get Bruiser to the surgical suite Stat!
bx	biopsy	This specimen is a bx of the ® thoracic lymph node.
lac	laceration	A 3-inch lac was found in the paralumbar fossa.

pt

PE

hx

YOB

wt

R/O

®

Ⓛ

CC

BAR

DDN

TPR

FUO

BW

BD/LD

dx

ddx

DOA

GSW

HBC

Stat

bx

lac

ANSWERS TO EXERCISES

Exercise 4-1

1. under
2. black
3. upper or outer
4. after-effects
5. disease
6. claws or nails
7. fat
8. skin and nerves
9. fat
10. across or through
11. hard or horn-like
12. skin
13. growth, development, or formation
14. muscle
15. horns

Exercise 4-2

1. epidermis
2. sudoriferous gland
3. dermis
4. dermis
5. adipose tissue
6. epidermis
7. hair follicle
8. sebaceous gland
9. epidermis
10. hypodermis
11. arrector pili muscle
12. sudoriferous gland
13. epidermis
14. epidermis
15. hair follicle
16. hypodermis
17. hair
18. adipose tissue
19. sebaceous gland
20. sudoriferous gland

Exercise 4-3

1. abrasion—a wound caused by rubbing or scraping
2. laceration—a wound produced by tearing the skin, as opposed to a cut or an incision
3. excoriate—lose or remove the outer layer of skin; flay
4. fissure—a crack-like lesion in the skin
5. incision—a cut or wound made by a sharp instrument
6. keloid—overgrowth of scar tissue at the site of injury
7. scar—a mark remaining after the healing of a wound caused by injury, illness, or surgery
8. proud flesh—overgrowth of granulation tissue developed during healing of large surface wounds
9. granulation tissue—new tissue formed in repair of wounds of soft tissue
10. cicatrix—a scar
11. papule—a small, solid elevation of the skin; does not contain pus
12. plaque—a solid elevation of the skin (papule) that is greater than 1 cm in diameter
13. wheal—elevated papule that is redder or paler than surrounding skin; usually accompanied by itching
14. pus—cells and cellular debris in a thin fluid, formed as a result of inflammation
15. abscess—localized collection of pus in a cavity
16. purulent—containing or forming pus
17. suppurate—to produce or discharge pus
18. furuncle—a boil or skin abscess, usually around follicles
19. carbuncle—a cluster of furuncles in adjacent hairs
20. boil—a furuncle
21. eschar—a scab; dry crust that results from trauma such as a burn; consists of dried serum, blood, and pus
22. ecchymosis—a bruise; blood leaking from a ruptured blood vessel into the skin; a "black and blue" mark
23. petechia—tiny, pinpoint, nonraised, round purplish red spots with the dermal layer; tiny ecchymoses
24. signalment—the part of the animal's history that deals with its age, sex, and distinguishing features
25. signs—observable indicators like body temperature or bleeding
26. symptoms—what the patient tells you is wrong
27. palliative—treating symptoms, but not curing the cause
28. tumor—any mass or swelling; new growth of tissue where cell multiplication is uncontrolled (a cancer)
29. ulcer—an open sore; crater-like lesion of the skin or mucous membrane
30. inflammation—tissue is injured; classic signs are heat, redness, swelling, pain, and loss of function

Exercise 4-4

1. F—A zoonotic disease is one that can be spread from animals to humans.
2. F—A prognosis is a prediction of the outcome of Holstein's disorder.
3. T
4. T
5. F—A laceration that is superficial is in the epidermis.
6. T
7. T
8. F—Holstein is a male feline.
9. T
10. T

Exercise 4-5

1. a castrated male
2. coronary band
3. a small part of the body
4. jagged tears
5. proud flesh
6. within the skin
7. at the side
8. near the hoof
9. dissolves in body fluids and disappears
10. a scrape

Exercise 4-6

1. dermatitis
2. hypothyroid
3. diagnosis
4. alopecia
5. dermatosis
6. pyoderma
7. bilateral symmetry
8. topical treatment

Exercise 4-7

1. pachyhematous—pertaining to or having thickened blood
2. epicranium—things (like the scalp and muscles) that cover the head
3. polychondritis—inflammation of many cartilages
4. pyohemothorax—pus and blood in the thorax
5. hyperliposis—abnormal condition of excess fat
6. neuroplasty—surgical repair of nerves
7. histohydria—pertaining to excess water in tissue
8. onychopathology—study of diseases of nails or claws
9. supraspinal—pertaining to something above the spine
10. atrichosis—abnormal condition of no hair (baldness)

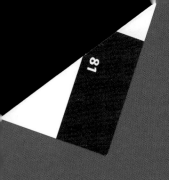

Chapter 5

The Skeletal System

The foot bone connected to the ankle bone, The ankle bone connected to the shin bone, The shin bone connected to the knee bone, The knee bone connected to the thigh bone, The thigh bone connected to the hip bone, the hip bone connected to the back bone, The back bone connected to the shoulder bone, The shoulder bone connected to the neck bone, The neck bone connected to the head bone.

Traditional Spiritual

WORD PARTS

ab-	ahb	cyan/o	**sī**-ahn-ō	leuk/o	**loo**-kō	plas/o	**plā**-zō
ad-	ahd	-cyte	sīt	lumb/o	**luhm**-bō	-plasm	plahzm
albin/o	ahl-**bī**-nō	dactyl/o	**dahk**-tihl-ō	mal-	mahl	pod/o	**pō**-dō
-algia	**ahl**-jē-ah	dia-	**dī**-ah	malac/o	mah-**lā**-shō	por/o	**pohr**-ō
ambi-	**ahm**-bē	digit/o	**dihg**-iht-ō	mandibul/o	mahn-**dihb**-ū-lō	post-	pōst
amphi-	**ahm**-fih	-dynia	**dihn**-ē-ah	maxill/o	mahck-**sih**-lō	pro-	prō
ankyl/o	**ahng**-kih-lō	end-	ehnd	melan/o	**mehl**-ah-nō	pub/o	**pehw**-bō
ante-	**ahn**-tē	endo-	**ehn**-dō	meta-	**meht**-ah	purpur/o	**pər**-pər-ō
arthr/o	**arth**-rō	epi-	**ehp**-ih	meta- + carp/o	**meht**-ah-**kahr**-pō	radi/o	**rā**-dē-ō
articul/o	ahr-**tihck**-yoo-lō	erythr/o	eh-**rihth**-rō	meta- + tars/o	**meht**-ah-**tahr**-sō	rubr/o	**rū**-brō
-blast	blahst	ex-	ehcks	myel/o	mī-**eh**-lō	sacr/o	**sā**-krō
brachi/o	**brā**-kē-ō	exo-	**ehcks**-ō	-oma	**ō**-mah	scapul/o	**skahp**-yoo-lō
carp/o	**karh**-pō	femor/o	**fehm**-ohr-ō	orth/o	**ohr**-thō	skelet/o	**skehl**-eh-tō
cervic/o	**sihr**-vih-cō	fibul/o	**fihb**-yoo-lō	os	ohs	spondyl/o	spohn-**dih**-lō
chlor/o	**klohr**-ō	gen/o	**jehn**-ō	osse/o	**ohs**-ē-ō	stern/o	**stər**-nō
chondr/o	**kohn**-drō	-genesis	**jehn**-eh-sihs	oste/o	**ohs**-tē-ō	syn-	sihn
chrom/o	**krō**-mō	gnath/o	**gnahth**-ō	pachy-	**pahck**-ē	tars/o	**tahr**-sō
cirrh/o	**sihr**-ō	humer/o	**hū**-mər-ō	patell/o	pah-**tehl**-ō	thorac/o	**thōr**-ah-cō
-clast	klahst	ile/o	**ihl**-ē-ō	pelv/i	**pehl**-vī	tibi/o	**tihb**-ē-ō
coccyg/o	kohck-**sihd**-jō	ili/o	**ihl**-ē-ō	pelvi/o	**pehl**-vē-ō	tuber/o	**too**-bər-ō
cost/o	**kohs**-tō	inter-	**ihn**-tər	peri-	**pehr**-ih	uln/o	**uhl**-nō
cox/o	**kohx**-ō	intra-	**ihn**-trah	phalang/o	fah-**lahn**-jō	vertebr/o	vehr-**tē**-brō
crani/o	**krā**-nē-ō	ischi/o	**ihs**-kē-ō	physi/o	**fihz**-ē-ō	xanth/o	**zahn**-thō

OUTLINE

LEARNING OBJECTIVES

When you have completed this chapter, you will be able to:

1 Understand the components and functions of the skeletal system.

2 Identify and recognize the meanings of word parts related to the skeletal system, using them to build or analyze words.

3 Apply your new knowledge of understanding clinical veterinary language in the context of medical reports.

CASE STUDY 5-1 #2010-98 KEVIN

Signalment and History: An 8-month-old M Rottweiler named Kevin was brought to the Frisbee Small Animal Veterinary Hospital for evaluation of a left rear limb lameness of 5 months' duration. Kevin had never walked completely normally and had a shifting rear limb lameness that had become worse in the past week. Kevin is still eating and drinking well but was reluctant to play with his littermate, who is owned by the same person.

Physical Examination and Diagnosis: On physical examination, Jess found that Kevin was mildly depressed and had a non–weight-bearing lameness of the left rear limb. Temperature, pulse, and respiration (TPR) were all within the expected reference ranges. Palpation of the left **coxofemoral** joint elicited signs of pain. X-rays of the pelvis showed a possible left coxofemoral joint **septic arthritis.** The **diaphyseal cortex** of the left femur was thin. Dr. Frisbee explained to the owner that the degeneration of the **femoral cortex** may have been a result of disuse **osteoporosis** and **myelitis.** Absence of the left **femoral epiphysis** indicated complete **lysis.** The right coxofemoral joint was shallow with **subluxation** of the **femoral head. Periarticular osteogenesis** also was evident at this site. Right coxofemoral joint **dysplasia** and degenerative **arthropathy** were diagnosed.

Thoracic X-rays revealed a **T4-T5 diskospondylitis** caused by **hematogenous** spread of an infection. The **T4 vertebra** was shortened with a decreased T4-T5 **intervertebral disk space.** Bridging **spondylosis** was also evident. The **caudal** aspect of the left **humeral head** was slightly flattened. These findings were consistent with **bilateral humeral osteochondrosis.**

Treatment: Kevin underwent surgery for a left femoral head and neck **ostectomy. Purulent** discharge present in and around the joint capsule was collected. The femur **fractured** during surgery at the junction of the **proximal** and middle thirds of the bone. The cortex of the femur was thin with necrotic (dead) marrow. After consultation with Dr. Frisbee, the owners elected to have the left limb amputated. Samples of the bone and joint capsule were sent for **histological** evaluation. Kevin recovered from surgery without incident. Histological evaluation revealed severe, **chronic,** active **osteomyelitis.** No evidence of **neoplasia** was present. The condition was **exacerbated** by the presence of bridging **spondylosis.** Culture test results revealed the cause as *Staphylococcus aureus* (a bacterium). Kevin was placed on antibiotics for 2 weeks.

Outcome: By 3 weeks **post surgery,** the owner noticed a considerable increase in overall activity of Kevin, the now amazing three-legged dog. The **prognosis** for complete recovery is good.

THE SKELETAL SYSTEM

Now that you have figured out the container for the prototype animal that you are building, it is time to start filling it. Can you envision a big burlap bag of bones with a nose, four legs, and a tail? *"Get that old bag of bones off the racetrack!" "That dog has lost so much weight he's just a bag of bones."* Animals are not made of burlap, but they are bags of bones if you think of the skin as a big bag.

Your prototype animal starts with the skeletal system, which will give it a basic shape. Say "skeleton" to someone, and he immediately thinks "bones." And he is mostly right. The skeletal *system,* however, is composed of three structures: bones, cartilages, and ligaments. Fortunately, the bones are held together by the cartilages and ligaments in a shape that we recognize as a horse, dog, camel, duck, mouse, and all other animals.

FUNCTIONS OF BONES

There are many different bones in a body, but they all function in one or more of the following ways.

Bones:
- help define the appearance of an animal through its shape

    Imagine what a strange animal you would have if the ankle bone was connected to the hip bone.
- act as storage depots for minerals, especially calcium and phosphorus

    An animal that does not get enough calcium in its diet will start using the calcium from its bones, resulting in soft bones that easily fracture. This can be seen in primates who are kept as pets and are fed only fruits and nuts; their bones may become so soft that you can bend them with your hands.
- allow mobility and movement in conjunction with the muscles and nerves of the body

    Muscles attach to bones. When muscles contract, bones move. If the bones in all four legs are moved at the same time in a coordinated sequence, the animal is walking or running.
- provide protection for what they are covering

    Most of the bones of the skull do not move, but think of what would happen to brains if the bones were not there. The same is true of the heart and lungs. What would happen if the ribs were gone?
- afford the site for blood cell production

    Not all bones participate in blood cell production. Only those bones with red bone marrow contain the necessary blood cell–producing cells.

BONE FORMATION AND GROWTH

Bone is living tissue made up of cells (**osteocytes** = bone cells; **osteoblasts** = bone-forming cells; **osteoclasts** = cells that "eat" or destroy bone tissue so new bone can be formed) and a matrix or framework. The matrix is what contains the mineralized calcium and phosphorus and gives bones their strength. Bones have a nerve supply and are fed by a series of blood vessels. They are covered by a dense membrane called the **periosteum,** which contains the nerves and blood vessels that are supplied to the bone.

Bone formation, or **osteogenesis,** initially takes place over cartilage rods that serve as templates in developing fetuses. The cartilage is replaced by bone through a process called **ossification** as the fetus develops. When a baby animal is born, most of the cartilage template has been **ossified,** but the bones are still soft because the matrix has not yet become totally mineralized.

The formation of the bones of the skull (cranium) is a little different. It occurs through a process called **intramembranous bone formation.** If you analyze *intramembranous,* you will deduce that the bone formation takes place within a membrane. This is exactly what happens. In the developing fetus, the skull bones are formed in the fibrous tissue membrane that covers the brain.

Bones grow. If they did not, animals would remain the same size as when they are born. For the bones to grow, they have to retain a cartilage growth site. A few cartilage sites remain in some of the bones until the animal has reached full size. In a typical long bone, these growth sites are found near the ends of the bone and are called **epiphyseal plates or growth plates.** When an animal is born, only the epiphyseal plates remain as sites of bone growth. As the bones grow longer from these growth plates, the animal grows (Figure 5-1).

ANATOMY OF THE SKELETAL SYSTEM

Bones, cartilages, and ligaments are the three components of the skeletal system and are often referred to collectively as the *skeleton.* The skeletons of most of the animals you will care for in veterinary medicine are termed **endoskeletons.** This means that the skeletons are located beneath the skin of the animal. If the skeleton is located on the outside of the animal (e.g., ticks, insects, spiders, crabs), it is called an **exoskeleton.** Endoskeletons are the focus of this chapter (Table 5-1).

skelet/o

oste/o

osse/o

os

myel/o

-cyte

-blast

-clast

gen/o

-genesis

epi-

TABLE 5-1	Word Parts Associated with the Skeletal System		
Word Part	**Meaning**	**Example and Definition**	**Word Parts**
skelet/o	skeleton, the bony and some of the cartilaginous framework of the body of animals	**skeletal** pertaining to the bony framework of the body of animals	skelet/o = skeleton -al = pertaining to
oste/o osse/o os	bone	**osteoarthritis** most common type of arthritis, characterized by inflammation, degeneration, and eventual loss of the cartilage of the joints	oste/o = bone arthr/o = joint -itis = inflammation
		osseous tissues bone tissue	osse/o = bone -ous = pertaining to
		os penis the bone in the penis of a dog	os = bone penis = penis, a biological feature of male animals
myel/o	bone marrow	**periosteomyelitis** inflammation of the entire bone, including the periosteum and the bone marrow ⚠ myel/o *also refers to the spinal cord. Depending on the context in which this combining form is used, you should know whether* myel/o *refers to bone marrow or to the spinal cord. The term* myelitis *is a very general term; it does not tell the location of the inflammation.* Periosteomyelitis *is much more specific.*	peri- = around, surrounding oste/o = bone myel/o = bone marrow -itis = inflammation
-cyte	cell	**osteocyte** bone cell	oste/o = bone -cyte = cell
-blast	bud, germinal, seed	**osteoblast** cell responsible for bone formation	oste/o = bone -blast = bud, germinal, seed
-clast	to break	**osteoclast** cell that breaks down bone	oste/o = bone -clast = to break
gen/o -genesis	formation or beginning	**hematogenous** originating or spread by blood	hemat/o = blood gen/o = formation or beginning -ous = pertaining to
		pathogenesis origin of a disease	path/o = disease -genesis = formation or beginning
epi-	on or upon	**epibiosis** living attached to another organism, such as a fungus	epi- = on or upon bi/o = life -osis = disease or abnormal condition

TABLE 5-1	Word Parts Associated with the Skeletal System—cont'd		
Word Part	**Meaning**	**Example and Definition**	**Word Parts**
physi/o	to make grow, to produce	**physiology** related to the study of natural functions	physi/o = to make grow, to produce -logy = to study, or to have knowledge of
endo- end-	within, inner	**endopelvic** within the pelvis	endo- = within, inner pelvi/o = pelvis -ic = pertaining to
		endosteoma tumor within bone	end- = within, inner oste/o = bone -oma = a tumor or abnormal new growth, a swelling
ex- exo-	out, outside, outer, away from	**excise** in surgery, the complete removal of an organ, tissue, or tumor from a body	ex- = out, outside, outer, away from -cise = to cut (e.g., an incision is a cut made into something, and incisors are the cutting teeth)
		exoskeletal pertaining to the outer hard framework that supports and protects the soft tissues of a body	exo- = out, outside, outer, away from skelet/o = skeleton -al = pertaining to
inter-	between, among	**intercostal** area between the ribs	inter- = between, among cost/o = ribs -al = pertaining to
intra-	within, inside	**intracranial** within the head (skull)	intra- = within, inside crani/o = head, skull -al = pertaining to
meta-	beyond, after, next	**metaplasm** the nonliving constituents, such as pigment granules, in the cytoplasm of a cell	meta- = beyond, after, next plasm = formed material (as of a cell or tissue)
peri-	around, surrounding	**periosteotomy** surgical incision through the periosteum (membrane surrounding bone)	peri- = around, surrounding oste/o = bone -tomy = surgical incision
tuber/o	rounded projection, knob	**tuberous** covered with tubers; knobby *The roots of the tuberous begonia are knobby, as are the tuber vegetables: potatoes and yams.*	tuber/o = rounded projection, knob -ous = pertaining to

physi/o

endo-

end-

ex-

exo-

inter-

intra-

meta-

peri-

tuber/o

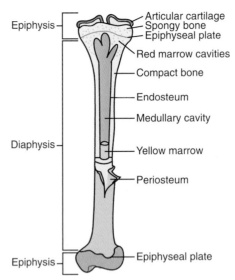

FIGURE 5-1 Schematic diagram of a longitudinal section of long bone (tibia) showing spongy (cancellous) and compact bone.

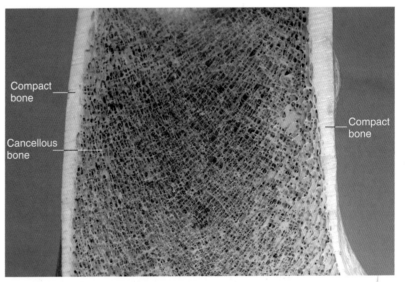

FIGURE 5-2 **Bone structure.** Cut surface of distal end of horse femur showing detail of compact and cancellous bone structure. (From Colville TP: *Clinical Anatomy and Physiology Laboratory Manual for Veterinary Technicians*, St Louis, 2009, Mosby.)

BONES

Bones form the physical framework of the skeleton. A "bone" is actually made up of two different types of bone: **compact bone** and **cancellous bone** (Figure 5-2).
- Compact bone
  - is also known as *cortical bone*
  - makes up the outer part of the bone, which is very strong and hard
  - contains mineralized calcium and phosphorus, which together form the second hardest material in the body after tooth enamel (if bones were solid compact bone, they would be heavy and a real pain to drag around)
- Cancellous bone
  - is also known as *spongy bone* because grossly, it looks like a sponge
  - has the same makeup as compact bone but is not as dense because it is made up of spicules (small, slender, needle-like pieces of bone) instead of solid

bone (thus the bones are lighter, making it easier for the animal to move around)

- provides space for bone marrow between the spicules

Bone Marrow

Bones are not solid. Within the outer compact bone shell, the cancellous bone is made up of spicules with spaces between them. These spaces are filled with **bone marrow.** In some bones (e.g., long bones), the mid portion of the shaft of the bone does not contain cancellous bone. It is a hollow cavity called the **medullary cavity** or the **marrow cavity** and is filled with bone marrow. Two types of bone marrow have been identified: red marrow and yellow marrow, which are named for what they look like. The function of red bone marrow is to produce blood cells from the primitive cells that live there. The marrow looks red because of the large number of red blood cells that are being produced. When an animal is born, almost all of its bone marrow is red bone marrow because the animal needs lots of blood cells to support growth and development. As the animal gets older, it does not need as great a supply of red marrow to maintain health, so some of the red marrow quits making blood cells and is replaced by fat cells. The fat appears pale yellow, hence the name *yellow bone marrow.* In an adult animal, red bone marrow is found primarily in flat bones (ribs, hip bone) and in the proximal ends of the femur (thigh bone) and humerus (brachium). In small animals, most bone marrow biopsy specimens are taken from the hip bone, the proximal humerus, or the proximal femur. In large animals, the sternum (breastbone) is biopsied.

EXERCISE 5-1 *Define It!*

Match the best answers from words in the right column to their descriptions on the left.

1. Red bone marrow red blood cell production starts here — ~~cancellous bone~~
2. Compact bone outer, hard part of bone — ~~compact bone~~
3. Endoskeleton skeleton within the skin of an animal — ~~cranium~~
4. ~~Periosteum~~ ligaments structure that holds bones together — ~~endoskeleton~~
5. Osteocytes living tissue composing bone — ~~epiphyses~~
6. Periosteum dense membrane covering bone — ~~exoskeleton~~
7. yellow bone fat cells in bones — ~~ligament~~
8. Cranium bones of the skull — ~~osteocytes~~
9. Osteogenesis formation of bones — ~~osteogenesis~~
10. epiphyses growth sites on long bones — ~~periosteum~~
11. cancellous bone tissue made of spicules — ~~red bone marrow~~
12. Exoskeleton skeleton on outside of animal — ~~yellow bone marrow~~

Check your answers at the end of the chapter, Answers to Exercises.

What Color?

Speaking of yellow and red bone marrow, you already know that there should be more combining forms in your new clinical veterinary language that indicate color in general, or a specific color. Table 5-2 lists the common color combining forms.

Bone Shapes

Look at a skeleton, and you will notice that all bones are not created equal. They come in a variety of shapes and sizes, but they can be classified as belonging to one of four shape categories:

- **Long bones** are longer than they are wide. Many of the bones of an animal's legs are long bones.
- **Short bones** are shaped roughly like cubes. The bones of the carpus (wrist) and tarsus (ankle) are examples of short bones.
- **Flat bones** are thin and flat. They are composed mostly of external compact bone with very little internal cancellous bone. The bones of the skull are flat bones. So are hip bones, ribs, and the sternum (breastbone).
- **Irregular bones** are bones that do not fit neatly into the other three categories. They come in a variety of shapes. The bones of the spine (**vertebrae**) are irregular bones. Another special group of bones called **sesamoid bones** (they look like sesame seeds) is also included in the irregular shape category. These bones are embedded in muscle tendons and act as "ball bearings" when the tendon moves over a joint. The kneecap (**patella***)* is the largest sesamoid bone in the body. But there are others; the horse has three sesamoid bones in each digit.

Parts of a Long Bone

Long bones are sometimes broken (fractured) as a result of trauma. It is important to be able to identify what part of the bone is affected, so bones are divided into anatomical parts. These parts are named on the basis of their location in relation to the epiphyseal plates (Figure 5-3).

- The **epiphyses** are located at both ends of the bone sitting upon the epiphyseal plates.
- The longest part of the bone is the shaft or **diaphysis.** It is located between the epiphyseal plates.
- The widest part of the diaphysis situated immediately next to the epiphyseal plates is the **metaphysis.**
- Other parts of the long bones that are found on and in most bones are:
  - the periosteum
  - the endosteum, a membrane that lines the medullary or marrow cavity of the bone

Bone Bumps, Humps, and Holes

Bones have many irregularities on their surfaces. Some stick up from the surface of the bone; others are depressed into the surface. These projections and depressions can be called a **head, condyle, process, trochanter, tuberosity, crest, wing,** or **spine,** depending on where they are located. However, no matter where they are located, these irregularities serve specific functions. For example, heads generally are found on the proximal ends of long bones, and condyles most often are found on the distal ends of long bones. Both have smooth surfaces and will form parts of joints (more about that later). The other projections have rough surfaces and are found at locations where muscles attach to bones. The larger the projection, the larger the muscle that attaches to it, and the more powerful the movement it produces.

Depressions in bones usually are called **foramina** (*singular* = foramen) or **fossas** (*singular* = fossa). A foramen is usually a hole through which a blood vessel or a nerve passes to enter or leave the bone. A fossa is a depression where a muscle is attached to the bone.

TABLE 5-2	Combining Forms for Colors		
Combining Form	**Colors**	**Example and Definition**	**Word Parts**
chrom/o	color	**achromodermic** pertaining to no color in the skin *On the piano/keyboard when you play all the black and white keys of an octave, you are playing the chromatic scale.*	a- = without, no, not chrom/o = color derm/o = skin -ic = pertaining to
albin/o	no color	**albinism** condition where the animal is unable to produce melanin; an albino is achromodermic and achromotrichic	albin/o = no color -ism = state, condition, action, process, result
melan/o	black, dark	**melanocyte** cell in the epidermis that produces the black pigment melanin	melan/o = black, dark -cyte = cell
leuk/o	white	**melanoleukoderma** marbled or mottled appearance of the skin	melan/o = black leuk/o = white derm/o = skin -a = structure, thing
purpur/o	purple	**purpura** purplish coloration, visible through the epidermis, and caused by blood leaking into the tissue—the "black and blue" bruise	purpur/o = purple -a = structure, thing
cyan/o	blue	**hypercyanosis** extreme bluish discoloration of the skin and mucous membranes *This is what can happen if you hold your breath way too long.*	hyper- = above, over, excess cyan/o = blue -osis = disease or abnormal condition
rubr/o erythr/o	red	**rubricity** redness *Think of the red ruby.*	rubr/o = red -ic = pertaining to -ity = state or condition
		erythrocyanosis mottled red and bluish colorations that appear on human skin, as in mild frostbite	erythr/o = red cyan/o = blue -osis = disease or abnormal condition
chlor/o	green	**chlorosis** rare form of anemia in women, that results in greenish skin *Is this a condition that results from severe envy?*	chlor/o = green -osis = disease or abnormal condition
cirrh/o	orange-yellow	**cirrhosis** a disease or abnormal condition (of the liver) *Symptoms of* cirrhosis *may include jaundice (yellow color in the skin, mucous membranes, or eyes).*	cirrh/o = orange-yellow -osis = disease or abnormal condition
xanth/o	yellow	**xanthoma** condition characterized by yellowish nodules in the skin; can be a sign of hyperliposis (abnormal condition of excess fat tissue)	xanth/o = yellow -oma = a tumor or abnormal growth, a swelling

chrom/o

albin/o

melan/o

leuk/o

purpur/o

cyan/o

rubr/o

erythr/o

chlor/o

cirrh/o

xanth/o

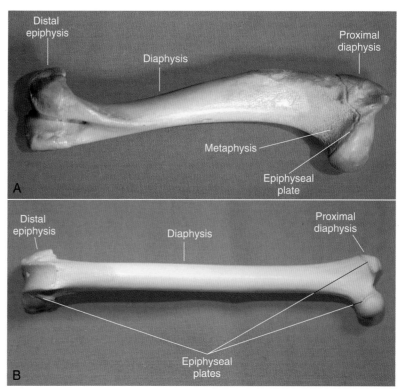

FIGURE 5-3 **External anatomy of long bones. A,** Tibia. **B,** Femur. (From Colville TP: *Clinical Anatomy and Physiology Laboratory Manual for Veterinary Technicians*, St Louis, 2009, Mosby.)

EXERCISE 5-2 *Understand It!*

Complete these statements by writing words in the blanks to complete the definitions.

1. The projection on the surface of a bone at its proximal end is its _head_.

2. A _formen_ is a hole through which blood vessels or nerves pass to enter or leave a bone.

3. Cartilage is replaced by bone in a process called bone _ossification_.

4. _peristieum_ is the membrane that covers bone. It contains _nerves_ and _blood vessels_.

5. The largest sesamoid bone in the body is the _patella_; it is inserted into the tendon that moves over the _Knee_ joint.

6. The irregularly shaped bones of the spine are collectively known as the _vertebrae_.

7. The red marrow that quits making blood cell cells is replaced by _fat cells_.

8. The growth plates found near the ends of long bones are the _Epiphyseal_.

9. The projection on the surface of a bone at its distal end is its _condyle_.

10. A _fossa_ is a depression where a muscle is attached to a bone.

Check your answers at the end of the chapter, Answers to Exercises.

AXIAL AND APPENDICULAR SKELETONS

An animal has just one complete skeleton. However, as you look at a skeleton, you will notice that the bones can be divided easily into two groups: the bones of the head and trunk (barrel, body) and the bones of the appendages (legs). If a bone is located in the head or trunk of an animal, it is part of the **axial skeleton** (Table 5-3). If a bone is located in one of the legs of an animal, it is part of the **appendicular skeleton** (Figure 5-4; Table 5-4).

TABLE 5-3	Combining Forms for Bones of the Axial Skeleton		
Combining Form	Meaning	Example and Definition	Word Parts
crani/o	cranium, skull	**cranioplasty** surgical repair of the skull *The cranium is located cranial (toward the head) to the neck!*	crani/o = cranium, skull -plasty = surgical repair
gnath/o	jaw	**prognathism** abnormal protrusion of one or both jaws, especially the lower jaw	pro- = before gnath/o = jaw -ism = state, condition, action, process, or result
mandibul/o	mandible (lower jaw)	**mandibulectomy** surgical removal of the lower jaw	mandibul/o = mandible -ectomy = surgical removal
maxill/o	maxilla (upper jaw)	**maxillotomy** surgical incision into the upper jaw	maxill/o = maxilla -tomy = surgical incision
vertebr/o	vertebra vertebrae (plural)	**intervertebral** between the vertebrae *A vertebra is any one of the separate bones that make up the spine (vertebral column).*	inter- = between, among vertebr/o = vertebra -al = pertaining to
spondyl/o	vertebral column, the spine	**spondylosis** a general term for degenerative changes in the spine	spondyl/o = vertebrae -osis = disease or abnormal condition
cervic/o	neck	**cervicodorsal** pertaining to the neck and the back *Cervical vertebrae are located in the neck, caudal to the skull and cranial to the thoracic vertebrae. They are named with the letter **C** and a number (e.g., C1). Seven cervical vertebrae are found in all common species.* *Only the two uppermost vertebrae have actual names. C1 is the **atlas,** and it supports the skull. It is named for the Greek god Atlas, who supported the pillars of heaven on his shoulders. C2 is the **axis,** and it makes it possible for the head to turn.* *The neck is any constricted portion. A neck holds up the head. The uterus also has a neck; it is called the cervix. A **cervicectomy** would certainly be performed on the neck of the uterus.*	cervic/o = neck dors/o = back -al = pertaining to cervic/o = neck -ectomy = surgical removal

crani/o

gnath/o

mandibul/o

maxill/o

vertebr/o

spondyl/o

cervic/o

Continued

thorac/o

lumb/o

sacr/o

coccyg/o

cost/o

stern/o

TABLE 5-3		Combining Forms for Bones of the Axial Skeleton—cont'd	
Combining Form	Meaning	Example and Definition	Word Parts
thorac/o	thorax	**thoracoscopy** procedure for examining the thorax, especially the chest cavity around the lungs; machine used is a thoracoscope *Thoracic vertebrae are located dorsal to the thorax, caudal to the cervical vertebrae, and proximal to the lumbar vertebrae. They are named with the letter **T** and a number (e.g., T1). The number of thoracic vertebrae varies with the species.*	thorac/o = thorax scop/o = examine, view -y = having the quality of
lumb/o	loin (lower part of the back between the hipbones and the ribs)	**lumbocostal** pertaining to the loin and the ribs—it is here that you might feel your lumbago *Lumbar vertebrae are dorsal to the abdomen, caudal to the thoracic vertebrae, and cranial to the sacral vertebrae. They are named with the letter **L** and a number (e.g., L1). The number of lumbar vertebrae varies with the species.*	lumb/o = loin cost/o = ribs -al = pertaining to
sacr/o	sacrum (bones lying dorsally between the two hip bones)	**sacrocaudal** pertaining to the sacrum and the tail *Sacral vertebrae are in the pelvic area, caudal to the lumbar vertebrae and cranial to the coccygeal vertebrae. They are named with the letter **S** and a number (e.g., S1). The number of sacral vertebrae varies with the species.*	sacr/o = sacrum caud/o = tail -al = pertaining to
coccyg/o	tail	**coccygectomy** surgical removal of the tail *Coccygeal vertebrae make up the tail; they are found caudal to the sacrum. They are named with the letters **Cy** or **Co** and a number (e.g., Cy1). The number of coccygeal vertebrae varies with the species.*	coccyg/o = tail -ectomy = surgical removal
cost/o	ribs	**cervicocostal** pertaining to the neck and the ribs	cervic/o = neck cost/o = ribs -al = pertaining to
stern/o	sternum	**costosternoplasty** surgical procedure to support the sternum by using a portion of a rib *The sternum is the breastbone. Do you remember sternal recumbency?*	cost/o = ribs stern/o = sternum -plasty = surgical repair

TABLE 5-4	Word Parts for the Appendicular Skeleton		
Word Part	**Meaning**	**Example and Definition**	**Word Parts**
scapul/o	scapula	**scapulopexy** surgical fixation of the scapula *The scapula is the shoulder blade, the flat triangular bone that forms the dorsal portion of the shoulder. It is located in the front leg, proximal to the humerus.*	scapul/o = scapula -pexy = surgical fixation, stabilization
brachi/o	brachium (front leg proximal to the humeroradial joint or elbow)	**cervicobrachial** pertaining to the neck and to the front leg above the humeroradial joint	cervic/o = neck brachi/o = brachium -al = pertaining to
ante-	before, in front of, prior to	**antebrachium** the front leg distal to the humeroradial joint; the forearm— an accepted veterinary anatomical term even though arm and forearm do not have common clinical usage related to animals *Anterior is in the front; Antebellum refers to that period before the American Civil War.*	ante- = before, in front of, prior to brachi/o = brachium; the front leg cranial to the humeroradial joint -um = structure, thing
humer/o	humerus	**scapulohumeral** pertaining to the scapula and the humerus *The humerus is the bone of the upper front leg and is located distal to the scapula and proximal to the radius and ulna. It is equivalent to the "upper arm" bone in humans.*	scapul/o = scapula humer/o = humerus -al = pertaining to
radi/o	radius	**radiohumeral** pertaining to the radius and the humerus *The radius is the cranial bone of the lower front leg. It is located distal to the humerus and proximal to the carpal bones. The radius is equivalent to the larger "lower arm" bone in humans.*	radi/o = radius humer/o = humerus -al = pertaining to
	radiation	*The combining form for radiation is also radi/o. The term for a dermatitis caused by excess exposure to X-rays is* **radiodermatitis,** *an inflammatory reaction to radiation. The inflammation could be anywhere on the skin, not necessarily associated with the area of the radius bone.*	radi/o = radiation dermat/o = skin -itis = inflammation

scapul/o

brachi/o

ante-

humer/o

radi/o

Continued

uln/o

carp/o

meta-   carp/o

phalang/o

TABLE 5-4	Word Parts for the Appendicular Skeleton—cont'd		
Word Part	**Meaning**	**Example and Definition**	**Word Parts**
uln/o	ulna	**ulnar** pertaining to the ulna or to any of the structures named from it (e.g., ulnar nerve and ulnar artery) *The ulna is the caudal bone of the lower front leg. It is located distal to the humerus and proximal to the carpal bones. The ulna is equivalent to the thinner "lower arm" bone in humans.* *The **olecranon** is the bony extension that forms the point of the elbow, at the proximal end of the ulna.*	uln/o = ulna -ar = pertaining to
carp/o	carpus	**intercarpal** pertaining to a place between two rows of carpal bones *The carpus typically consists of six to eight bones (depending on the species) arranged in two rows. It is distal to the radius and the ulna, and proximal to the metacarpal bones. The carpus is equivalent to the wrist in humans. It is also called the wrist in dogs and cats, but the knee in horses and cattle.*	inter- = between, among carp/o = carpus -al = pertaining to
meta- + carp/o	metacarpal bones	**metacarpectomy** surgical removal of a metacarpal bone *Remember the prefix meta- (meaning beyond or after)? The metacarpal bones are located distal to (beyond or after) the carpus and proximal to the phalanges. They are equivalent to the hand bones in humans.*	meta- = beyond, after carp/o = carpus -ectomy = surgical removal
phalang/o	phalanges	**metacarpophalangeal** pertaining to a joint between the metacarpal bones and the phalanges; the *fetlock* of equines *The phalanges bones are found on both the front and rear legs of animals. In the front leg, they are distal to the metacarpal bones. These phalanges are equivalent to the finger bones in humans. In the rear leg, the phalanges are distal to the metatarsal bones and are equivalent to the toe bones in humans.* *Phalanx is singular for phalanges; it is a single bone. In the front leg, a phalanx is equivalent to <u>one bone</u> in the finger in humans. In the rear leg, a phalanx is equivalent to <u>one bone</u> in the toe in humans.*	meta- = beyond, after carp/o = carpus phalang/o = phalange -al = pertaining to

TABLE 5-4　Word Parts for the Appendicular Skeleton—cont'd

Word Part	Meaning	Example and Definition	Word Parts
digit/o	digit, finger, toe	**interdigital** pertaining to a place between the digits	inter- = between, among digit/o = digit, a finger or toe -al = pertaining to
dactyl/o	dactyl	**polydactyly** presence of more than the normal number of dactyls (or digits); occurs as an inherited defect in cattle, horses, cats, and some breeds of dogs *A digit (or a dactyl) is a toe in cats, dogs, and chickens; a foot in a horse; and a cleat in cattle, sheep, goats, and pigs. Digits consist of a set of two or three phalanges. They are found on both the front and rear legs. In the front leg, they are distal to the metacarpal bones and are equivalent to a finger in humans.*	poly- = much or many dactyl/o = digit, a finger or toe -y = made up of, characterized by
cox/o	hip	**coxofemoral** pertaining to the hip and the thigh; the hip joint	cox/o = hip femor/o = femur -al = pertaining to
pelv/i pelvi/o	pelvis	**pelviscope** an endoscope (*endo-* = within, inner) used to examine the pelvic organs of a female	pelv/i = pelvis -scope = instrument for examining or viewing
		pelvioplasty surgical enlargement of the pelvic outlet to facilitate birthing *The pelvis is the caudal portion of the body forming a basin bounded ventrally and laterally by the hip bones and dorsally by the sacrum and coccygeal vertebrae. The pelvic canal is a natural hole in the pelvis through which certain viscera (e.g., colon) pass to reach the external environment to deposit their contents (e.g., feces).*	pelvi/o = pelvis -plasty = surgical repair
ili/o	ilium	**iliocostal** pertaining to the ilium and the ribs *The ilium is one of three bones that make up the pelvis—the cranial portion of the hip bone.*	ili/o = ilium (bone in the pelvis) cost/o = ribs -al = pertaining to
		The ilium (part of the pelvis) sounds the same as the ileum (the distal portion of the small intestine). The combining form for the ileum is ile/o, as found in **ileostomy.** *Think of the letter e in ile/o as like the e in eat, while the second i in ili/o is like the i in hip.*	ile/o = ileum (distal portion of the small intestine) -stomy = surgical creation of a new permanent opening

digit/o

dactyl/o

cox/o

pelv/i

pelvi/o

ili/o

ile/o

Continued

ischi/o

pub/o

femor/o

patell/o

tibi/o

fibul/o

TABLE 5-4 Word Parts for the Appendicular Skeleton—cont'd

Word Part	Meaning	Example and Definition	Word Parts
ischi/o	ischium	**ischiococcygeal** pertaining to the ischium and the coccyx *The ischium is one of three bones that make up the pelvis—the caudal dorsal portion. When you sit down, most of your weight rests on your ischium.*	ischi/o = ischium coccyg/o = coccyx -al = pertaining to
pub/o	pubis	**pubocaudal muscles** the more caudal muscles attached to the pubis *The pubis is one of three bones that make up the pelvis—its cranioventral portion. (Think of the location of pubic hair that appears at puberty in humans.)*	pub/o = pubis caud/o = tail -al = pertaining to
femor/o	femur	**pubofemoral** pertaining to the pubis and the femur *The femur is the bone of the upper rear leg. It is located distal to the pelvis; its head on the proximal end fits into the hip socket to form the hip joint. The femur is equivalent to the* thigh *bone in humans.*	pub/o = pubis femor/o = femur -al = pertaining to
patell/o	patella	**patellectomy** surgical removal of the patella *The patella is an irregularly shaped sesamoid bone embedded in a muscle tendon. It protects the cranial surface of the stifle joint. The patella is equivalent to the* kneecap *in humans.*	patell/o = patella -ectomy = surgical removal
tibi/o	tibia	**femorotibial** pertaining to the femur and the tibia; the area of the *stifle* joint of the rear leg, equivalent to the human *knee* *The tibia is the larger of two long bones of the lower rear leg. It is located distal to the femur and proximal to the tarsal bones. The tibia is equivalent to the* shin *bone in humans.*	femor/o = femur tibi/o = tibia -al = pertaining to
fibul/o	fibula	**tibiofibular** pertaining to the tibia and the fibula *The fibula is the thinner of two long bones of the lower rear leg. It is located distal to the femur and proximal to the tarsal bones. The fibula is equivalent to one of the two "lower leg" bones in humans.*	tibi/o = tibia fibul/o = fibula -ar = pertaining to

TABLE 5-4	Word Parts for the Appendicular Skeleton—cont'd		
Word Part	**Meaning**	**Example and Definition**	**Word Parts**
tars/o	tarsus	**tibiotarsal** pertaining to the tibia and the tarsus; the area of the *hock* joint of the rear leg, equivalent to the *ankle* in humans *The tarsus consists of up to seven bones. It is distal to the tibia and fibula and proximal to the metatarsal bones. The tarsus is sometimes referred to as the* hock *and is equivalent to the* ankle *in humans.*	tibi/o = tibia tars/o = tarsus -al = pertaining to	tars/o
pod/o	foot	**pododerm** portion of the skin that lies under the hooves of animals; the *corium* (remember that word?)	pod/o = foot derm/o = skin	pod/o
meta- + tars/o	metatarsal bones	**metatarsophalangeal** pertaining to an area between the metatarsal bones and the phalanges on the rear leg; the *fetlock* of equines *Remember meta- (meaning "beyond," "after")? The metatarsal bones are located distal to (beyond) the tarsus, and proximal to the phalanges. They are equivalent to the* foot *bones in humans.* *Horses walk on what would be the equivalent of the tip of your middle finger or toe. For example, the horse's rear leg below the hock is equivalent to your middle metatarsal (foot) bone, and the horse is walking on the tip of the end phalanx.*	meta- = beyond, after, next tars/o = tarsus phalang/o = phalange -(e)al = pertaining to	meta- tars/o

The bones of the word skeleton (Figure 5-5) are the more clinically important bones of the skeleton. You will need to know where bones are located for two reasons: (1) They are directly involved in medical/surgical conditions and procedures; and (2) they serve as landmarks for other tissues or organs.

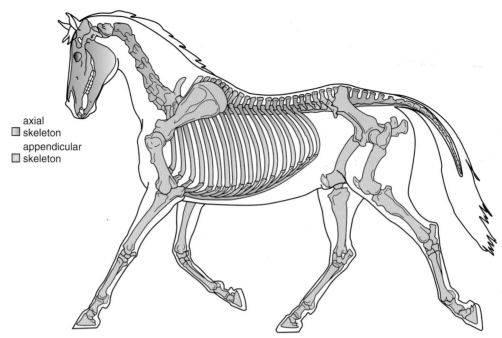

FIGURE 5-4 **Axial and appendicular portions of the skeleton.** (Adapted from Colville TP: *Clinical Anatomy and Physiology Laboratory Manual for Veterinary Technicians*, St Louis, 2009, Mosby.)

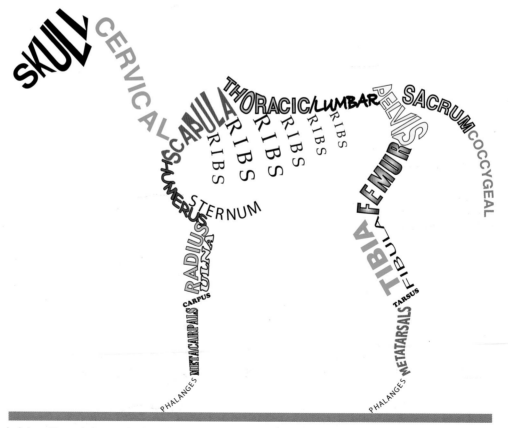

FIGURE 5-5 **Word skeleton.** The main bones of axial and appendicular portions of the skeleton. (From Colville TP: *Clinical Anatomy and Physiology Laboratory Manual for Veterinary Technicians*, St Louis, 2009, Mosby.)

EXERCISE 5-3 *Position It!*

The front leg is often referred to as the thoracic limb; the rear leg is the pelvic limb. Choose from the list of bones on the left to name the bones for each limb in order from proximal to distal.

1. Thoracic Limb
   (proximal)

   Scalpula
   humerus
   Radius/ulna
   Carpus
   metaCarpus
   phalanges

   (distal)

2. Pelvic Limb
   (proximal)

   pelvis
   ~~femur patella~~
   ~~tibia/fibula~~ femur
   ~~Tarsus~~ patella
   ~~Metatarsals~~
   tarsus
   metatarsal bones
   phalanges

   (distal)

carpus

femur

fibula

humerus

metacarpal bones _tibia/fibula_

metatarsal bones

patella

pelvis

phalanges

radius

scapula

tarsus

tibia

ulna

Check your answers at the end of the chapter, Answers to Exercises.

VISCERAL SKELETON

There is another group of bones that is not part of either the axial or the appendicular skeleton. These bones are called the **visceral skeleton.** They are embedded in soft organs. Examples of these bones are found in Table 5-5.

TABLE 5-5	Bones of the Visceral Skeleton		
Word Part	**Meaning**	**Example**	**Definition and Location**
os	bone	**os penis**	bone in the penis of carnivores and many other groups
		os cordis	bone in the heart of some species, such as the bovine
		os rostri	bone in the nose of the porcine, at the rostral end of the snout

os

EXERCISE 5-4 *Choose It!*

Circle the best answer for each statement:

1. The mandible and the maxilla are bones of the (cranium), (vertebrae), or (ribs).

2. You would look for coxitis in the area of the (shoulder), (spine), or (hip).

3. Which bone is not found on the foreleg? (humerus), (ulna), (femur), or (radius)

4. Carpal bones in animals are located (at the knee), (at the stifle), or (at the fetlock).

5. A combining form for the spine is (vertebr/o), (spondyl/o), or (both vertebr/o and spondyl/o).

6. Ilium, ischium, and pubis make up the (coccyx), (tarsus), or (pelvis).

7. A vertebra is any of the separate bones that make up the (foreleg), (spine), or (digit).

8. Surgical incision into the front leg above the knee is a (humerectomy), (carpostomy), or (brachiotomy).

9. Which bone is found on the hind leg? (patella), (radius), or (atlas).

10. The pelvis is located in this position in the body: (cranial), (proximal), or (caudal).

11. A set of two or three phalanges is called (a digit), (a phalanx), or (a tarsus).

12. This bone is located where the foreleg attaches to the spinal column: (ilium), (humerus), or (scapula).

13. These bones are equivalent to the wrist in humans: (metacarpal), (carpal), or (tarsal).

14. The axis is a (cervical), (thoracic), or (lumbar) vertebra.

15. Phalanges are found on (front legs only), (rear legs only), or (both front and rear legs).

16. The sternum is located (dorsal to the thorax and ribs), (ventral to the thorax and ribs), or (caudal to the thorax and ribs).

17. Lumbar vertebrae are found in the (loin), (thorax), or (sacrum).

18. The bone that attaches the rear leg to the axial skeleton is the (femur), (ilium), or (metatarsal).

19. C7 refers to the seventh (coccygeal vertebra), (rib), or (cervical vertebra).

20. Osteoneuromyelitis is an inflammation of bone, nerves, and (muscle), (bone marrow), or (spinal column).

Check your answers at the end of the chapter, Answers to Exercises.

JOINTS OR ARTICULATIONS

When two (or more) bones meet on the skeleton, they form a **joint** (Table 5-6). You will learn about many different types of joints in your anatomy/physiology course.

TABLE 5-6	Word Parts Associated with Joints		
Word Part	**Meaning**	**Example and Definition**	**Word Parts**
arthr/o	joint	**arthrodysplasia** hereditary congenital defect of joint development	arthr/o = joint dys- = bad, defective, painful, or difficult plas/o = growth, development, or formation -ia = pertaining to
articul/o	joint	**articular** pertaining to a joint	articul/o = joint -ar = pertaining to
dia-	through, between, apart, across	**diadermic** a reference to penetration through the skin	dia- = through, between, apart, across derm/o = skin -ic = pertaining to
ab-	away from	**abnormal** irregular, unusual, or unexpected; not normal or typical *To abdicate is to formally give up one's responsibility; to abduct a child is to take it away.*	ab- = away from normal = usual, expected
ad-	toward	**adneural** directed toward a nerve *An adhesive is a substance used to unite or bond things toward each other.*	ad- = toward neur/o = nerve -al = pertaining to
syn-	together, joined	**synchondrosis** type of joint in which the cartilage is usually converted into bone before adult life *Think of the syndicate; they work together to get a job done.*	syn- = together, joined chondr/o = joint -osis = disease or abnormal condition
amphi-	both, on both sides	**amphicranitis** inflammation affecting both sides of the head *Remember ambidextrous, a term for "one who can use both hands with equal ease"?* *Each of the prefixes ambi- and amphi- mean "both," or "on both sides." It just depends on whether a word is based on its Latin or Greek origins, as to which prefix is used.*	amphi- = both, on both sides crani/o = head, skull -(i)tis = inflammation
pro-	before, anterior, in front of	**prognosis** a medical opinion as to the likely course and outcome of a disease	pro- = before, in front of -gnosis = knowledge
post-	after, behind, later	**postinfection** period following an infection	post- = after, behind, later infection = infection

arthr/o

articul/o

dia-

ab-

ad-

syn-

amphi-

ambi-

pro-

post-

Generally, joints fall into one of three categories:
* fibrous joints or **synarthroses**

    These joints provide stability and do not allow any movement. An example is the joints between bones in the skull. They are called **sutures** and are very tightly connected to provide protection to the brain and to shape the face.
* cartilaginous joints or amphiarthroses

    These joints are connected by cartilage and provide limited movement. Examples are the **intervertebral disks** and the joints that connect the two halves of the pelvis or the two halves of the mandible.
* synovial joints or diarthroses

    These joints provide full movement and are the joints with which you are probably most familiar. Examples of synovial joints are the elbow, shoulder, hip, and stifle joints.

Synovial Joints

The function of synovial joints is to allow movement. Imagine how hard it would be to walk if your hip, knee, and ankle joints did not move. But synovial joint movements are not haphazard. In fact, these joints can move in only six directions (Figure 5-6):
* flexion—*decreases* the angle between two bones

    When you do arm curls at the gym, you are flexing your elbow joint as you lift the weight.
* extension—*increases* the angle between two bones

    This movement is the opposite of flexion. When you lower the weight after one arm curl, you extend your elbow joint.
* abduction—moves a limb *away* from the median plane

    It is like when someone is kidnapped or abducted; she is carried *away*.
* adduction—moves a limb *toward* the median plane

    This movement is the opposite of abduction.
* rotation—twists a bone on its own axis

    Hold your arm out in front of you with your palm up. Now turn your arm so your palm is down. You have just rotated your forearm.
* circumduction—moves the distal end of an appendage in a circle

    Hold your leg out in front of you just high enough so your foot is not touching the ground. Draw the letter "O" with your heel while keeping your knee locked. You have just moved your leg in a *circum*ference around a circle.

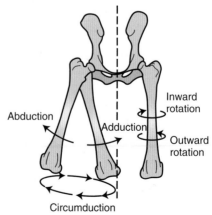

FIGURE 5-6 Movements of the canine femurs. Cranial view. (From Colville TP: *Clinical Anatomy and Physiology Laboratory Manual for Veterinary Technicians*, St Louis, 2009, Mosby.)

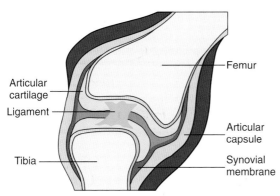

FIGURE 5-7 Canine stifle joint. The articular surfaces. (Adapted from Colville TP: *Clinical Anatomy and Physiology Laboratory Manual for Veterinary Technicians*, St Louis, 2009, Mosby.)

A synovial joint is made up of three structures (Figure 5-7):

- articular capsule

    This is a continuation of the periosteum. It encloses the area where the ends of the two adjoining bones meet.

- articular cartilage

    This is hyaline cartilage that covers the smooth joint surfaces of the adjoining bones and acts as smooth "ball bearings" and shock absorbers.

- synovial membrane

    This is what forms the inner surface of the articular capsule and produces a thick lubricating fluid called **synovial fluid.** The condition of the synovial fluid can be an indicator of bleeding, inflammation, or infection in a joint. The fluid can be withdrawn with a needle and syringe **(aspirated)** from the joint and examined microscopically.

EXERCISE 5-5 *Picture It!*

These drawings represent four movements of the equine front leg. The dotted line shows the leg after it moves. Answer the following questions about these drawings.

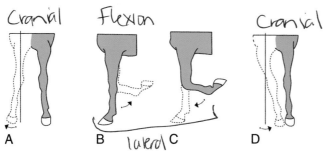

Movements of the equine front leg. (Adapted from Colville TP: *Clinical Anatomy and Physiology Laboratory Manual for Veterinary Technicians*, St Louis, 2009, Mosby.)

1. Which drawing shows flexion of a joint? _B_

2. In drawing D, the arrow is pointing to (the right leg) or (the left leg). _Right_

3. Drawing A is an example of _Abduction_ movement.

4. Which two drawings show a lateral view? _B_ and _C_

5. In drawings B and C, name the joint involved in movement. _Carpus_

6. Drawing D is an example of _Adduction_ movement.

7. Which drawing shows adduction? _D_

8. _horses_ are members of the equine family.

9. Which two drawings show a cranial view? _A_ and _D_

10. True or False: The brachium is visible in all four drawings. _True_

11. Name two long bones that meet in the joint that is flexed. _humerus_ and _radius_

Check your answers at the end of the chapter, Answers to Exercises.

CASE STUDY 5-2 #2008-8104 LUCKY DANCER

Signalment and History: A 6-year-old Thoroughbred **gelding** was brought to the Frisbee Large Animal Veterinary Hospital because of **left forelimb** lameness of 12 days' duration. The horse, Lucky Dancer, was in training and racing, and the **etiology** of the lameness was suspected to be an **inflammatory** lesion of the **interosseous ligament.**

Physical Examination: Lucky Dancer was bright, alert, and responsive **(BAR).** His temperature, pulse, and respiratory rate **(TPR)** were within the expected range. He appeared to be in good physical condition, but when he was walked, he favored his left front leg. The left **metacarpophalangeal joint** was swollen and was warm to the touch, suggesting that **inflammation** was present.

Diagnosis and Treatment: A tentative **diagnosis** of inflammation of the left metacarpophalangeal joint was made by Dr. Murdoch. **Antibiotics** and other medications were injected into the ligament. Lucky Dancer was released and, against Dr. Murdoch's advice, was raced once more. He was then rested for 3 weeks. The owner reported that the response to treatment was minimal.

Follow-up Examination: When Lucky Dancer was brought back to the veterinary hospital a month later, he was still limping on his left front leg. The left metacarpophalangeal joint was more **inflamed** than when it was previously examined. An **arthrocentesis** of the left metacarpophalangeal joint was performed to withdraw **synovial fluid. Microscopic** examination of the joint fluid did not reveal any evidence of bacteria. Lucky Dancer was hospitalized for further evaluation and treatment. Within 24 hours after arthrocentesis, the metacarpophalangeal joint had become grossly distended.

Outcome: Because of the rapid progression of the lesions involving the left metacarpophalangeal joint, the lack of response to treatment, and the poor **prognosis,** Lucky Dancer was **euthanized** (humanely put to death).

When the joint was opened and examined at necropsy, severe **arthritis** and degenerative **osteomyelitis** of the left metacarpophalangeal joint were seen. **Cartilage** on the **distal** end of the third **metacarpal bone** and on the **proximal** end of the proximal **phalanx** was eroded in a number of areas. Erosions extended through the **articular cartilage** into the **subchondral** bone, and bone under the articular cartilage was degenerative and **osteolytic.** Articular cartilage of the proximal **sesamoid bones** also was eroded in several areas, and degeneration and **osteolysis** of the subchondral bone were noted. The distal part of the third metacarpal bone adjacent to the proximal sesamoid bones was undergoing degeneration and **osteolysis.** The metacarpophalangeal joint contained less fluid than normal, and the **left forefoot** had evidence of mild inflammation. Other joints and bones were not affected, and no clinically important gross or **histological** lesions of any other organs were seen. The joint fluid was cultured for microorganisms. A fungus was isolated and was considered the likely cause of the bony lesions. Clinical and gross **pathological** findings were consistent with a diagnosis of **septic** osteomyelitis and arthritis.

EXERCISE 5-6 *Case It!*

The following words are all highlighted in Case Study 5-2. Using the system that you have learned for analyzing clinical veterinary language, identify the respective word parts to which you have already been introduced. Then define the word part. You will <u>not</u> define all the word parts for each word.

1. **interosseous**

   prefix = *Inter*   meaning *between*

2. **metacarpophalangeal**

   prefix = *meta*   meaning *beyond*

   combining form = *capp/o*   meaning *carpus*

   word root = *phalang*   meaning *phalanges*

3. **diagnosis**

   prefix = *Dia*   meaning *through*

   suffix = *gnosis*   meaning *Knowledge*

4. **antibiotic**

   combining form = *bi/o*   meaning *life*

5. **arthrocentesis**

   combining form = *arthro*   meaning *joint*

   suffix = *tesis*   meaning *Surgical puncture*

6. **synovial**

   prefix = *Syn*   meaning *together*

7. **arthritis**

   suffix = *itis*   meaning *inflammation*

8. **osteomyelitis**

   combining form = *osteo*   meaning *bone*

   word root = *my/el*   meaning *Bone marrow*

9. **subchondral**

   prefix = *sub*   meaning *below*

   word root = *chondr*   meaning *cartilage*

10. **histologic**

    combining form = *hist/o*   meaning *tissue*

    word root = *log*   meaning *to study*

11. **pathologic**

    combining form = *path/o*   meaning *disease*

    word root = *log/o*   meaning *to study*

Check your answers at the end of the chapter, Answers to Exercises.

Naming Joints

Joints are named with the names of the bones that come together to make the joint. For instance, the joint in the front leg at the shoulder between the scapula and humerus bones is the **scapulohumeral joint** (Figure 5-8). When naming the joint, start with the most proximal or cranial bone (Table 5-7).

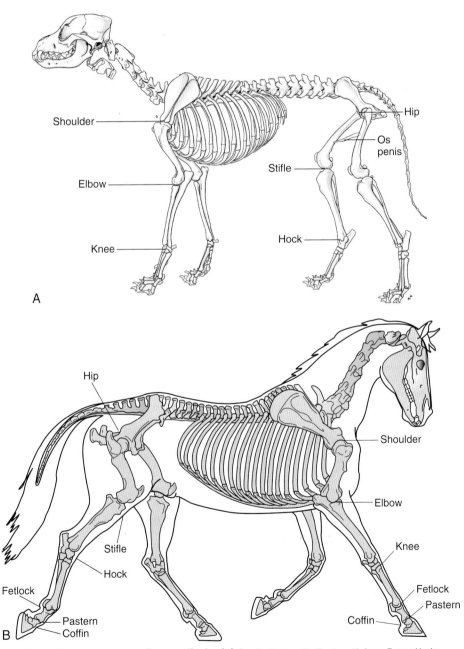

FIGURE 5-8 **Common names of appendicular joints. A,** Canine. **B,** Equine. (A from Evans H, de Lahunta A: *Guide to the Dissection of the Dog,* ed 7, St Louis, 2010, Saunders; B adapted from Colville TP: *Clinical Anatomy and Physiology Laboratory Manual for Veterinary Technicians,* St Louis, 2009, Mosby.)

TABLE 5-7	Common Joint Names		
Common Name	**Anatomical Name**	**Location**	**Human Equivalent**
shoulder	scapulohumeral joint	front leg between the scapula and the humerus	shoulder
knee	radiocarpal joint	front leg between the radius and carpal bones	wrist
hip	coxofemoral joint	rear leg attachment to the axial skeleton	hip
stifle	femorotibial joint	rear leg between the femur and the tibia	knee joint
hock	tibiotarsal joint	rear leg between the tibia and tarsal bones	ankle joint
fetlock (equine)	metacarpophalangeal or metatarsophalangeal joint	all legs of equines between the metacarpal or metatarsal bones and the phalanges	knuckle
pastern (equine)	interphalangeal joint	all legs of equines between the proximal and middle phalanges	knuckle
coffin (equine)	interphalangeal joint	all legs of equines between the middle and distal phalanges	knuckle

EXERCISE 5-7 *Sing It!*

The foot bone connected to the ankle bone, The ankle bone connected to the shin bone, The shin bone connected to the knee bone, The knee bone connected to the thigh bone, The thigh bone connected to the hip bone, The hip bone connected to the back bone, The back bone connected to the shoulder bone, The shoulder bone connected to the neck bone, The neck bone connected to the head bone.

Traditional Spiritual

Now that you know bone names, rewrite the words to "Dem Bones" using the anatomical names of the bones in animals and the anatomical descriptions of the joints formed by the connection of the bones. The first line of the song will start as follows—

I. The foot bone connected to the ankle bone

the metatarsal bone connected to the tarsal bone at the tarsometatarsal joint

2. The ankle bone connected to the shin bone

The tarsal bone connected to the tibia at the tibotarsal joint

3. The shin bone connected to the knee bone

The tibia connected to the patella at the patellatibia joint

4. The knee bone connected to the thigh bone

The patella bone con to the femur at the femur patellar joint

5. The thigh bone connected to the hip bone

The femur bone connected to the illium at the ileoformal joint

6. The hip bone connected to the back bone

illium bone con to the sacrum, Sacnillael joint

7. The back bone connected to the shoulder bone

Thorax vertebrae con to scalpula, at the thoracovertebro, scapular joint

8. The shoulder bone connected to the neck bone

Scalpula con to the cervical vertabrae at the cervicoscapular joint

9. The neck bone connected to the head bone

The cervical vertebrae con to the cranium at the craniocervical joint.

Unfortunately it is not easy to sing in this format. Nor does it make anatomical sense. Such is music.

Check your answers at the end of the chapter, Answers to Exercises.

CASE STUDY 5-3 POLYARTHRITIS IN A HOLSTEIN COW

Signalment and History: A first-lactation Holstein **cow** was submitted to the Frisbee Veterinary Hospital on July 18 because of swelling of the **carpal** joints, diffuse **subcutaneous** buildup of fluid between the cells (edema) extending from the carpal to the **metacarpophalangeal** joints, and **forelimb** lameness. The cow (tag #32747) had **calved** twins approximately 15 days earlier. The **freemartin** calf died within 24 hours after birth. The cow had died during transit to the hospital.

Carcass Examination: Necropsy revealed that the cow weighed 386 kg (850 lb) and had poor body condition. **Abscesses** were detected in the right lung. Subcutaneous edema and **suppurative polyarthritis** of both **forelimbs** and the right hind limb were evident, with the subcutaneous edema extending from the carpal joints to the metacarpophalangeal joints of both forelimbs. The left **humeroradial** joint was distended and contained cloudy fluid with fibrin strands. Both **tarsometatarsal** joints were distended with yellow fluid that contained small amounts of fibrin, and the right **metatarsophalangeal** joint was distended with blood-tinged **purulent exudate.** The underlying **cartilage** of the third and fourth **metatarsal** bones was eroded and showed signs of **synovitis.** Hardening of the **articular cartilage** was evident on the **radial head of the left humeroradial joint.** The **synovial capsules and membranes** were **erythematous** and swollen. **Microscopic, histological** examination revealed indications of synovial cell **hyperplasia.** The **synovial fluid** was cultured, and *Mycoplasma bovis* (a microorganism that is neither a bacterium nor a virus) was isolated. *Mycoplasma bovis* is the most frequently isolated *Mycoplasma* **pathogen** of **bovine arthritis.**

EXERCISE 5-8 *Case It!*

Read Case Study 5-3. Then circle the correct word or phrase in the parentheses that makes each statement true.

1. A <u>first-lactation</u> cow means that she was a (heifer) or (cow) before she calved.

2. <u>Suppurative</u> polyarthritis means that (pus) (blood), or (synovial fluid) was present.

3. Suppurative <u>polyarthritis</u> indicates (new growth), (tumor), or (inflammation).

4. You would look for swelling of the <u>carpal</u> joint in the cow's (neck) (foreleg) or (rear leg).

5. An <u>agent</u> that causes disease is (an inflammation), (a pathogen), or (a membrane).

6. Arthritis that affects <u>cows</u> is (equine), (ovine), or (bovine).

7. A <u>freemartin</u> is the (female) (first-born), or (male) calf of the twin calves.

8. The cow's right lung <u>abscess</u> involved (signs of localized pus), (a wound caused by tearing), or (a scar).

9. <u>Articular</u> cartilage is found (in the arteries), (in the skin), or (in the joints).

10. The common name for the <u>carpal</u> joint in animals is (hock) (knee) or (stifle).

11. The radial <u>head</u> refers to which end of the bone? (proximal) (medial), or (distal)

12. Something erythematous is (white), (blue), or (red)

13. Fluid that has escaped from blood vessels and has been deposited <u>in tissues</u> or on tissue surfaces as a result of inflammation is (an abscess) (an exudate), or (synovial fluid).

14. Hyperplasia involves (excess growth) (poor growth), or (deficient growth).

15. Which of the following joints is <u>not found</u> on a foreleg? (humeroradial), (metacarpophalangeal), or (tarsometatarsal)

Check your answers at the end of the chapter, Answers to Exercises.

CARTILAGE

Cartilage is a tough, somewhat flexible connective tissue that is found in numerous parts of the body. It is called *gristle* when you try to eat it. Your ears, nose, vocal cords, and windpipe all contain cartilages that provide structure and support. Cartilage also is found covering the joint surfaces of long bones (epiphyses).

Functions of Cartilage

Cartilage

- provides a smooth joint surface so the bones can move freely over one another
- acts as a shock absorber for joints such as the intervertebral joints of the spinal column, where movement is limited but a lot of stress is present
- forms a template over which bones grow in a developing fetus
- makes up epiphyseal plates that are sites of long bone growth as an animal ages

Anatomy of Cartilage

Cartilage is composed of cells **(chondrocytes)** and a matrix similar to bones. Unlike bones, however, it does not have its own nerve and blood supply. Cartilage relies on a thin covering membrane **(perichondrium)** that contains many tiny blood vessels to provide it with nutrients. The cartilage matrix does not get as hard as the bone matrix, so cartilage has a little flexibility to it.

Three types of cartilage are found in the body:

- hyaline cartilage
    This is the most common cartilage. It is composed mainly of dense protein **(collagen)** fibers that make it rigid. Hyaline cartilage is found on the surfaces of bones that form joints, in the nose, and where the ribs join to the sternum.
- elastic cartilage
    This cartilage is similar to hyaline cartilage with the addition of some elastic fibers to give the cartilage more flexibility. As a result, elastic cartilage can be bent numerous times without damage. Elastic cartilage is not found in the skeletal system. You will meet up with it in later chapters.
- **fibrocartilage** (note this is one word)
    This cartilage contains more collagen than hyaline cartilage and is very tough. Fibrocartilage is ideal in places of frequent stress such as intervertebral disks.

LIGAMENTS

Ligaments are strips of tough, fibrous connective tissue that connect bones and cartilages to provide stability and strength for a joint. The ligament with which you are probably most familiar is the ACL, or anterior cruciate ligament, which is often damaged in human athletes. The same ligament is known as the cranial cruciate ligament, or CCL, in clinical veterinary language. The CCL helps to stabilize the stifle joint in animals, just as the ACL is one of the ligaments that stabilize the knee joint in humans.

Not all joints have or need ligaments for support. When a ligament is stretched or torn, the joint becomes unstable and very painful. A joint with stretched or torn ligaments is sometimes called a **sprained** joint.

Tendons

Tendons are not the same thing as ligaments even though both are made up of strips of tough, fibrous connective tissue. Tendons connect muscles to bones, and ligaments connect bone/cartilage to bone/cartilage. You will learn more about tendons in the muscular system chapter, Chapter 6.

CONDITIONS INVOLVING THE SKELETAL SYSTEM

Table 5-8 lists some word parts that are used to denote certain conditions that affect bones, cartilage, and ligaments. They are used with the skeletal system, as well as with other systems.

| mal- |

TABLE 5-8   Word Parts for Abnormal Skeletal Conditions

Word Part	Meaning	Example and Definition	Word Parts
mal-	diseased, bad, abnormal, defective	**malformation** faulty formation or structure of parts, especially of a living body *Malignant is the "bad" kind of cancer, tending to become progressively worse and leading to death. Malpractice is definitely "bad" medical treatment. A malady is any disease or illness.* *Before people knew that mosquitoes carried malaria, they thought it was caused by "bad air."*	mal- = diseased, bad, abnormal, defective formation = formation
malac/o	soft, softening	**osteomalacia** condition of softening of the bones	oste/o = bone malac/o = softening -ia = pertaining to
-oma	a tumor or abnormal growth, a swelling	**multiple myeloma** collections of abnormal cells accumulate in bones and in the bone marrow, where they interfere with the production of normal blood cells	myel/o = bone marrow -oma = a tumor or abnormal new growth, a swelling
orth/o	straight, normal, correct	**orthodigitia** pertaining to the art of correcting deformities of the "toes and fingers"	orth/o = straight, normal correct digit/o = digit, a set of two or three phalanges -ia = pertaining to
		Originally, the term orthopedic meant "to straighten a child," but it has come to mean "to straighten or correct abnormalities of the skeletal system."	orth/o = straight, normal, correct ped/o = child -ic = pertaining to
pachy-	thick	**pachydermia** pertaining to thickened skin *Remember the elephant from Chapter 4?*	pachy- = thick derm/o = skin -ia = pertaining to
-plasm	formed material (as of a cell or tissue)	**cytoplasm** the living substance surrounding the nucleus of a cell	cyt/o = cell -plasm = formed material (as of a cell or tissue)
plas/o	growth, development, or formation	**hypoplasia** incomplete development or underdevelopment of an organ or tissue	hypo- = under, beneath, below plas/o = growth, development, formation -ia = pertaining to
por/o	a pore, small opening, or cavity	**osteoporosis** thinning of bones with a reduction in bone mass due to depletion of calcium and bone protein	oste/o = bone por/o = a pore, small opening, or cavity -osis = disease or abnormal condition
ankyl/o	stiff, not movable, bent, crooked	**ankylosis** condition of stiffness	ankyl/o = stiffness -osis = disease or abnormal condition

| malac/o |
| -oma |
| orth/o |
| pachy- |
| -plasm |
| plas/o |
| por/o |
| ankyl/o |

TABLE 5-8	Word Parts for Abnormal Skeletal Conditions—cont'd		
Word Part	**Meaning**	**Example and Definition**	**Word Parts**
-algia	pain	**analgia** no pain *Analgesics are drugs like aspirin, opium, and morphine. They all relieve pain. Can you see "no pain" in analgesic?*	an- = without, no, not -algia = pain
-dynia	pain	**ischiodynia** pain in the ischium	ischi/o = ischium -dynia = pain
		-dynia and -algia are usually interchangeable. Are all these new words giving you **craniodynia?** *A headache.*	crani/o = head, skull -dynia = pain

-algia

-dynia

BOX 5-1   Terms That Defy Word Analysis

- callus—a bridge that forms as part of the healing process across the two halves of a bone fracture; composed of cartilage that becomes ossified over time
- cannon bone—the lay term for the third metacarpal or metatarsal bone in four-legged mammals such as cattle and horses; located between the hock and fetlock joints
- condyle—smooth end of a bone that forms part of a joint
- crest—a raised ridge along the surface of a bone
- cull—take out an animal (especially an inferior one) from a herd; or reduce the size of a herd or flock by removing a proportion of its members
- exacerbation—an increase in the severity of a disease or any of its clinical signs
- foramen—small opening or perforation
- fossa (from the Latin for *ditch*—so remember, fossils are dug up from a ditch)—a depression, trench, or hollow area
- fracture—a break or rupture
- head—rounded proximal end of a bone (e.g., femur); also the end of a muscle nearest the origin
- luxation—a joint dislocation where the joint is displaced or goes out of alignment
- olecranon—large process on the proximal end of the ulna that forms the point of the elbow; literally means "the head of the elbow"
- oosik—the os penis of a walrus
- pin bones and hook bones—in cattle, the two prominent raised areas on either side of the tailhead and backbone; the caudal raised area is the pin bone, and the cranial raised area is the hook bone
- process—a natural outgrowth or projection
- spine—a hard, pointed process that runs the length of the lateral surface of the scapula
- sprain or strain—the result of stretching or tearing a ligament, which connects bone/cartilage to bone/cartilage
- subluxation—a partial dislocation of a joint
- suture—the line of junction of two bones forming an immovable joint
- trochanter—two knobs at the proximal end of the femur where muscles of the thigh and pelvis attach
- tuberosity—a rough projection on a bone; usually an area of muscle attachment
- wings—transverse processes on the first cervical vertebra (atlas) so named because they give the appearance of wings on the bone

CASE STUDY 5-1 #2010-98 KEVIN

Signalment and History: An 8-month-old M Rottweiler named Kevin was brought to the Frisbee Small Animal Veterinary Hospital for evaluation of a left rear limb lameness of 5 months' duration. Kevin had never walked completely normally and had a shifting rear limb lameness that had become worse in the past week. Kevin is still eating and drinking well but was reluctant to play with his littermate, who is owned by the same person.

Physical Examination and Diagnosis: On physical examination, Jess found that Kevin was mildly depressed and had a non–weight-bearing lameness of the left rear limb. Temperature, pulse, and respiration (TPR) were all within the expected reference ranges. Palpation of the left **coxofemoral** joint elicited signs of pain. X-rays of the pelvis showed a possible left coxofemoral joint **septic arthritis**. The **diaphyseal cortex** of the left femur was thin. Dr. Frisbee explained to the owner that the degeneration of the **femoral cortex** may have been a result of disuse **osteoporosis** and **myelitis**. Absence of the left **femoral epiphysis** indicated complete **lysis**. The right coxofemoral joint was shallow with **subluxation** of the **femoral head. Periarticular osteogenesis** also was evident at this site. Right coxofemoral joint **dysplasia** and degenerative **arthropathy** were diagnosed.

Thoracic X-rays revealed a **T4-T5 diskospondylitis**. The **etiology** was **hematogenous** spread of an infection. The **T4 vertebra** was shortened with a decreased T4-T5 **intervertebral disk space**. Bridging **spondylosis** was also evident. The **caudal** aspect of the left **humeral head** was slightly flattened. These findings were consistent with **bilateral humeral osteochondrosis**.

Treatment: Kevin underwent surgery for a left femoral head and neck **ostectomy. Purulent** synovial fluid present in and around the joint capsule was collected. The femur **fractured** during surgery at the junction of the **proximal** and middle thirds of the bone. The cortex of the femur was thin with necrotic (dead) marrow. After consultation with Dr. Frisbee, the owners elected to have the left limb amputated. Samples of the bone and joint capsule were sent for **histological** evaluation. Kevin recovered from surgery without incident. Histological evaluation revealed severe, **chronic,** active **osteomyelitis.** No evidence of **sarcoma** or other **neoplasia** was present. The condition was **exacerbated** by the presence of bridging **spondylosis.** Culture test results revealed the cause as *Staphylococcus aureus* (a bacterium). Kevin was placed on antibiotics for 2 weeks.

Outcome: By 3 weeks **post surgery,** the owner noticed a considerable increase in overall activity of Kevin, the now amazing three-legged dog. The **prognosis** for complete recovery is good.

EXERCISE 5-9 *Case It!*

Several words used in Case Study 5-1 are highlighted with bold type. With practice, most words should get easier to dissect to comprehend their definitions. Match the words listed in the left column to their definitions on the right.

1. *hematogenous* produced in the blood system

2. *head* proximal end of the femur

3. *periarticular* occurring around a joint

4. *dysplasia* bad or defective development

5. *spondylosis* diseased or abnormal condition of the spine

6. *vertebrae* T4-T5

7. *Arthropathy* disease affecting the joints

8. *purulent* containing or forming pus

9. *Coxofemoral* joint between the pelvis and the rear leg

10. *Osteoctomy* surgical removal of bone

11. *Bilateral* occurring on two sides

12. *Septic* presence of pathogenic organisms in blood or tissues

13. *Exacerbation* increase in the severity of a disease or any of its clinical signs

14. *Chronic* persisting for a long time

15. *Osteomyelitis* inflammation affecting bone and bone marrow

16. *histological* study of tissues

17. *intervertebral* between the bones of the spinal column

18. *fracture* a break or a rupture

19. *Thorax* the area of the chest

20. *Neoplasia* new growth or formation

21. *etiology* science studying the causes of diseases

22. *Sarcoma* a malignant neoplasm arising in bone, cartilage, or striated muscle that spreads into neighboring tissue or by way of the bloodstream

23. *Subluxation* partial dislocation of a joint

24. *prognosis* forecast of probable outcome of disease

25. *Disk* pad of fibrocartilage present in some joints

26. *lysis* destruction or decomposition of a substance

27. *Caudal* referring to toward the tail end

28. *proximal* nearer to the center or to the attachment to the body

29. *Synovial* pertaining to the fluid excreted in joint cavities that provide full movement

30. *osteochondrosis* abnormal condition affecting bone and cartilage

arthropathy
bilateral
caudal
chronic
coxofemoral
disk
dysplasia
etiology
exacerbation
fracture
head
hematogenous
histological
intervertebral
lysis
neoplasia
ostectomy
osteochondrosis
osteomyelitis
periarticular
prognosis
proximal
purulent
sarcoma
septic
spondylosis
subluxation
synovial
thorax
vertebrae

Check your answers at the end of the chapter, Answers to Exercises.

Table 5-9 lists more abbreviations used in clinical veterinary language.

TABLE 5-9	Abbreviations	
Abbreviation	**Meaning**	**Example**
CCL	cranial cruciate ligament	Rumbles, the grossly overweight M(C) Basset Hound, jumped off the couch, landed wrong, and tore his CCL.
fx	fracture, broken bone	Roxie suffered a fx of the Ⓛ humerus as a result of an HBC incident.
sx	surgery	Roxie will have sx on Thursday to set her fx.

CCL

fx

sx

ANSWERS TO EXERCISES

Exercise 5-1
1. red bone marrow
2. compact bone
3. endoskeleton
4. ligament
5. osteocytes
6. periosteum
7. yellow bone marrow
8. cranium
9. osteogenesis
10. epiphyses
11. cancellous bone
12. exoskeleton

Exercise 5-2
1. head
2. foramen
3. ossification
4. periosteum; nerves; blood vessels
5. patella; knee
6. vertebrae
7. fat cells
8. epiphyses
9. condyle
10. fossa

Exercise 5-3
1. Thoracic limb: scapula, humerus, radius/ulna, carpus, metacarpal bones, phalanges
2. Pelvic limb: pelvis, femur, patella, tibia/fibula, tarsus, metatarsal bones, phalanges

Exercise 5-4
1. cranium
2. hip
3. femur
4. at the knee
5. both vertebr/o and spondyl/o
6. pelvis
7. spine
8. brachiotomy
9. patella
10. caudal
11. digit
12. scapula
13. carpal
14. cervical
15. both front and rear legs
16. ventral to the thorax and ribs
17. loin
18. ilium
19. cervical vertebra
20. bone marrow

Exercise 5-5
1. B
2. right
3. abduction
4. B and C
5. knee (or carpus)
6. adduction
7. D
8. horses
9. A and D
10. True
11. humerus; radius or ulna

Exercise 5-6
1. inter-; between, among
2. meta-; beyond, after, next; carp/o; carpus; phalang; phalanges
3. dia-; across, through; -gnosis; knowledge
4. bi/o; life
5. arthr/o; joint; -centesis; surgical puncture
6. syn-; together, joined
7. -itis; inflammation
8. oste/o; bone; myel; bone marrow
9. sub-; below, decrease, under; chondr; cartilage
10. hist/o; tissue; log; to study, or to have knowledge of
11. path/o; disease; logo; to study, or to have knowledge of

Exercise 5-7
1. the metatarsal bone connected to the tarsal bone at the tarsometatarsal joint
2. the tarsal bone connected to the tibia at the tibiotarsal joint
3. the tibia connected to the patella at the patellotibial joint
4. the patella connected to the femur at the femoropatellar joint
5. the femur connected to the ilium at the iliofemoral joint
6. the ilium connected to the sacrum at the sacroiliac joint
7. the thoracic vertebra connected to the scapula at the thoracovertebroscapular joint
8. the scapula connected to the cervical vertebra at the cervicoscapular joint
9. the cervical vertebra (atlas) connected to the cranium at the craniocervical joint

Exercise 5-8

1. heifer
2. pus
3. inflammation
4. foreleg
5. a pathogen
6. bovine
7. female
8. signs of localized pus
9. in the joints
10. knee
11. proximal
12. red
13. exudate
14. excess growth
15. tarsometatarsal

Exercise 5-9

1. hematogenous
2. head
3. periarticular
4. dysplasia
5. spondylosis
6. vertebrae
7. arthropathy
8. purulent
9. coxofemoral
10. ostectomy
11. bilateral
12. septic
13. exacerbation
14. chronic
15. osteomyelitis
16. histological
17. intervertebral
18. fracture
19. thorax
20. neoplasia
21. etiology
22. sarcoma
23. subluxation
24. prognosis
25. disk
26. lysis
27. caudal
28. proximal
29. synovial
30. osteochondrosis

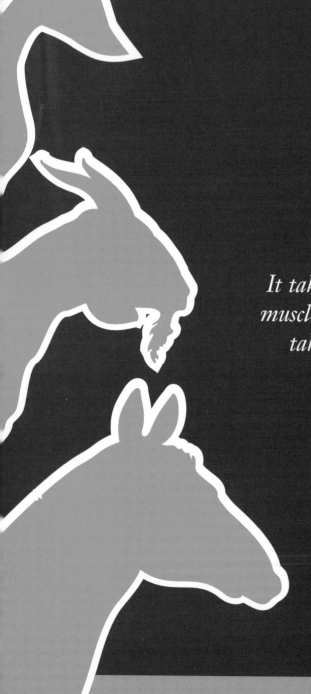

The Muscular System

It takes seventeen muscles to smile and forty-three muscles to frown; but when someone annoys you, it takes only four muscles to extend your arm and smack him on the head.

Anonymous

WORD PARTS

a-	ah *or* ā	electr/o	ē-**lehck**-trō	muscul/o	**muhs**-kyoo-lō	rhab	
ab-	ahb	erg/o	ər-gō	my/o	**mī**-ō	sar	
ad-	ahd	fibr/o	**fib**-rō	nano-	**nah**-nō	semi-	
an-	ahn	-gram	grahm	-oid	oyd	spasm/o	**sp**
bi-	bī	-graph	grahf	pan-	pahn	syn-	sihn
bi/o	**bī**-ō	-graphy	**grahf**-ē	par-	pehr	ten/o	**tehn**-ō
cardi/o	**kahr**-dē-ō	hemi-	**hehm**-ih	para-	**pehr**-ah	tendin/o	**tehn**-dihn-ō
cata-	**kaht**-ah	ipsi-	**ihp**-sē	-paresis	pah-**rē**-sihs	tendon/o	**tehn**-dohn-ō
centi-	**sehnt**-ah	kilo-	**kihl**-ō	path/o	**pahth**-ō	tenont/o	**tehn**-ohnt-ō
cep	sehp	kinesi/o	kih-**nē**-sē-ō	-pathy	**pahth**-ē	tetra-	**teht**-rah
cephal/o	**seh**-fahl-ō	lys/o	**lī**-sō	pico-	**pī**-cō	therm/o	**thər**-mō
contra-	**kohn**-trah	-meter	**mē**-tər	plas/o	**plā**-zō	ton/o	**tō**-nō
cry/o	**krī**-ō	metr/o	**meh**-trō	-plegia	**plē**-jē-ah	tri-	trī
de-	dē	micro-	**mī**-krō	poly-	**pohl**-ē	-trophy	**trō**-phē
deci-	**deh**-sih	milli-	**mihl**-ih	pyr/o	**pī**-rō	uni-	**ū**-nah
di-	dī	mono-	**mohn**-ō	pyrex/o	pī-**rehx**-ō		
dynam/o	**dī**-nah-mō	multi-	**muhl**-tī	quadri-	**kwohd**-rih		

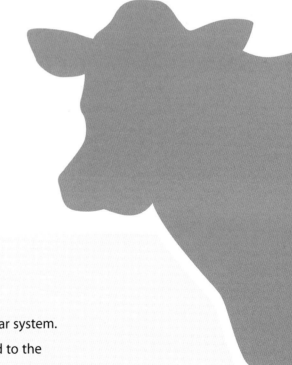

OUTLINE

THE MUSCULAR SYSTEM

PHYSIOLOGY OF SKELETAL MUSCLES

HOW MANY, HOW MUCH
  Learning the Names of Muscles

PHYSIOLOGY OF CARDIAC MUSCLE

PHYSIOLOGY OF SMOOTH MUSCLE

LEARNING OBJECTIVES

When you have completed this chapter, you will be able to:

1 Understand the components and functions of the muscular system.

2 Identify and recognize the meanings of word parts related to the muscular system, using them to build or analyze words.

3 Apply your new knowledge and understanding of clinical veterinary language in the context of medical records.

CASE STUDY 6-1 | #1999-87 ANNABELLE

Signalment and History: A 4-year-old domestic shorthair **queen** named Annabelle was brought to the Frisbee Small Animal Clinic because of a 1-week history of shifting limb lameness that had progressed to **tetraparesis**. She was not eating well but was still drinking plenty of water. Her level of activity was greatly diminished.

Physical Examination: Physical examination revealed a normal TPR and a depressed level of activity. Dr. Frisbee found that generalized **muscle atrophy** and signs of discomfort were elicited when the muscles of the **appendicular skeleton** were palpated. Neurological examination revealed diminished **myotatic** (-tatic = stretch reflex) and withdrawal reflexes in both **thoracic** and **pelvic** limbs.

Diagnosis and Treatment: Annabelle was anesthetized and an **electromyography procedure** (EMG) was performed. Nerve and muscle **bx** specimens were obtained while she was still anesthetized. **Histological examination** of the specimens revealed severe **myositis** and **neuritis**. Immune-mediated **polymyositis** and neuritis was the tentative diagnosis because no other signs of **pathology** could be identified. The **etiology** was unknown. A daily dose of an **anti-inflammatory** medication was prescribed. Dr. Frisbee thought that the **prognosis** for recovery was excellent with long-term treatment but warned the owner that there was a chance of recurrence.

Four months after the initial diagnosis of immune-mediated polymyositis and neuritis, Annabelle had been gradually taken off her anti-inflammatory medication and was doing well. Her appetite and energy had returned, and there was no sign of recurrence.

THE MUSCULAR SYSTEM

Your prototype animal is now a bag of skin fashioned into a recognizable shape by bones, cartilage, and ligaments. If all it wanted to do was to stand still, this would be fine, but movement is necessary for survival, so muscles have to be added.

Muscle is one of the four basic tissues in the body (Table 6-1). The other three are epithelium, connective tissue, and nervous tissue. When you think "muscle," you most likely think of the external muscles that move the body. Muscles make walking, running, trotting, and galloping possible. They allow animals to open their mouths and close their eyes. Have you ever run around in a pasture and tried to catch a horse that does not want to be caught? That is muscles of the thoracic and pelvic limbs at work. Put medication in a dog's ear and it is the muscles of the head and neck that allow the dog to shake its head and spray the medication all over you. Try to restrain an unhappy cat and it is the pelvic limb muscles that extend the hind leg with enough force to embed the cat's claws into your arm.

Not all muscle action is dire. There are many muscles in the body that also perform work that is important. Animals use muscles to chew food and vocalize. Other muscles move food through the digestive tract and ultimately force the elimination of waste material through a bowel movement. Muscles are necessary to empty the urinary bladder. The heart consists almost entirely of muscle tissue. Blood is distributed throughout the body by the action of muscles. When a cow is calving, many muscles are used to bring the calf into the world. When your Golden Retriever smiles at you, the face muscles are at work. So the bottom line is that movement depends on muscle. The amazing thing is that muscle accomplishes all this movement with only one action; it takes energy and turns it into motion through contraction.

TABLE 6-1	Word Parts Associated with the Muscular System		
Word Part	**Meaning**	**Example and Definition**	**Word Parts**
my/o muscul/o	muscle	**myopathology** study of muscle diseases	my/o = muscle path/o = disease -logy = to study or to have knowledge of
		cervicomuscular related to or affecting the muscles of the neck	cervic/o = neck muscul/o = muscle -ar = pertaining to
rhabd/o	rod, cylinder	**rhabdomyoma** rare benign tumor derived from striated muscle	rhabd/o = rod, cylinder my/o = muscle -oma = tumor or abnormal growth, a swelling
sarc/o	flesh	**rhabdomyosarcoma** malignant tumor that starts in muscle *In Chapter 2, you learned that a sarcoma is a malignant neoplasm arising in bone, cartilage, or striated muscle that spreads into neighboring tissue or by way of the bloodstream.*	rhabd/o = rod, cylinder my/o = muscle sarc/o = flesh -oma = tumor or abnormal new growth, a swelling
fibr/o	fiber	**myofibrosis** abnormal condition of muscle fibers	my/o = muscle fibr/o = fiber -osis = disease or abnormal condition
spasm/o	spasm (intermittent involuntary abnormal muscle contractions)	**myospasm** spasm of a muscle	my/o = muscle spasm = intermittent involuntary abnormal muscle contractions
ton/o	pressure, tension	**myotonia** symptom of disorders where muscles are slow to relax	my/o = muscle ton/o = pressure, tension -ia = pertains to
-meter	measure, a device to measure	**cytometer** device that measures and counts cells	cyt/o = cell -meter = measure, a device to measure
metr/o	measure	**metric system** decimal system of weights and measures based on the meter and the kilogram	metr/o = measure -ic = pertaining to
-gram	written record produced; something recorded or written	**arthrogram** X-ray of a joint, which usually implies the introduction of a contrast agent into the joint capsule *The definition of this suffix is easier to remember when you think of the telegram, telegraph, and telegraphy from Chapter 4.*	arthr/o = joint -gram = written record produced; something recorded or written
-graph	instrument used to write or record	**polygraph** the lie detector; an instrument for simultaneously recording tracings of several different pulsations (as of pulse, blood pressure, and respiration)	poly- = much or many -graph = instrument used to write or record

Continued

-graphy

electr/o

Word Part	Meaning	Example and Definition	Word Parts
TABLE 6-1	Word Parts Associated with the Muscular System—cont'd		
-graphy	method of recording	**autobiography** method of recording one's life, usually in written form	aut/o = self bi/o = life -graphy = method of recording
electr/o	electricity	**electromyography (EMG)** technique for evaluating and recording the electrical activity produced by skeletal muscles *Normally when a muscle is at rest, it is electrically silent. When a muscle is active, an electrical current is generated. In an EMG, this electrical activity is detected by needle electrodes, which are inserted into the muscle.*	electr/o = electricity my/o = muscle -graphy = method of recording

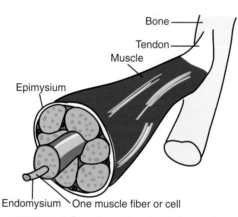

FIGURE 6-1 **Structure of a skeletal muscle.**

A muscle is made up of many cells called **muscle fibers** that look like long rods or cylinders. The **endomysium** is a connective tissue membrane that surrounds each muscle fiber. The **epimysium** is a connective tissue membrane that covers and defines the entire muscle. It is there to protect the muscle.

Three unique types of muscles are found in an animal's body: skeletal, cardiac, and smooth. Each performs specific functions for which it was developed.

In talking about a muscle at the cellular level, the word root is *sarc/o*. A tumor of skeletal muscle cells (or fibers) is a **sarcoma**; however, a muscle disease is a **myopathy.**

Figure 6-1 illustrates the anatomy of a skeletal muscle. When viewed microscopically, the muscle cells appear to be striped or striated. For this reason, skeletal muscle is also known as **striated muscle.** These striations are not visible without a microscope.

PHYSIOLOGY OF SKELETAL MUSCLES

To perform properly, muscles must have energy from the circulatory system and direction and coordination from the nervous system. Skeletal muscles will not operate unless they are stimulated by a nerve (see Chapter 11). This message from a nerve acts like an electrical current traveling along a fine wire.

When a muscle is in its relaxed state, its fibers overlap just a little. When stimulated by a nerve, the fibers slide over each other, shortening the muscle. This is what is called a **muscle contraction.** An individual muscle fiber will contract completely, or it will not contract at all. Small movements require only a few muscle fibers to contract; larger and more powerful movements require the contraction of many muscle fibers. Some muscle fibers are contracting while others are relaxing. **Relaxation** is a recovery from the contraction and is more passive. So when all the muscle fiber activity is averaged out, even and sustained movement results.

Muscle tone is the continuous and partial contraction of the entire muscle (not individual fibers) or the muscle's resistance to stretching during its resting state. The muscles that hold a dog's jaw shut keep it in position with continuous partial contraction. When the dog is sleeping, you will find the jaw relaxed and easily opened if he does not wake up. Muscle tone is a good thing. However, physical disorders can result in abnormally low (hypotonia) or high (hypertonia) muscle tone.

A sharp and unconscious muscle contraction is known as a cramp or a **spasm.** (A "charley horse" is a popular term for painful spasms in the leg muscles. Dogs can experience sudden leg spasms after overactivity or abrupt movement.) Spasms can occur suddenly, usually resolve quickly, and are often painful. A **tonic spasm** consists of a continued muscular contraction; a **clonic spasm** involves alternating spasm and muscle relaxation.

CASE STUDY 6-2   #2011-1408 ROSIE

Signalment and History: A **geriatric** F(S) **canine** named Rosie was evaluated at the Frisbee SA Clinic for acute intermittent **tonic muscle spasms** and a stiff gait. There was no history of trauma. She was not eating well and had bouts of salivation, vomiting, and diarrhea.

Physical Examination: Rosie was lethargic when brought into the exam room. On physical examination, multiple **subcutaneous lipomas** on the **lateral** and **ventral** surfaces of the **thoracic** and **abdominal** regions of the **trunk** were noted. Tapping on the **proximal appendicular muscles** with a reflex hammer resulted in formation of dimples consistent with **myotonia.** Dr. Frisbee suspected a toxicity, but the **etiology** was unknown. Rosie was admitted to the hospital for further evaluation.

Diagnosis and Treatment: Electromyography identified **myotonic** potentials. Blood and urine samples were collected and were sent to a reference laboratory to check for toxin residues. The results confirmed toxicity; residues of 2,4-dichlorophenoxyacetic acid herbicide (2,4-D) were detected in both serum and urine, which led Dr. Frisbee to a **diagnosis** of 2,4-D toxicity.

Outcome: Rosie was treated with intravenous fluid therapy for 36 hours, and her **clinical signs** improved dramatically. The **prognosis** was good. The source of the 2,4-D remains unknown. The lipomas were considered **nonpathological** old-age **tumors.** Four days after admission, Rosie was sent home. One month later, Rosie's owner reported that Rosie was doing well.

EXERCISE **6-1** *Case It!*

Read Case Study 6-2. Then circle the correct answer to complete each statement.

1. The patient is a (cat), (cow), or (dog).

2. Etiology has to do with the (outcome of the disease), (cause of the disease), or (symptoms of the disease).

3. Sharp and unconscious muscle contractions are (muscle spasms), (muscle tone), or (muscle diseases).

4. Tumors of (skin), (fat), or (muscle) were present on Rosie.

5. The most proximal appendicular muscles would be found (along the spine), (near the hoof), or (at the knee).

6. Electromyography is a procedure performed on (electricity), (muscles), or (joints).

7. Nonpathological tumors are (benign), (malignant), or (not diseased).

8. The patient's tumors were (on the surface of the skin), (deep in the skin), or (in the sweat glands).

9. Myotonia is a sign of disorders characterized by (slow relaxation of muscles), (slow contraction of muscles), or (slow movement of a joint).

10. Rosie's tumors were located on the (sides and belly), (sides and back), or (head and belly).

Check your answers at the end of the chapter, Answers to Exercises.

Muscles are built onto the skeleton in several layers. The **skeletal muscles** you can "see" and feel under an animal's skin are the **superficial muscles.** These are the muscles that work together in groups to move the limbs, head, neck, body, and tail of an animal. Other muscles **(deep muscles)** are hidden under the superficial muscles, farther away from the skin. Some are used as **intramuscular (IM)** injection sites for medications. These injections go deeper than **subcutaneous (SQ, subq)** injections and are absorbed into the body more quickly.

Figures 6-2 and 6-3 show the superficial muscles of a horse and a cat. Notice that in both animals (actually in every animal) the muscles run in many different directions. Consequently, when a number of muscles contract, a unique movement may result. If all of the muscles ran in the same direction, very little movement would result when muscles contracted and relaxed.

Some skeletal muscle contractions and relaxations enable an animal to move all or a part of its body. All these movements are under voluntary control of the conscious mind by way of the nervous system. If a cow wants to kick you, she will receive a message from her brain to tell the proper muscles of her rear leg to contract, so her leg can shoot straight back. If your brain is quick enough, it will tell your leg muscles to jump you out of the way. In other words, the brain tells the muscles what to do by sending messages through nerves. Skeletal muscle is therefore a **voluntary, striated muscle.**

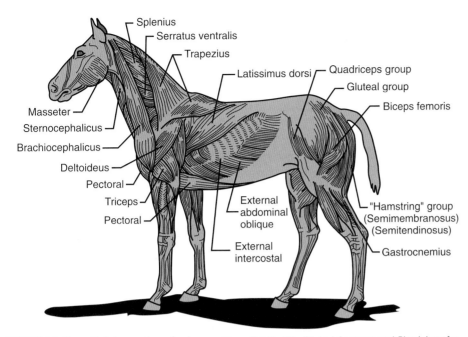

FIGURE 6-2 Superficial muscles of a horse. (From Colville TP: *Clinical Anatomy and Physiology for Veterinary Technicians,* ed 2, St Louis, 2009, Mosby.)

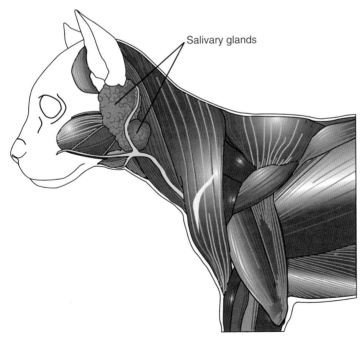

FIGURE 6-3 Superficial muscles of a cat. (Adapted from Colville TP: *Clinical Anatomy and Physiology for Veterinary Technicians,* ed 2, St Louis, 2009, Mosby.)

Other skeletal muscle actions make it possible for an animal to breathe, swallow saliva, and keep its body upright. These bodily functions go on, usually without conscious thought about them. However, the muscles involved can also be controlled by conscious thought. Have you ever tried to pick up a dog and she just goes limp? With conscious thought, she has gone from standing to a lump of wiggly gelatin.

CASE STUDY 6-3 #2007-598 LADY

Signalment and History: A 3-year-old Quarter Horse **mare** named Lady was admitted to the Frisbee Large Animal Hospital because of recurrent muscular stiffness, **myalgia,** sweating, and reluctance to move. Additionally, the owner noticed that the **gluteal muscles** became hard during these episodes. After more questioning, the owner revealed that the signs most often occur within 20 minutes after they start to exercise Lady.

Physical Examination: After unloading Lady from the trailer, Dr. Murdoch performed a thorough examination. He could find nothing physically wrong except possible muscle **atrophy** in her hind quarters. Lady was BAR, and her TPR were within the normal reference range. A blood sample was drawn and was submitted to the lab. Dr. Murdoch suspected a **diagnosis** of **equine polysaccharide** storage **myopathy** or **exertional rhabdomyolysis** and ordered an exercise tolerance test. For the next 15 minutes, Lady was walked and trotted around the indoor arena. Toward the end of the 15 minutes, Lady was starting to look sluggish in her walk, was sweating profusely, and was beginning to show signs of **neuromuscular** weakness with an abnormal **pelvic limb** gait. At this point, she was put in a box stall and was hosed off to reduce her body temperature; she was given small sips of water containing electrolytes over the next 2 hours. Another blood sample was drawn and was sent to the lab.

The results of the **hematology** tests in both blood samples showed that Lady had persistently high levels of an enzyme that indicates muscle **pathology.** This ruled out exertional rhabdomyolysis, which would have shown an increased enzyme blood level only **post-exercise.** To confirm his diagnosis, Dr. Murdoch took a muscle **bx** and sent it to an outside lab for confirmation. The results came back positive for equine polysaccharide storage myopathy. The other method of confirming the diagnosis would have been through a **necropsy,** but that was not needed in this case.

Diagnosis and Treatment: Equine polysaccharide storage myopathy (PSSM) is a disease that is associated with a high-carbohydrate diet (this was confirmed by Lady's owner), so Dr. Murdoch recommended that all grain, sweet feed, and molasses be eliminated from Lady's diet. Fresh water was to be always available. Additionally, forced exercise was to be eliminated until Lady's blood enzyme level returned to normal, which should happen once carbohydrates were eliminated from her diet. Free choice exercise was recommended rather than keeping Lady in a box stall.

Outcome: Four months after the initial diagnosis, Lady was reportedly doing well, with no further episodes of myopathy. Dr. Murdoch went to Lady's ranch and drew a blood sample. The results revealed a blood enzyme level within the expected reference range.

EXERCISE 6-2 *Case It!*

Read Case Study 6-3, and decide whether each of the following statements is True or False. Rewrite to correct the false statements on the lines below.

T F   1. This case study is about what can happen to equines after unaccustomed exercise while they are on a heavy-carbohydrate diet.

T **F**   2. Necropsy studies are performed under anesthesia.

T F   3. A disorder that is recurrent returns after a period that could consist of weeks or months.

T **F**   4. Neuromuscular weakness is a sign that something is wrong with the muscles of the heart.

T **F**   5. Muscle atrophy means that the muscles have become swollen and painful.

T F   6. Polysaccharide storage tells you that many carbohydrates are involved.

T **F**   7. The abnormal gait reported in Lady occurred in the front limbs.

T F   8. Exertional rhabdomyolysis refers to a situation where muscles become immobile during exercise.

T F   9. Grain, sweet feed, and molasses all are high in carbohydrates.

T F   10. Gait is the manner or style of walking.

2. Necro means dead

4. false muscles nerves

7. hind legs

Check your answers at the end of the chapter, Answers to Exercises.

To create a movement, each end of a skeletal muscle must be attached to a different bone of the skeleton (Table 6-2). This can be done in a couple of ways: (1) an **aponeurosis** (a broad fibrous connective tissue *sheet*), or (2) a **tendon** (a tough fibrous connective tissue *cord*, also known as a **sinew**).

The **tendon of origin** (or muscle origin) usually attaches a muscle to a bone that is more stable. That bone usually is located at the more proximal end of a limb. When a muscle contracts, this bone moves the least. From its origin, a muscle travels over one or more joints to its point of insertion on another bone. The **tendon of insertion** (or muscle insertion) usually attaches a muscle to a bone that is more movable. That bone is usually located at the more distal end of a limb. When a muscle contracts, this bone moves the most.

Tendons allow a muscle to exert its force from a distance. For example, muscles of the lower leg have long tendons to control the foot. If the carpus or the tarsus had to depend on its own muscles to move it, the joint would have to be many times its size.

One muscle rarely acts alone. It depends on its companions to accomplish a move. Try this on your **brachium** (upper arm). Hold your arm close to your body and flex your elbow; the biceps muscle is contracting and the triceps muscle is relaxed, moving your radius and ulna closer to your humerus. Your humerus should not have moved. Now extend your elbow; the triceps muscle is contracting and the biceps muscle is relaxed, causing your arm to straighten. Again, your humerus did not move. Both the biceps and triceps muscles originate on the humerus and insert on the radius and ulna. These two muscles, which are located on opposite sides of your arm, produce opposite movements when they contract. If you try to contract both your triceps and biceps muscles at the same time ("flex" your muscles), your **antebrachium** (forearm) will stay still. Many muscles work in pairs because muscles can only contract to produce their actions. They pull, but they cannot push to reverse their actions.

ten/o

tendin/o

tendon/o

tenont/o

kinesi/o

erg/o

syn-

dynam/o

ab-

ad-

ipsi-

contra-

TABLE 6-2		Word Parts Related to Muscle Movements	
Word Part	**Meaning**	**Example and Definition**	**Word Parts**
ten/o tendin/o tendon/o tenont/o	tendon	**tenotomy** surgical incision into a tendon	ten/o = tendon -tomy = surgical incision
		polytendinitis inflammation of multiple tendons	poly- = much or many tendin/o = tendon -itis = inflammation
		tendonitis inflammation of a tendon	tendon/o = tendon -itis = inflammation
		tenontomyoplasty surgical repair of a tendon and muscle	tenont/o = tendon my/o = muscle -plasty = surgical repair
kinesi/o	movement	**kinesiology** study of the mechanics of movement	kinesi/o = movement -logy = to study or to have knowledge of
erg/o	work	**ergometer** an instrument that measures muscle power *In Physics, an erg is a unit to measure work, just as pounds are used to measure flour and gallons are used to measure gasoline.*	erg/o = work -meter = measure, a device to measure
syn-	together, joined	**synergic muscles** muscles that work together	syn- = together, joined erg/o = work -ic = pertaining to
dynam/o	force, energy	**dynamoscope** a modified stethoscope for listening for sounds of the muscles *A dynamo is a machine that changes mechanical energy into electricity, or the term may be used to describe a hard-working, tirelessly energetic person with a lot of determination and energy. Dynamite definitely has force and energy.*	dynam/o = force, energy -scope = instrument for examining or viewing
ab-	away from	**abnormal** irregular, unusual, or unexpected; not normal or typical	ab- = away from normal = usual, expected ab- = away from
		abductor muscles muscles that move a limb away from the body	duct/o = to take, to lead -or = a person or a thing that does something specified
ad-	toward	**admaxillary** near or connected to the maxilla or jawbone	ad- = toward maxill/o = maxilla -ar = pertaining to -y = made up of, characterized by
		adductor muscles muscles that move a limb toward the body	ad- = toward duct/o = to take, to lead -or = a person or a thing that does something specified
ipsi-	same, self	**ipsilateral** located on or affecting the same side of the body	ipsi- = same, self later/o = side -al = pertaining to
contra-	against, contrary, opposing	**contralateral** on the opposite side of the body	contra- = against, contrary, opposing later/o = side -al = pertaining to

EXERCISE 6-3 *Define It!*

Below is a diagram of the hind limb of a canine. This diagram will help you with the answers to the following questions.

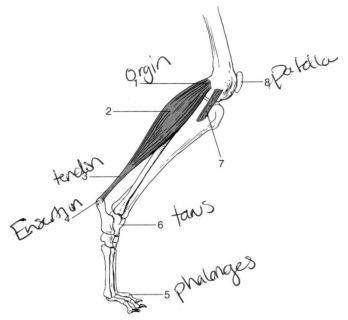

orgin 1

Patella 8

2

7

tendon 3

Ensertion 4

6 *tarus*

5 *phalanges*

Hind limb of a canine. (Adapted from McBride DF: *Learning Veterinary Terminology,* St Louis, 2002, Mosby.)

1. The movable bone to which a muscle is attached is known as the bone of ___Ensertion___ . (# _4_)

2. The immovable bone to which a muscle is attached is known as the bone of ___orgin___ . (# _1_)

3. (# _2_) is a muscle. It produces movement by ___Contraction___ and ___relaxation___ .

4. The tough fibrous connective tissue cord that connects muscles to bone is called a ___tendon___ .
   (# _3_)

5. #8 depicts the kneecap or ___Patella___ bone; it is located cranial to
   the ___femur___ bone.

6. The tendon of origin is located on the ___femur___ bone. (# _1_).

7. The study of muscles is called ___Myology___ .

8. The joint depicted at #6 is the ___tarus___ , commonly called
   the ___hock___ joint.

9. The bones depicted at #5 are known as ___phalanges___ .

10. The bones located between #6 and #5 are known as the ___Metacarsals___ .

11. #7 is a ligament. It connects the ___femur___ bone to the ___tibia___ bone at
    the ___Stifle___ joint.

12. The muscle action that causes this joint (see question 11) to bend is called ___flexion___ . The
    foot will move forward or backward? ___Backward___

Check your answers at the end of the chapter, Answers to Exercises.

HOW MANY, HOW MUCH

Before you continue on to learn how muscles are named, it will be helpful to know the prefixes that are used to denote numbers—like how many and how much. Number prefixes use their Greek and Latin origins. Many of these prefixes have already become familiar to you through common usage. For example, the prefix for "two" is *bi-*. Think *bi*cycle and how many wheels it has. The prefix for "three" is *tri-*. Now think *tri*cycle. Table 6-3 lists the common prefixes denoting numbers. Table 6-4 is a good place to review the prefixes used in the metric system. These prefixes are used primarily in naming units of measurement; however, you will also find them used in describing something biological.

TABLE 6-3	Prefixes Used in Counting and Measuring		
Prefix	**Meaning**	**Example and Definition**	**Word Parts**
hemi- semi-	half, partial	**hemialgia** pain affecting half the body	hemi- = half -algia = pain
		semiconscious only half awake *Our globe is divided into North and South hemispheres; a semiprivate hospital room is only half-private. Is a "semi" just half of a truck?*	semi- = half conscious = awake and aware
uni- mono-	one, single	**unicellular** made up of only one cell (e.g., bacteria)	uni- = one cellul/o = cell -ar = pertaining to
		mononeuropathy disease affecting only one nerve	mono- = one neur/o = nerve -pathy = disease
bi- di-	two	**bicaudal** having two tails	bi- = two caud/o = tail -al = pertaining to
		Do not confuse the prefix bi- *with the combining form* bi/o, *meaning "life" (as in* **biology,** *the study of life).*	bi/o = life -logy = to study, or to have knowledge of
		dichromic having two colors	di- = two chrom/o = color -ic = pertaining to
tri-	three	**triphalangia** pertaining to a malformation in which three bones are present (where normally there are only two—as in the dewclaw on the front legs of dogs) **Triage** *(trē ahzh) is the screening and classification of patients to determine priority needs and thereby ensure the most efficient use of medical and surgical manpower, equipment, and facilities. Triage has <u>no connection</u> with the Greek-Latin element* tri-.	tri- = three phalang/o = phalange -ia = pertaining to

hemi-

semi-

uni-

mono-

bi-

bi/o

di-

tri-

TABLE 6-3 Prefixes Used in Counting and Measuring—cont'd

Prefix	Meaning	Example and Definition	Word Parts
quadri- tetra-	four	**quadrilateral** having four sides	quadri- = four later/o = side -al = pertaining to
		tetradactyly the presence of four digits on a foot	tetra- = four dactyl/o = a digit or a toe -y = made up of, characterized by
multi- poly-	much or many	**multiarticular** pertaining to many joints	multi- = much or many articul/o = joint -ar = pertaining to
		polypathia presence of many diseases at the same time	poly- = much or many path/o = disease -ia = pertaining to
pan-	all	**panosteitis** inflammation of all bones or inflammation of every part of one bone *A pandemic is a widespread epidemic; a panacea is a remedy for all diseases.*	pan- = all oste/o = bone -itis = inflammation

TABLE 6-4 Prefixes Used in Metric Measurements

Prefix	Meaning	Example and Definition	Word Parts
kilo-	one thousand; written as 10^3 or 1000	**kilosecond** one thousand seconds (16 minutes and 40 seconds)	kilo- = one thousand second = unit of time equal to one-sixtieth of a minute
deci-	one-tenth; written as 1×10^{-1} or 0.1	**decibel** common measure of sound intensity that is one-tenth of a "bel"	deci- = one-tenth bel = unit of sound intensity used in acoustics, electronics, etc.
centi-	one-hundredth; written as 1×10^{-2} or 0.01 OR one hundred; written as 100	**centimeter** a unit of length in the metric system, equal to one-hundredth of a meter	centi- = one-hundredth meter = unit of length in the metric system equal to 3.28 feet
		centigrade a scale and a unit of measurement for temperature, based on 100 "steps" between the freezing point of water and the boiling point of water *The bicentennial is celebrated in 200 years.*	centi- = one hundred grade = the position in a scale of ranks or qualities
milli-	one-thousandth; written as 1×10^{-3} or 0.001	**milligram** a unit of weight in the metric system, equal to one- thousandth of a gram *The prefix milli- is confusing. It seems to mean one-thousandth only in reference to the metric system. When you think of a millennium, it is the reference to a period of one thousand (1000) years. And, a millionaire has 1000 times 1000 dollars.*	milli- = one-thousandth gram = a unit of weight in the metric system

quadri-

tetra-

multi-

poly-

pan-

kilo-

deci-

centi-

milli-

Continued

micro-

nano-

pico-

TABLE 6-4	Prefixes Used in Metric Measurements—cont'd		
Prefix	Meaning	Example and Definition	Word Parts
micro-	one-millionth; written as 1×10^{-6} or 0.000001 OR small, very small	**microcurie** one-millionth of a curie; a common measure of radioactivity	micro- = one-millionth curie = unit of radioactivity based on the activity of 1 gram of radium per second
		microbiologist person who specializes in the study of small organisms such as bacteria, rickettsiae, viruses, fungi, and protozoa	micro- = small, very small bi/o = life log/o = to study, or to have knowledge of -ist = a person or thing that does something specific
		A microbiologist uses the **microscope,** an instrument used to view something that is extremely small or that is not large enough to be seen with the naked eye.	micro- = small, very small -scope = instrument for examining or viewing
nano-	one-billionth; written as 1×10^{-9} or 0.000000001 OR extremely small	**nanosecond** one-billionth of a second; popular term for an extremely short time; a common measurement of the time to read or write to random access memory (RAM) on computer hard disks	nano- = one-billionth second = unit of time equal to one-sixtieth of a minute
		nanocranous pertaining to an extremely small head	nano- = extremely small crani/o = skull -ous = pertaining to
pico-	one-trillionth; written as 1×10^{-12} OR 0.000000000001	**picoliter** one-trillionth of a liter; a measure of the size (2 to 25 picoliters) of ink droplets that inkjet printers typically use (the smaller the droplet, the higher the resolution of images)	pico- = one-trillionth liter = a unit of liquid volume in the metric system (a liter is equal to 1.06 quarts)

EXERCISE 6-4   *Number It!*

You supply the "number" to complete the following definitions.

1. Tricostal means ___Three___ ribs.

2. Tetrabrachius is an individual with ___four___ arms.

3. A micrometer is an instrument for precise measurement

    of ___small___ distances.

4. Hemiatrophy is the wasting away of ___half___ of a body, an organ, or a part.

5. Polysyndactyly is the webbing of ___many___ fingers or toes.

6. Quadrilateral means having ___four___ sides.

7. A millimeter is a unit of length that is ___one thousandths___ of a meter.

8. A monopathy is _____ one _____ uncomplicated disease, or a

   disease affecting _____ one _____ part of the body.

9. Something that occurs bihourly occurs once every

   _____ two _____ hours.

10. _____ one billionth _____ of a volt is a nanovolt.

Check your answers at the end of the chapter, Answers to Exercises.

TABLE 6-5	Word Parts Used in Muscle Names		
Word Part	**Meaning**	**Example and Definition**	**Word Parts**
cephal/o	head, skull	**cephalocaudal** pertaining to a direction from the skull to the tail	cephal/o = head, skull caud/o = tail -al = pertaining to
cep	head, origin of a muscle	**biceps** muscle on brachium with two heads (two origins)	bi- = two cep = head, origin of a muscle -s = makes the word plural
cardi/o	heart	**cardiomyopathy** a general diagnostic term designating disease of the heart muscle of an unknown cause	cardi/o = heart my/o = muscle -pathy = disease
-oid	resembling	**myoid** resembling muscle	my/o = muscle -oid = resembling

cephal/o

cep

cardi/o

-oid

Learning the Names of Muscles

Learning the names of muscles can initially look like a daunting task, but it is really not that bad (Table 6-5). Many times, the name of a muscle will give you a hint as to where it is located because skeletal muscles are frequently named by their attachment sites. Muscles are also named for their actions, the number of divisions (or heads) that constitute them, or their shapes. Following is a list of terms that are used to indicate location when naming muscles. You will recognize familiar word roots in many of the names.

oris = oral = mouth
oculi = ocular = eye
abdominis = abdomen
brachii = brachium = upper foreleg
femoris = femur = thigh
tibialis = tibia = shin bone
digitorum = digit
costals = rib
carpi = carpus = wrist
spinalis = spine = backbone
scapularis = scapula = shoulder blade

Here are some examples of descriptive muscle names.
- sternocephalicus
  - This muscle is named for its attachment sites. The first part of the name tells you where the muscle originates, and the second part tells you where it inserts. The sternocephalicus muscle originates on the cranial end of the **sternum** and inserts into two places on the skull.

- When this muscle contracts, it flexes the neck, turns the head, and opens the mouth. Drop your chin to your chest, turn your head to the left, and open your mouth. An amazing muscle, the sternocephalicus muscle!
- extensor carpi radialis
  - This muscle is named for its action, but not for its sites of attachment. When it contracts, it extends **(extensor)** the wrist (carpi or carpus). The radialis part indicates its location over the radius as it travels from its origin on the humerus. There is also an **extensor carpi ulnaris.**
  - Bend your wrist as if you are going to "high five" with your dog (or a real person). Both of you can thank your two extensor carpi muscles that you can do that.
- biceps brachii
  - This muscle has two heads. The tendons of origin attach to the scapula. The two heads travel over the humerus (area of the **brachium**), and the tendons of insertion insert on the radius.
  - When the biceps brachii muscle contracts, it helps flex the elbow and rotate the antebrachium. Lifting weights and hitchhiking are two activities that you can perform with your biceps brachii muscle.
- **deltoideus** (also known as the **deltoid** muscle)
  - This muscle was named by early anatomists, who noticed that it was triangle-shaped (delta).
  - The tendon of origin of the deltoid muscle attaches to the scapula. The muscle travels over the shoulder joint, and the tendon of insertion attaches to the humerus.
  - When the deltoideus muscle contracts, it flexes the shoulder.

Many important functions in the body are carried out by groups of skeletal muscles, rather than by a single muscle. A few examples of muscles that perform as a part of group are given here:

- cutaneous muscles
  - These muscles are located in the connective tissue below the skin. They have no bone-to-bone attachment.
  - When they contract, they twitch the skin. This is a handy function when the animal is besieged with irritating insects.
- abdominal muscles
  - The four layers of these muscles aid in any action that requires straining. The muscles involved are:
    - external abdominal oblique muscles
    - internal abdominal oblique muscles
    - rectus abdominis muscles
    - transverse abdominis muscles
  - The name of each muscle group tells you about the location of the muscles (external, internal, abdominal) and the direction in which the muscle fibers run (oblique, **rectus** [*rectus* = straight], transverse).
  - The four abdominal muscles from each side of the abdomen meet on the ventral midline of the body to form a large aponeurosis called the **linea alba** (white line). The linea alba is a common incision site for abdominal surgery or exploration because the aponeurosis contains very few blood vessels or nerves.
- thoracic muscles
  - These muscles are used primarily for breathing.
  - When an animal breathes in (inspiration), the **diaphragm** and **external intercostal muscles** are working to expand the thorax.
  - Breathing out requires the work of the abdominal muscles and the **internal intercostal muscles.**
- muscles of the thoracic and pelvic limbs
  - **Extrinsic muscles** attach the limb to the body.

- **Intrinsic muscles** originate and insert on the limb.
- **Adductor muscles** move the limb toward the body.
- **Abductor muscles** move the limb away from the body.
- Numerous **flexor** and **extensor muscles** work together to flex and extend the various joints.
- Groups of muscles on the pelvic limbs that have been given names are:
  - glutes or **gluteal** muscles—three muscles that form the rump of the animal and work together to extend the hip joint (move the thigh backward)
  - **hamstring** muscles—a group of four muscles on the caudal aspect of the rear leg that is used to flex the stifle joint and extend the hip joint (move the thigh backward)
  - quads or **quadriceps** muscle—really one muscle with four heads (each with a separate name) that extend the stifle joint
  - **triceps surae** ("three-headed calf")—the primary muscle that covers the caudal surface of the rear leg over the stifle joint
  - two muscles: the **gastrocnemius** muscle with its lateral and medial heads, and the single-headed **superficial digital flexor muscle** (sometimes called the *soleus muscle*).
    - Their combined actions are to extend the hock (tarsal joint) and flex the digits.
    - The tendons of insertion of these muscles form the Achilles tendon.

> Sometimes you cannot get much information from the name of a muscle. The **gastrocnemius** muscle is a good example of this. You cannot tell where it is located, what it does, where the attachments are located, or how many heads it has. It was so named because to the ancient Greeks, the muscle looked like a stomach bulge (gastr/o = stomach) in the area of the calf of the leg (knem = area between the knee and the ankle).

EXERCISE 6-5 *Muscle It!*

This exercise involves descriptive muscle names. Your knowledge of muscles will amaze you as you look for the word parts in each muscle name to answer questions about the various muscles in the following groups.

adductor femoris   biceps femoris   caudofemoralis   rectus femoris

1. What bone is involved with all four muscles? *adductor femoris*

2. Which muscle would you look for near the tail end of the animal? *caudo ~~rectus~~ femoralis*

3. Does the adductor femoris muscle move the bone toward the body, or away from the body? *toward the body*

4. Which muscle has two heads? *biceps femoris*

5. Which muscle's fibers run straight? *rectus femoris*

brachiocephalicus   pectoantebrachialis   triceps brachialis

6. On which limbs of the body would you look for these muscles? *forelimbs*

7. Which muscle has a point of insertion in the skull? *brachiocephalicus*

8. How many heads does the triceps brachialis muscle have? *three*

9. The *ante* in pectoantebrachialis tells you that the muscle is located where? *in front*

extensor digitorum longus   **palmaris longus**

10. Are these muscles found on the axial or appendicular skeleton? _appendicular_

11. The action of the extensor muscle is to _increase angle between bones_

12. True or False? Both of these muscles are long. _true_

13. Both of these muscles could be found on which limbs of an animal? _forelimbs_

14. Which muscle would be the more distal of the two? _extensor_

interossei   **interspinales**   **transversospinalis**   **transversus thoracis**

15. The *inter-* in the first two muscle names indicates that these muscles are located _Between_

16. The *trans-* in the other two muscle names indicates that these muscles travel in what direction? _across the body_

17. Interossei could be found anywhere in the body, but interspinales will be located on the (dorsal) or (ventral) aspect of an animal? _Dorsal_

18. Which muscle is more ventral—the transversospinalis or the transversus thoracis? _transversus_

spinalis dorsi   **latissimus dorsi**   **gluteus medius**   **vastus lateralis**

19. Which muscle is huge? _vastus lateralis_

20. *Dorsi* refers to which location in an animal? _Back of the head_

21. Which two muscles would you expect to find on the side of an animal? _latissimus dorsi_

sternocleidomastoid   **sternothyroid**   **subscapularis**

22. Which muscle is found on the underside of a bone? _subscapularis_

23. Sternocleidomastoid and sternothyroid muscles both have an attachment on which bone? _Sternum_

orbicularis oculi	trapezius	rhomboid major	pronator quadratus

24. Which muscle is named for its action? _____ *pronator quadradus*

25. Which muscle has four heads? _____ *pronator quadradus*

26. Which muscles are named for their shapes? _____ *trapezius* and _____ *rhomboid major*

27. Which muscle is near the eye? _____ *orbicularis oculi*

Check your answers at the end of the chapter, Answers to Exercises.

PHYSIOLOGY OF CARDIAC MUSCLE

A second type of muscle is **cardiac muscle.** It is found in only one place in an animal's body: the heart. The only function of heart muscle **(myocardium)** is to contract and relax for the entire life of the animal. When viewed microscopically, cardiac muscle has stripes (striations) similar to skeletal muscle, so cardiac muscle is also known as *striated muscle.* Because the animal has no conscious control over how the heart muscle contracts, cardiac muscle is an involuntary muscle and is classified as an **involuntary, striated muscle.**

PHYSIOLOGY OF SMOOTH MUSCLE

The third type of muscle is **smooth muscle.** It is not as easily visible as skeletal muscle because it does not exist in distinct muscle masses. When viewed microscopically, no stripes (striations) are discernible, so it is called *smooth muscle.* Smooth muscle is also an involuntary muscle. Therefore, it is classified as an **involuntary, nonstriated muscle.**

Throughout an animal's body, smooth muscle is found in two forms: visceral and multiunit. Large sheets of smooth muscle cells are found in the walls of many hollow organs (e.g., intestines, stomach, uterus, urinary bladder). This smooth muscle in organ walls is classified as **visceral smooth muscle.** It contracts in large, rhythmic waves that create propelling movements. No delicate movements are produced from visceral smooth muscle contractions. If the organ is stretched, the waves become stronger. This is why food moves along the digestive tract, babies are born, and urine is released only when the bladder is full. (*Note:* Animals that are housebroken can control urination through a voluntary sphincter, much as humans who are toilet-trained do.)

Multiunit smooth muscle is made up of individual smooth muscle cells or small groups of cells. When these cells contract, they create delicate movements like dilating and contracting pupils in the eye or adjusting the diameter of small blood vessels. These movements are involuntary actions but are not automatic; they require specific autonomic (self-governing) nerve stimulation.

Table 6-6 presents word parts associated with medical conditions of the muscular system. Combining these word parts with word parts from previous chapters will allow you to build words that describe muscular medical conditions.

TABLE 6-6	Word Parts for Medical Conditions of Muscles		
Word Part	**Meaning**	**Example and Definition**	**Word Parts**
a- an-	without, no, not	**amyoplasia** lack of muscle formation or development	a- = without, no, not my/o = muscle plas/o = growth, development, or formation -ia = pertaining to
		anerythroplasia condition in which there is no formation of red blood cells; absence of red blood cell formation in the bone marrow	an- = without, no, not erythr/o = red plas/o = growth, development, or formation -ia = pertaining to
cata-	down, reverse, backward, degenerative	**catabiosis** degenerative biological changes occurring in cells as they age after their maturity A cata*clysm is a violent disruption or breaking up, a terrible disaster or accident.*	cata- = down, reverse, backward, degenerative bi/o = life -osis = disease or abnormal condition
de-	removal, separation, reduction	**deoxygenation** process of removing oxygen	de- = removal, separation, reduction oxygen = oxygen -ation = state, condition, action, process, or result
par-	other than, abnormal	**paresthesia** abnormal sensations of stinging, tingling, burning, crawling, etc., of the skin for no apparent cause	par- = other than, abnormal esthesia = sensations
para-	near, beside, abnormal, apart from	**paranuclear** beside the nucleus	para- = near, beside, abnormal, apart from nucle/o = nucleus -ar = pertaining to
path/o -pathy	disease	**myopathologist** a specialist in the study of any disease of muscle	my/o = muscle path/o = disease log/o = to study, or to have knowledge of -ist = a person or a thing that does something specified
		myopathy any disease of a muscle	my/o = muscle -pathy = disease
-paresis	partial paralysis, weakness	**hemiparesis** muscular weakness or partial paralysis restricted to one side of the body	hemi- = half -paresis = partial paralysis, weakness
-plegia	paralysis	**myoplegia** paralysis of muscles	my/o = muscle -plegia = paralysis

a-

an-

cata-

de-

par-

para-

path/o

-pathy

-paresis

-plegia

TABLE 6-6	Word Parts for Medical Conditions of Muscles—cont'd		
Word Part	**Meaning**	**Example and Definition**	**Word Parts**
plas/o	growth, development, or formation	**hypoplasia** underdevelopment or incomplete development of a tissue or organ	hypo- = under, beneath, below plas/o = growth, development, or formation -ia = pertaining to
-trophy	growth	**hypertrophy** increase in the volume of an organ or tissue due to enlargement of its component cells (an example of hypertrophy occurs when skeletal muscles respond to strength training)	hyper- = above, over, or excess -trophy = growth
		⚠ *Hypertrophy should be distinguished from* **hyperplasia,** *in which the cells remain approximately the same size but increase in number.*	hyper- = above, over, or excess plas/o = growth, development, or formation -ia = pertaining to
lys/o	destruction, dissolution, dissolving, breakage	**rhabdomyolysis** destruction of the rod-shaped muscle cells 💡 *A good marketing ploy—is this how* Lysol *gets its name?*	rhabd/o = rod, cylinder my/o = muscle lys/o = destruction, dissolution, dissolving, breakage -is = structure, thing
cry/o	freezing, icy cold	**cryotherapy** treatment with an icy cold substance	cry/o = freezing, icy cold therapy = treatment
pyr/o pyrex/o	heat, high temperature	**pyrogen** an agent that causes heat	pyr/o = heat, high temperature gen/o = formation or beginning
		pyrexia a fever 💡 Pyrex *dishes are oven-proof and can withstand high temperatures.*	pyrex/o = heat, high temperature -ia = pertaining to
therm/o	heat	**catathermal** falling temperature or lowering of heat 💡 *A* thermo*meter is a device for measuring heat.*	cata- = down, reverse, backward, degenerative therm/o = heat -al = pertaining to

plas/o

-trophy

lys/o

cry/o

pyr/o

pyrex/o

therm/o

EXERCISE 6-6 *Analyze It!*

This exercise will give you a chance to dissect "new to you" clinical veterinary language containing word parts introduced in this chapter. Match each "new" word with its definition.

New Words

catathermometer

diathermy

ergograph

fibrolipoma

hypermyatrophy

kinesialgia

myodystonia

myonecrosis

paracentesis

tenomyotomy

1. _Myodystonia_ disorder of muscle, whereby the muscle cannot relax

2. _Kinesialgia_ pain upon moving any sore or injured part of the body

3. _tenomyotomy_ surgical incision into a muscle and tendon

4. _myonecrosis_ condition of death of muscle cells

5. _hypermyatrophy_ excessive wasting away of many muscles

6. _diathermy_ method of sending heat through tissue for therapeutic purposes, commonly used for muscle relaxation

7. _ergograph_ an instrument for recording the amount of work done during muscular activity

8. _fibrolipoma_ a fatty tumor containing an excess of fibrous tissue

9. _Catathermometer_ device that measures how quickly air is cooling

10. _paracentesis_ surgical procedure whereby a body cavity is punctured from the outside for the purpose of removing fluid for analysis as an aid to diagnosis

Check your answers at the end of the chapter, Answers to Exercises.

BOX 6-1 **Terms That Defy Word Analysis**

- aponeurosis—sheet-like dense fibrous collagenous connective tissue that binds muscles together or connects muscle to bone; the linea alba is an aponeurosis
- avulsion—an acute tendon injury in which the tendon is forcibly torn away from its attachment site on the bone
- fatigue—muscle contractions get feebler under repeated stimulation until they stop altogether
- rigor mortis—temporary muscular stiffening that follows death, resulting from lack of energy to allow muscle fibers to relax
- shivers—rapid involuntary muscle contractions that release waste heat, which will warm the animal's body; seen in response to a cold environment
- spasm—an acute involuntary muscle contraction
- tonic spasm—a continuous spasm
- clonic spasm—alternating spasm and muscle relaxation
- tetanus—painful, sustained muscle contractions caused by toxins released from the *Clostridium tetani* bacteria
- tetany—intermittent, painful, sustained muscle contractions related to defective calcium metabolism

Shivers is the name given to a neuromuscular syndrome that is found primarily in draft horses. The signs involve one or both hind legs and the tail. Horses experience intermittent involuntary muscle spasms of varying intensity. The tail is held upright, and the horse has difficulty backing up. The etiology is unknown and no treatment is available.

EXERCISE 6-7 *Recall It!*

Repetitive use of terms that defy word analysis will help you commit them to memory. Write a word or a group of words in each blank to complete the following statements. You will find some terms here that were introduced in previous chapters.

1. _Idiopathic_ pertains to a disease of unknown origin.

2. A sprain or a strain is the result of stretching or tearing a/an _ligament_ that connects bone/cartilage to bone/cartilage.

3. The tissue response to injury or destruction, with signs of pain and swelling, redness, and a feeling of warmth, is called a/an _inflammation_.

4. An acute involuntary muscle contraction is a/an _spasm_.

5. A cancer is called _malignant_ when it becomes progressively worse and leads to death.

6. Poor calcium metabolism leads to the condition of _tetany_—intermittent and painful muscle contractions.

7. Another name for a scar is a/an _cicatrix_.

8. _Signs_ provide objective evidence of disease; they are observable indicators, like body temperature and bleeding.

9. In _fatigue_, muscle contractions get weaker from repeated stimulation until they stop altogether.

10. *Purulent* refers to containing or consisting of ___pus___.

11. The ___callus___ is a bridge that forms when a fracture heals.

12. A laceration is a/an ___skin tear___.

13. An eschar is a/an ___scab___.

14. Exacerbation is the ___worsening___ of a disease.

15. Granulation tissue is new tissue that grows where? ___wound defect___ (fills in)

16. ___luxation___ is when the joint goes out of alignment. Partial dislocation is called ___subluxation___.

17. The pastern in horses and cattle is located between which two other structures? ___fetlock, hoof___

18. Avulsion is an acute injury in which the ___tendon___ is torn away from its attachment to the ___bone___.

19. A continuous spasm is a/an ___tonic___ spasm.

20. The species of murines consist of ___rats and mice___.

Check your answers at the end of the chapter, Answers to Exercises.

EXERCISE 6-8   *Case It!*

Here is the case study from the beginning of the chapter, rewritten in everyday language. Now, rewrite each underlined word or set of words from the case study on the line that corresponds to its term.

CASE STUDY 6-1   **#1999-87 ANNABELLE**

Signalment and History: A 4-year-old domestic shorthair <u>intact female cat who has not been spayed/neutered</u> named Annabelle was brought to the Frisbee Small Animal Clinic because of a 1-week history of shifting limb lameness that had progressed to <u>muscular weakness in all four limbs</u>. She was not eating well, but was still drinking plenty of water. Her level of activity was greatly diminished.

Physical Examination: Physical examination revealed a normal <u>temperature, pulse, and respiration</u>. A depressed level of activity was also noted. Dr. Frisbee found generalized <u>wasting away</u> of the muscles, and signs of discomfort were elicited when the muscles of <u>all four limbs</u> were <u>examined by touching and feeling</u>. <u>Study of nervous system</u> signs revealed diminished <u>muscle stretch</u> reflex and withdrawal reflexes in both thoracic and pelvic limbs.

Diagnosis and Treatment: The <u>cat</u> was <u>given drugs to bring about a loss of sensation</u>, and a <u>recording of the electricity in the muscles</u> was performed. Nerve and muscle <u>bx</u> specimens were obtained while she was still anesthetized. <u>Study of tissue</u> specimens revealed severe <u>inflammation of muscles</u> and <u>inflammation of nerves</u>. Immune-mediated <u>inflammation of many muscles</u> and neuritis was the tentative diagnosis because no other signs of pathology could be identified. The <u>cause of this condition</u> was unknown. A daily dose of a <u>medication to counteract the inflammation</u> was pre-scribed. Dr. Frisbee thought there was an excellent <u>probable outcome of the disease</u>, i.e., recovery with long-term treatment. But Dr. Frisbee warned the owner that there was also a chance of recurrence.

Four months after the initial diagnosis of <u>a condition that occurs when a cat's immune system overreacts and attacks its body</u>, Annabelle had been gradually taken off her anti-inflammatory medication and was doing well. Her appetite and energy had returned, and there was no sign of recurrence.

1. anesthetized = Given drugs loss of sensation
2. anti-inflammatory = Counteract inflamation Reduce
3. appendicular skeleton = All four limbs
4. atrophy = wasting away
5. biopsy = bx
6. electromyography = Recording of electricity
7. etiology = Cause condition
8. feline = cat
9. histological = Study of tissue
10. immune-mediated = immune System cats overreacts attacks body
11. myositis = infla of muscles
12. myotatic = muscle stretch
13. neuritis = infl of nerves
14. neurological = study of nervous system
15. palpated = examend by touching feeling
16. polymyositis = inflamation of muscles
17. prognosis = outcome of disease
18. queen = intact female cat not neutered
19. tetraparesis = Muscular weakness in all four limbs
20. TPR = Temp, pulse, rate.

Check your answers at the end of the chapter, Answers to Exercises.

EMG

bid

tid

qid

qh

q*x*h

q24h

sid

oid

PO

NPO

tx

med

cap

tab

Rx

ad lib

TABLE 6-7	Abbreviations	
Abbreviation	Meaning	Example
EMG	electromyography, electromyograph, and electromyogram	Sparky had his EMG, and the EMG report has been read by the veterinarian.
bid	twice a day	Sparky is supposed to take two tablets bid for 7 days. How many tablets a day is that?
tid	3 times a day	Sparky gets physical therapy tid in the hydrotherapy pool.
qid	4 times a day	Bruiser is to have his wound examined qid for the next 3 days.
qh	every hour	Dudley, the cat, wants to eat qh, and his weight indicates that he does.
q*x*h	every *x* number of hours (e.g., q4h is every 4 hours)	A blood sample was drawn q8h for 3 days and then q12h for the next 4 days.
q24h sid oid	once a day	Dudley has vomited at least q24h for the past week. Dudley should be fed sid for the next month and then have his weight rechecked. Give Dudley one antiemetic tablet oid while he is hospitalized.
PO	by mouth	Never give medications PO to an animal suffering from emesis.
NPO	nothing by mouth	In other words, vomiting animals should get NPO.
tx	treatment	tx: Feed boiled ground beef and cooked rice tid for 3 days.
med	medication	To Dudley's owner: This med should be taken for the entire prescribed duration, even if Dudley looks better.
cap	capsule	Licorice's med instructions are 1 cap q4h for 14 days.
tab	tablet	Dr. Frisbee could not find a tab with the needed strength of med, so she had to prescribe 18 tabs bid for 7 days.
Rx	prescription	Rx: Ampicillin 7 mg/lb q24h and metronidazole ½ tab bid for 5 days.
ad lib	as much as needed	In this case, you give as much as you need to for the desired result. There is no prescribed amount to give.

TABLE 6-7	Abbreviations—cont'd	
Abbreviation	**Meaning**	**Example**
L or l *In the United States, Canada, and Australia, the capital **L** is preferred, but most other nations use the lowercase **l**.*	liter or litre *The spellings* liter *and* litre *are both correct. In the United States, the* liter *spelling is mainly used. In most other nations, the* litre *spelling is used.*	Normal saline or 0.9% NaCl consists of 154 mmol/L of Na^+ and 154 mmol/L of Cl^-. (A mole is the molecular weight of a substance in grams. 1 mmol = 1 millimole.)
mL or ml	milliliter	The average value for systemic clearance of theophylline in Daisy was 0.780 mL/kg/min after IV administration.
dL or dl	deciliter	There are 20.2 teaspoons in a dL. How many teaspoons are present in a L?
m	meter or metre *The spellings of* meter *and* metre *are both correct. In the United States, the* meter *spelling is used nearly all the time. In most other nations, the* metre *spelling is used.*	A sheep's small intestine measures just over 15 m long.
cm	centimeter	A mass measuring 3 cm by 4 cm was removed from Midnight's abdomen along the ventral midline.
mm	millimeter	If the GSW had been 4 mm more caudal, Sherman would be dead.
cc	cubic centimeter (equivalent to 1 mL)	Each cc of TKX contains 50 mg of tiletamine, 50 mg of zolazepam, 80 mg of ketamine, and 20 mg of xylazine.
g	gram	Roxie's Hgb value today is 15 g/dL.
mg	milligram	Silver was treated IV with phenylbutazone at 4.4 mg/kg q24h for 4 days.
mcg µg	microgram *The mcg is preferred in the medical field because the hand-written µg looks almost exactly like mg and is therefore a frequent cause of overdose.*	Sundance's breathing was improved after administration of 1000 mcg of beclomethasone.
kg	kilogram	Brahman (cattle) calves weigh between 30 and 33 kg at birth. By comparison, kittens weigh about 100 g at birth.
IA	intra-arterial	You must be very careful when administering IV medications, so you do not accidentally administer them IA.

Continued

ID

IM

IP

IV

SQ

subq

SC

subcu

TABLE 6-7	Abbreviations—cont'd	
Abbreviation	**Meaning**	**Example**
ID	intradermal	ID testing is used to test for tuberculosis in animals.
IM	intramuscular	You want to avoid hitting nerves and blood vessels when administering medications IM.
IP	intraperitoneal	IP blood transfusion can be used as a rapid, safe, and efficient procedure for blood replacement in dogs.
IV	intravenous	An IV injection is the fastest way to distribute a drug throughout the body.
SQ subq SC subcu	subcutaneous	There are four abbreviations for subcutaneous. SQ and subq are used most often; SC and subcu are rarely used. The abbreviations are most often used in conjunction with a route of drug administration.

ANSWERS TO EXERCISES

Exercise 6-1
1. dog
2. cause of disease
3. muscle spasms
4. fat
5. at the knee
6. muscles
7. not diseased
8. deep in the skin
9. slow relaxation of muscles
10. sides and belly

Exercise 6-2
1. T
2. F—Necropsy studies are performed after death.
3. T
4. F—Neuromuscular weakness is a sign that something is wrong with muscles and nerves.
5. F—Muscle atrophy means that the muscles are wasting away.
6. T
7. F—The weakness reported in Lady occurred in the rear limbs.
8. T
9. T
10. T

Exercise 6-3
1. insertion; #4
2. origin; #1
3. #2; contraction and relaxation
4. tendon; #3
5. patella; femur
6. femur; #1
7. myology
8. tarsus; hock
9. phalanges
10. metatarsals
11. femur; tibia; stifle (femorotibial)
12. flexion; backward

Exercise 6-4
1. three
2. four
3. very small
4. one-half
5. many
6. four
7. one-thousandth
8. one; one
9. two
10. one-billionth

Exercise 6-5
1. femur
2. caudofemoralis
3. toward the body
4. biceps femoris
5. rectus femoris
6. forelimbs
7. brachiocephalicus
8. three
9. in front
10. appendicular
11. increase the angle between two bones
12. True
13. forelimbs
14. extensor digitorum longus
15. between bones
16. across the bone
17. dorsal
18. transversus thoracis
19. vastus lateralis
20. dorsal surface, the back of the animal, the area of the spine
21. latissimus dorsi and vastus lateralis
22. subscapularis
23. sternum
24. pronator quadratus
25. pronator quadratus
26. trapezius and rhomboid major
27. orbicularis oculi

Exercise 6-6
1. myodystonia
2. kinesialgia
3. tenomyotomy
4. myonecrosis
5. hypermyatrophy
6. diathermy
7. ergograph
8. fibrolipoma
9. catathermometer
10. paracentesis

Exercise 6-7

1. idiopathic
2. ligament
3. inflammation
4. spasm
5. malignant
6. tetany
7. cicatrix
8. signs
9. fatigue
10. pus
11. callus
12. rough or jagged skin tear
13. scab
14. worsening severity
15. it fills in a wound defect
16. luxation; subluxation
17. between the fetlock and the hoof
18. tendon; bone
19. tonic
20. rats and mice

Exercise 6-8

1. anesthetized = given drugs to bring about a loss of sensation
2. anti-inflammatory = medication to counteract the inflammation
3. appendicular skeleton = all four limbs
4. atrophy = wasting away
5. biopsy = bx
6. electromyography = recording of the electricity in the muscles
7. etiology = cause of this condition
8. feline = cat
9. histological = study of tissue
10. immune-mediated = a condition that occurs when a cat's immune system overreacts and attacks its body
11. myositis = inflammation of muscles
12. myotatic = muscle stretch
13. neuritis = inflammation of nerves
14. neurological = study of nervous system
15. palpated = examined by touching and feeling
16. polymyositis = inflammation of many muscles
17. prognosis = probable outcome of the disease
18. queen = intact female cat who has not been spayed/neutered
19. tetraparesis = muscular weakness in all four limbs
20. TPR = temperature, pulse, and respiration

Chapter 7

The Cardiovascular System

Once I had brains and a heart also; so having tried them both, I should much rather have a heart.

Tin Man, The Wizard of Oz

WORD PARTS

ang/o	**ahn**-jō	coron/o	**kohr**-ō-nō	necr/o	**neh**-krō	-stasis	**stā**-sihs
angi/o	**ahn**-jē-ō	dis-	dihs	phil/o	**fihl**-ō	sten/o	**stehn**-ō
aort/o	ā-**ohr**-tō	echo-	**ehck**-ō	-philia	**fihl**-ē-ah	steth/o	**stehth**-ō
arter/o	ahr-**tehr**-ō	edem/o	eh-**dē**-mō	phleb/o	**flē**-bō	tachy-	**tahck**-ē
arteri/o	ahr-**tehr**-ē-ō	electr/o	ē-**lehck**-trō	-phobia	**fō**-bē-ah	valvul/o	**vahl**-vū-lō
atri/o	ā-**trē**-ō	-emia	ē-**mē**-ah	pulmon/o	**puhl**-mohn-ō	vas/o	**vahs**-ō
auricul/o	aw-**rihck**-ū-lō	isch/o	**ihs**-kō	rhythm/o	**rihth**-mō	vascul/o	**vahsk**-yoo-lō
brady-	**brā**-dē	mega-	**mehg**-ah	-rrhage	rihdj	ven/o	**vē**-nō
cardi/o	**kahr**-dē-ō	megal/o	**mehg**-ah-lō	-rrhexis	**rehx**-sihs	ventricul/o	vehn-**trih**-kū-lō
-centesis	sehn-**tē**-sihs	my/o	**mī**-ō	scler/o	**sklehr**-ō		

OUTLINE

THE CARDIOVASCULAR SYSTEM

FUNCTION OF THE CARDIOVASCULAR SYSTEM
    External Anatomy of the Heart
    Internal Anatomy of the Heart

ANATOMY OF BLOOD VESSELS

CIRCULATION AND THE HEARTBEAT
    The Cardiac Cycle
    Blood Pressure

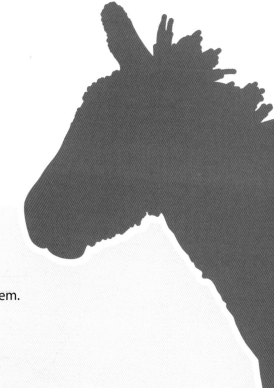

LEARNING OBJECTIVES

When you have completed this chapter, you will be able to:

1 Understand the components and functions of the cardiovascular system.

2 Identify and recognize the meanings of word parts related to the cardiovascular system, using them to build or analyze words.

3 Apply your new knowledge and understanding of clinical veterinary language in the context of medical reports.

CASE STUDY 7-1 **COW RFID TAG #985120008191595**

Signalment and History: A 1675-lb 4-year-old Holstein **cow** with an **acute** history of **brisket edema** was examined at the Frisbee LA Hospital. At the time of evaluation, the cow was 6 months into her **gestation** period. The owner reported that the brisket edema had progressed to **ventral abdominal edema** the day before. The cow was not eating and was listless.

Physical Examination: At the time of examination, Dr. Murdoch noted the following abnormalities: **tachycardia** (100 to 120 bpm), muffled **heart sounds, ventral abdominal and limb edema,** and **jugular vein distention.** The cow had a mild fever (103.5° F). **Electrocardiography** (ECG) revealed **sinus tachycardia. Echocardiography** revealed a large volume of **pericardial fluid** and moderate **bilateral pleural effusion. Right atrium** and **right ventricle** collapse during **diastole** was also detected on echocardiography. The cow was admitted to the hospital.

(See the rest of the story at the end of this chapter.)

THE CARDIOVASCULAR SYSTEM

As you continue to build your prototype animal, you now find that you have a bag of skin being shaped into a familiar animal form by muscles, bones, ligaments, and tendons and having the capability of moving by using its muscles. You pretty much have an animal mannequin made up of gazillions of cells that are hungry, thirsty, and in need of oxygen. But you want a healthy, functioning animal. So what is missing? Well, for one thing, as the Tin Man from *The Wizard of Oz* lamented, "If I only had a heart"—your animal needs a cardiovascular system.

The heart and the blood vessels form the cardiovascular system, which is the transport system for what the cells need. They make sure all living cells in the body receive the substances essential for life.

FUNCTION OF THE CARDIOVASCULAR SYSTEM

Remember myocytes, chondrocytes, dermatocytes, lipocytes, melanocytes, myelocytes, and osteocytes? These and all the other living cells in an animal's body need a blood supply to bring the oxygen and nutrients necessary to fuel cellular metabolism. Blood also is necessary to carry away the waste products of cellular metabolism, which primarily consist of carbon dioxide. This exchange of oxygen for carbon dioxide takes place at the cellular level throughout the body. The exchange of carbon dioxide for oxygen takes place in the lungs.

Take a deep breath and blow it out. That was simple enough. But between those two actions, something amazing happened in your body. You breathed in air rich in oxygen and blew out air rich in carbon dioxide. How did that happen? At the microscopic level in the lungs, the oxygen contained in the air you breathed in was exchanged for the carbon dioxide that was waiting in the blood to be eliminated. This exchange happened across two thin membranes lying next to each other: one lining a microscopic lung sac and one lining a capillary, the smallest blood vessel of the cardiovascular system. The blood then traveled through the heart and on to the cells in the body, where the exchange of oxygen and carbon dioxide was reversed.

For all these exchanges to take place, there has to be a force that moves the blood throughout the body. This force is initially provided by the heart, the pump of the cardiovascular system. It propels blood into the lungs to get oxygenated, and then into the rest of the body to deliver oxygen, pick up and deliver nutrients, and carry away carbon dioxide.

All blood vessels in the body are branches of blood vessels that connect directly to the heart. The nonstriated involuntary smooth muscles that are found in blood vessel walls help direct how and where blood flows in the body by adjusting the size of the vessels. When the blood vessel muscles contract, the vessel diameter gets smaller and less blood flows through, resulting in less blood supply to the cells the vessel supplies.

Blood is constantly flowing or circulating in the blood vessels in a continuous loop through the heart. This is the **cardiovascular system—a closed loop that has** no beginning and no end (Table 7-1). For the sake of this chapter, the heart pumping blood will represent the beginning of the loop (Figure 7-1).

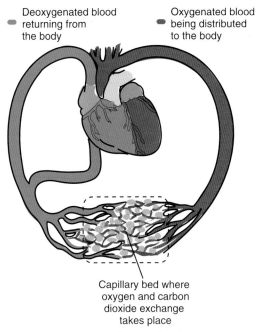

Deoxygenated blood returning from the body

Oxygenated blood being distributed to the body

Capillary bed where oxygen and carbon dioxide exchange takes place

FIGURE 7-1 **The cardiac loop.**

TABLE 7-1   Word Parts for Cardiovascular Anatomy

Word Part	Meaning	Example and Definition	Word Parts	
cardi/o	heart	**acardia** absence of the heart	a- = without, no, not cardi/o = heart -ia = pertaining to	cardi/o
my/o	muscle	**cardiomyopathy** disease affecting the muscles of the heart	cardi/o = heart my/o = muscle -pathy = disease	my/o
auricul/o	auricle of the heart, or the ear flap	**auricular hyperplasia** excessive growth of the auricles	auricul/o = auricle of the heart (or the ear flap) -ar = pertaining to hyper-= above, over, or excess plas/o = growth, development, or formation -ia = pertaining to	auricul/o
		auricular mange an infestation with ear mites	auricul/o = ear flap (or the auricle of the heart) -ar = pertaining to mange = mite-infested skin disease	
vascul/o	blood vessel, tube that conveys or circulates blood	**cardiovascular** pertaining to the heart and to the blood vessels	cardi/o = heart vascul/o = blood vessel, tube that conveys or circulates blood -ar = pertaining to	vascul/o

Continued

TABLE 7-1   Word Parts for Cardiovascular Anatomy—cont'd

Word Part	Meaning	Example and Definition	Word Parts
dis-	apart, away from, separation	**disease** any deviation from or interruption of the normal structure or function of any body part, organ, or system that is manifested by characteristic signs, and whose etiology, pathology, and prognosis may be known or unknown	dis- = apart, away from, separation ease = freedom from pain or discomfort or sickness
atri/o	atrium (upper chamber of the heart) (*plural* = atria)	**atriotomy** surgical incision into the upper chamber of the heart	atri/o = atrium -tomy = surgical incision
ventricul/o	ventricle (lower chamber of the heart)	**atrioventricular** pertaining to the upper and lower chambers of the heart	atri/o = atrium ventricul/o = ventricle -ar = pertaining to
pulmon/o	lung	**pulmonologist** a skilled specialist who has expert knowledge about lung conditions and diseases	pulmon/o = lung log/o = to study, or to have knowledge of -ist = a person or a thing that does something specified
valvul/o	valve	**valvulosis** diseased condition of a valve, especially a valve of the heart	valvul/o = valve -osis = disease or abnormal condition
necr/o	death	**avascular necrosis** death of body tissue because the blood supply has been cut off	a- = without, no, not vascul/o = tubes that convey or circulate fluids -ar = pertaining to necr/o = death -osis= disease or abnormal condition
coron/o	crown	**coronary** pertaining to one of the blood vessels that circle the heart like a crown *To help you remember coron/o, think of the crown you will receive at your coronation!*	coron/o = crown -ar = pertaining to -y = made up of, characterized by
-emia	blood condition (usually abnormal)	**hydremia** disorder in which there is excess fluid (water) in the blood; opposite of dehydration	hydr/o = water -emia = blood condition (usually abnormal)
isch/o	stop, keep back, suppress	**ischemia** inadequate supply of blood to a part of the body; caused by partial or total blockage of an artery *Do not confuse isch/o with ischi/o, the combining form for the ischium bone in the hip.*	isch/o = stop, keep back, suppress -emia = blood condition (usually abnormal)

atri/o

ventricul/o

pulmon/o

valvul/o

necr/o

coron/o

-emia

isch/o

EXERCISE 7-1 *Define It!*

Now that you are able to identify and recognize even more word parts, complete these definitions by writing in the blank the word or words that correspond to the underlined word parts.

1. A hyper<u>emia</u> is an unusually high level of _____Blood_____ in som part of the body.

2. Cardio<u>dynamics is</u> the mechanics of the heart's _____energy_____.

3. Cardio<u>dynia is</u> _____pain_____ in the heart or heart region.

4. <u>Cryocardioplegia</u> is the ~~freezing~~ paralysis of the heart that results

   from hypothermia (or ~~endothermic~~ cold _____)

5. <u>Leuko</u>necrosis is a _____white_____ gangrene.

6. The inside lining of the heart and heart valves

   is _____Inflamation_____ in an endocard<u>itis</u>. this means inflamation

7. The procedure <u>ergo</u>cardiography records

   the _____work_____ activities of heartbeats.

8. A necro<u>meter</u> is an _____measurement_____ of a dead body or any of its parts or organs.

9. Any disease of the _____heart muscle_____ is called a <u>myocardio</u>pathy.

10. <u>Pan</u>carditis is an inflammation of _____all the structures_____ of the heart.

11. <u>Dextro</u>cardia is a birth defect whereby the heart is

    placed _____Right side of body_____

Check your answers at the end of the chapter, Answers to Exercises.

External Anatomy of the Heart

When the heart is in the body, it is enclosed in a multilayered sac called the **pericardial** sac. The outer layer of the pericardial sac is the fibrous layer. It is made up of tough, fibrous connective tissue that does not stretch. It protects the heart. The inner layer of the pericardial sac is the **epicardium,** which lies directly on the heart as a clear membrane. It is more flexible than the fibrous layer. Fluid between these two layers acts as a lubricant as the heart expands and contracts (beats). Figure 7-2 shows the heart on the right with the pericardial sac partially removed on the left. What is most visible is the fibrous layer. The epicardium is still tightly attached to the **myocardium,** the middle and thickest layer of the heart. Myocardium makes up the bulk of the heart.

The heart is sort of heart-shaped. It is wider on the top than the bottom. The wide top of the heart is called the **base** of the heart. The narrower, pointed bottom of the heart is called the **apex** of the heart. If that seems upside down to you, you are not alone.

The heart is usually described as having a right side and a left side. The two sides are further subdivided into chambers: the **atria** (*singular = atrium*) and the **ventricles.** The hearts of mammals and birds have four chambers, and reptile hearts have only three chambers.

Figure 7-3 shows an external view of a preserved sheep heart. The areas labeled "base" and "left and right ventricle" show the cardiac muscle. The **auricles** are the flaps that lay on top of the heart. Anatomists with vivid imaginations thought these external pouches looked like ear flaps (also known as auricles), so naturally they had to call them *auricles*. These outpouching auricles are part of the atria (upper heart chambers) inside the heart.

The area labeled **interventricular groove** (or **sulcus**) is the demarcation line that separates the left and right ventricles (lower heart chambers) of the heart. This groove shows the location of the **interventricular septum** inside the heart. The left ventricle makes up the apex of the heart, is larger, and has a thicker myocardium because it has to propel blood with greater force. The blood from the left ventricle goes to the body. The right ventricle is smaller and has a narrower myocardial layer. Blood from the right ventricle is pumped into the lungs.

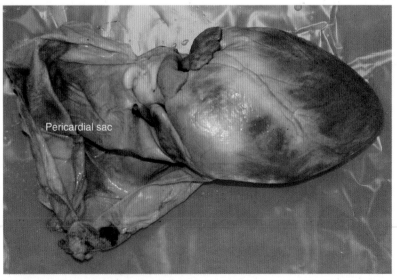

Pericardial sac

FIGURE 7-2 **Heart with pericardial sac removed.** (Adapted from Colville TP: *Clinical Anatomy and Physiology Laboratory Manual for Veterinary Technicians,* ed 2, St Louis, 2009, Mosby.)

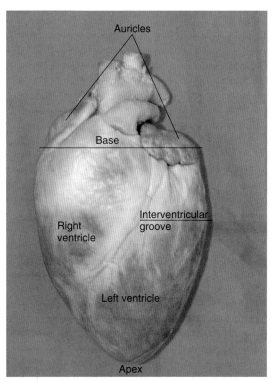

FIGURE 7-3 External view of a sheep heart. (Adapted from Colville TP: *Clinical Anatomy and Physiology Laboratory Manual for Veterinary Technicians,* ed 2, St Louis, 2009, Mosby.)

The big, pipe-looking objects coming out of the top of the heart are arteries. The one in front, the **pulmonary artery,** carries blood to the lungs. The arched one in back, shown with two smaller vessels branching off its top, is the **aorta.** It will eventually branch into all the blood vessels that carry blood to all parts of the body, except to the lungs.

Although they are not labeled in Figure 7-3, **coronary blood vessels** are present in the groove and branching out into the myocardium. These vessels provide the blood supply to the **myocardial cells.** Just like the other cells in the body, myocardial cells need a good blood supply to deliver oxygen and nutrients and to take away waste materials for the individual to remain alive and healthy. Each branch of the coronary artery supplies blood to a specific area of the myocardium. If any branch of the coronary artery becomes *totally plugged* for whatever reason (say a blood clot), the area of myocardium supplied by the artery suffers from a decreased blood supply **(ischemia).** If the ischemia lasts long enough and/or is severe enough, the affected area of myocardium undergoes death **(necrosis)** and becomes a localized area of dead tissue **(infarct).** This is known as a **myocardial infarct.** In humans, this causes a heart attack. **Coronary artery disease** involves a buildup of **plaque** in the lumen of a coronary artery, *decreasing* the blood supply to areas of myocardium. If enough of the myocardium is affected and if the effect is severe enough, the heart can go into **cardiac arrest,** in which case it stops beating and death results if the situation is not corrected.

Internal Anatomy of the Heart

The inside surface of the chambers of the heart is lined by a thin membrane called the **endocardium.** The heart in Figure 7-4 is divided into right and left halves by muscular interventricular and interatrial septa; each half has two chambers. The chambers include:

- right atrium (upper)
- right ventricle (lower)
- left atrium (upper)
- left ventricle (lower)

MYTHBUSTER

Dogs, cats, horses, cattle, and other domestic animals rarely suffer from "heart attacks." If they do suffer myocardial infarcts, it is usually because of a blockage in a coronary artery caused by a blood clot and not because of a buildup of plaque. In humans, the most common cause of heart attacks is a buildup of waxy plaque in coronary arteries.

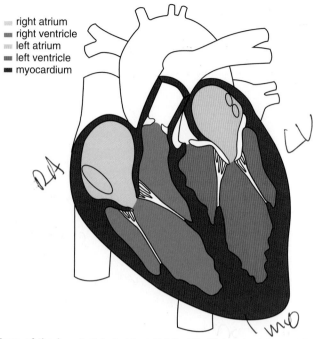

right atrium
right ventricle
left atrium
left ventricle
myocardium

FIGURE 7-4 Chambers of the heart. (Adapted from Colville TP: *Clinical Anatomy and Physiology Laboratory Manual for Veterinary Technicians,* ed 2, St Louis, 2009, Mosby.)

Each heart chamber has an intake opening and an outlet opening that can be opened and closed with a one-way valve. Blood enters the heart through the atria and flows through a healthy heart in one direction only. As blood passes from one chamber to another, a valve snaps shut to prevent the blood from flowing back into the chamber it just left. The four cardiac valves are labeled in Figure 7-5. These valves are listed here:

- right atrioventricular valve (right A-V valve)
  - known as the **tricuspid** valve because it has three flaps or cusps
  - open when the right atrium is contracting to force blood into the right ventricle
  - closed when the right ventricle is contracting
- pulmonary valve
  - known as one of two cardiac **semilunar valves** because its flaps look like half-moons or crescents
  - open when the right ventricle is contracting and is forcing blood into the lungs for oxygenation
  - closed as the right ventricle relaxes and refills
- left atrioventricular valve (left A-V valve)
  - a **bicuspid** valve, also known as the **mitral** valve because it has two flaps that reminded anatomists of a bishop's miter or hat
  - open when the left atrium is contracting and is forcing blood into the left ventricle
  - closed when the left ventricle is contracting
- aortic valve
  - the second cardiac semilunar valve
  - open when the left ventricle is contracting and is forcing blood into the aorta for distribution throughout the body
  - closed as the left ventricle relaxes and refills

Look again at Figure 7-5. You should notice a couple more things. First, all the valves are positioned close to one another. This will be important when you learn to listen to heartbeats. Second, the tricuspid and mitral valves are attached to the walls of their respective ventricles by cord-like bands called *chordae tendineae*. These bands prevent their valves from opening backward and allowing blood to flow back into their respective atria.

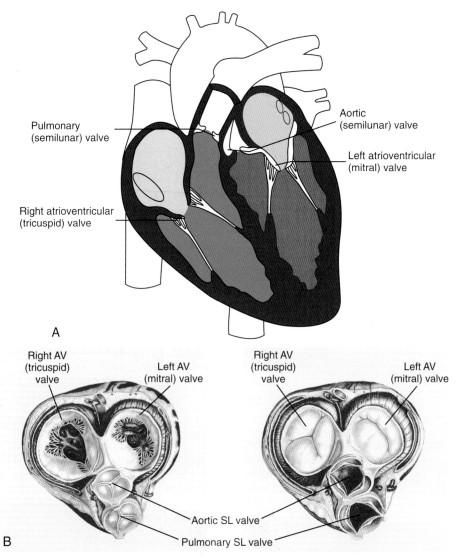

A

B

FIGURE 7-5 Valves in the heart. A, Longitudinal slice through the heart. **B,** Cross section of the heart. AV, Atrioventricular; SL, semilunar. (A adapted from Colville TP: *Clinical Anatomy and Physiology Laboratory Manual for Veterinary Technicians,* ed 2, St Louis, 2009, Mosby; B adapted from Thibodeau D: *Structure and Function of the Body,* ed 14, St Louis, 2012, Mosby.)

EXERCISE 7-2 *Define It!*

Decide whether each of the following statements is True or False. Rewrite to correct the false statements on the lines below.

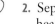
T F   **1.** The buildup of plaque can cause ischemia.

T **F**   **2.** Separate chambers in the heart ensure that blood passes through a healthy heart in one direction only.

T F   **3.** Blood enters the heart through atria and leaves through ventricles.

Relaxed

T F 4. A ventricle is refilling with blood when it contracts. *Blood is returned*

T **F** 5. Blood from the left ventricle is pumped to the lungs.

T F 6. Blood is constantly circulating in the blood vessels in a continuous loop through the heart.

T F 7. Blood travels through the lungs to exchange oxygen in the blood for carbon dioxide in the air. *Oxygen in air*

T F 8. The capillary is the smallest blood vessel in the body.

T **F** 9. Muscles direct how and where blood flows in the body.

T F 10. When you listen to a heartbeat, you are hearing the valves close.

Right ventricle lungs

closed loop

5)

Check your answers at the end of the chapter, Answers to Exercises.

TABLE 7-2	Word Parts Associated with Blood Vessels		
Word Part	**Meaning**	**Example and Definition**	**Word Parts**
ang/o angi/o	vessel, often a blood vessel	**periangitis** inflammation of the outer coat of or the tissues around a blood vessel	peri- = around, surrounding ang/o = vessel, often a blood vessel -itis = inflammation
		hemangioma benign tumor composed of newly formed blood vessels	hem/o = blood angi/o = vessel, often a blood vessel -oma = a tumor or abnormal new growth, a swelling
vas/o	vessel (for blood or other fluids)	**vasodilation** widening of the blood vessels, leading to increased blood flow or reduced blood pressure *A general combining form for a vessel is* angi/o *or* vas/o. *To specifically indicate a blood vessel, use the combining form* vascul/o.	vas/o = vessel (for blood or other fluids) dilation = an enlargement or expansion in bulk, the opposite of contraction
arter/o arteri/o	artery, vessel that carries blood away from the heart	**panarteritis** medium and small arteries that carry blood to the organs of the body become swollen and damaged (inflammation)	pan- = all arter/o = artery -itis = inflammation
		arteriospasm spasm of an artery or arteries *The early Greeks thought that the tubes they discovered in their corpses piped air, not blood. So they named the tubes appropriately. The word artery in Greek roughly translates as "I carry air."*	arteri/o = artery spasm/o = spasm (intermittent involuntary abnormal muscle contractions)

ang/o

angi/o

vas/o

arter/o

arteri/o

TABLE 7-2 Word Parts Associated with Blood Vessels—cont'd

Word Part	Meaning	Example and Definition	Word Parts
aort/o	aorta, the largest artery in the body	**aortectomy** surgical removal of a portion of the largest blood vessel in the body	aort/o = aorta -ectomy = surgical removal
ven/o	vein, vessel that carries blood toward the heart	**intravenous** within a vein or administered by means of a vein, such as an injection	intra- = within, inside ven/o = vein -ous = pertaining to
phleb/o	vein, vessel that carries blood toward the heart	**phlebotomy** surgical incision into a vein— when you stick a needle into a vein to collect a blood sample, you are the phlebotomist performing a phlebotomy Phlebotomy *was thought to be the cure for most diseases of the 18th century. Today, phlebotomy is one of the first procedures performed in disease diagnosis.*	phleb/o = vein -tomy = surgical incision
-stasis	stopping, slowing, or a stable state	**venostasis** slowing or stopping the flow of blood in a vein, as happens when a tourniquet is applied before a phlebotomy or when a vein is "held off"	ven/o = vein -stasis = stopping, slowing, or a stable state
		arteriostasis slowing or stopping the flow of blood in an artery *Prolonged arteriostasis could result in ischemia of the part of the body that gets its blood supply from that artery.*	arteri/o = artery -stasis = stopping, slowing, or a stable state
-rrhexis	to break, rupture	**arteriorrhexis** rupture of an artery	arteri/o = artery -rrhexis = to break, rupture
-rrhage	excessive flow	**hemorrhage** abnormal severe internal or external discharge of blood *Hemorrhage may be from arteries, veins, or capillaries. Venous blood is dark red, and its flow is continuous. Arterial blood is bright red, and it surges in spurts. Capillary blood is reddish, and it oozes from the tissues.*	hem/o = blood -rrhage = excessive flow

aort/o

ven/o

phleb/o

-stasis

-rrhexis

-rrhage

ANATOMY OF BLOOD VESSELS

TRICK QUESTION !

Which vessel in the body carries deoxygenated blood like a vein but carries it away from the heart?

A general term for blood vessel may include the combining form of *angi/o* or *vas/o* or *vascul/o*. However, the specific blood vessels are arteries, arterioles, capillaries, veins, and venules (Table 7-2). If you were a drop of blood circulating in the cardiovascular system loop, the various structures through which you would travel, in order, are as follows:

heart → artery → arteriole → capillary → venule → vein → heart

- heart
  - is the pump of the cardiovascular system
  - blood passes through on its way to the lungs for oxygenation
  - blood passes through on its way to be delivered to the rest of the body
- arteries
  - carry blood away from the heart
  - aorta
    - is the largest artery in an animal's body
    - comes directly off the heart
    - carries oxygenated blood away from the heart
  - pulmonary artery
    - comes directly off the heart
    - carries deoxygenated blood to the lungs only
  - diameters of the arteries get smaller with each branching to become medium and small arteries
- arterioles
  - are branches of small arteries
  - have smaller diameters than arteries
- capillaries
  - have walls that are only one cell thick
  - have smallest diameters of all blood vessels
  - exchange of oxygen and nutrients for carbon dioxide and other waste materials occurs here
- venules
  - are formed from the convergence of capillaries
  - have larger diameters than capillaries but smaller diameters than veins
  - converge to form veins
- veins
  - carry blood back to the heart
  - are formed from convergence of venules
  - have larger diameters than venules
  - converge to form larger veins
  - vena cava
    - largest vein in an animal's body
    - carries deoxygenated blood toward the heart
    - enters directly into the heart
  - pulmonary vein
    - carries oxygenated blood from lungs to the heart
- heart

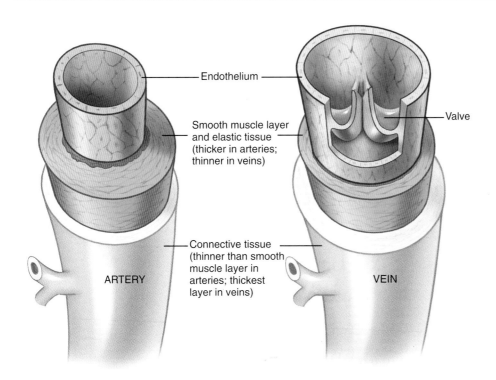

Endothelium

Valve

Smooth muscle layer and elastic tissue (thicker in arteries; thinner in veins)

Connective tissue (thinner than smooth muscle layer in arteries; thickest layer in veins)

ARTERY

VEIN

FIGURE 7-6 Anatomy of arteries and veins. (Adapted from Thibodeau D: *Structure and Function of the Body,* ed 14, St Louis, 2012, Mosby.)

The structure of arteries and veins is similar but not identical. Figure 7-6 shows a comparison of the two kinds of blood vessels. Large arteries closer to the heart have mostly elastic connective tissue in their walls to allow them to expand as blood is propelled through them. This is necessary because of the strength with which blood is forced out of the heart. If the arteries could not expand, they could burst. Veins do not need the same elasticity as large arteries because the blood flowing through them is not under as much pressure.

As the artery size decreases, fewer elastic fibers and more muscle fibers are found in the wall. Smaller arteries and most veins have this smooth muscle layer; it is thicker in arteries. The inner lining of arteries and veins is a thin, smooth membrane called the **endothelium.**

Small and medium veins have bicuspid valves in their lumens that keep blood flowing in one direction only. There is not a lot of blood pressure in veins; so if there were no valves, gravity could pull blood away from the heart, especially blood in veins ventral to the heart.

Arteries are often named for the part of the body to which they carry blood. And because an animal's body is **bilaterally symmetrical,** arteries are most often found in pairs with the same name. For example, the femoral artery supplies blood to the tissues around the femur, but because the animal has a right and a left femur, there has to be a right and a left femoral artery. The same is true for the right and left ovarian artery, which provide blood to the right and left ovaries.

Veins are usually paired with arteries. They are named for the area of the body from which the blood drains. For example, the right and left femoral arteries have companion right and left femoral veins; and the right and left ovarian arteries have companion right and left ovarian veins located in close proximity.

EXERCISE 7-3 *Have Fun with It!*

You could say that a big-hearted person suffers from **cardiomegaly,** a soft-hearted person suffers from **cardiomalacia,** and a person who wears her heart on her sleeve suffers from **extracardiosis.** Have some fun; be creative as you make up some fictional clinical veterinary language for the following heart "situations."

1. heart-sore   Cardialgia

2. heart-sick   Cardiosis

3. heart-broken   Cardiorrhexis

4. stony-hearted   lithocardia

5. heartless   Acardia

6. heartwarming   cardiothermia

7. heart-diseased   Cardioapathy

8. heartbeat   Cardio rhythmia

9. cold-hearted   cryocardia

10. half-hearted   hemicardia

11. burning heart   pyrexocadia

12. wholehearted   pancardia

13. heart-shaped   cardioid

14. hairy-hearted   trichocardia

15. black-hearted   Melanocardia

16. chicken-hearted   Cardiorooster

17. downhearted   catacardiosis

18. purple heart   purpurocardia

19. weak-hearted   cardioparesis

20. small-hearted   Cardiole

21. heart-stopping   Cardiostasis

22. heart-stabbing   cardiotomy

23. hard-hearted   Cardiosclerosis

24. my heart in your hands   metacarpocardia

Check your answers at the end of the chapter, Answers to Exercises.

CASE STUDY 7-2 #2001-45 SPICER

Signalment and History: An 8-year old **M(C)** Boxer named Spicer was brought to the Frisbee Small Animal Clinic because of a history of **chronic** weakness and collapse with associated fainting spells **(syncope)**. A history of coughing and **dyspnea** was described.

Physical Examination: On physical examination, Dr. Frisbee found a mild **tachycardia** of 145 beats per minute with a low-grade **systolic murmur** heard at the left **cardiac apex.** Thoracic X-rays showed marked generalized **cardiomegaly, edema,** and **engorged pulmonary veins.** Electrocardiography (ECG) revealed evidence of left **atrial** enlargement. **Echocardiography** was performed and revealed dilated cardiomyopathy of the left **atrium** and left **ventricle. Mitral** and **tricuspid valve insufficiencies** were noted.

Diagnosis: The diagnosis consisted of left-sided **congestive heart failure (CHF),** **syncope** resulting from severe **ventricular arrhythmias,** and **dilated cardiomyopa-thy.** Dr. Frisbee noted that dilated cardiomyopathy has a low **morbidity rate** but a high **mortality rate,** especially in middle-aged, male, large-breed dogs.

Treatment and Outcome: Appropriate medications were provided to control the con-gestive edema and cardiomyopathy. Over the next couple of weeks, Spicer's condition improved only slightly. After a month of treatment, Spicer's owners elected to have him humanely **euthanized.**

Note: This condition in Boxers is sometimes referred to as **arrhythmogenic right ventricular cardiomyopathy** (ARVC) because of its similarity to the same disease in humans. Boxers can also develop a cardiomyopathy that is characterized by congestive heart failure with frequent **tachyarrhythmias.**

EXERCISE 7-4 *Case It!*

Dilated cardiomyopathy is a disease of the heart muscle that primarily affects the heart's main pumping chamber (left ventricle). The left ventricle becomes enlarged (dilated) and cannot pump blood to the body with as much force as a healthy heart can.

When you have written the medical term to correspond to each definition below, you will know that you understand Spicer's disease as reported in Case Study 7-2.

1. _Cardiomyopathy_ disease of heart muscle

2. _Cardiomegaly_   an enlarged heart

3. _Chronic_   slow onset, or condition that lasts a long time

4. _Ventricle_   one of the lower chambers of the heart

5. _Signalment_   the part of an animal's history that deals with its age, sex, and distinguishing features

6. _mitral_   heart valve between left atrium and left ventricle

7. _insufficiency_   leaking of a heart valve that allows blood to flow in the reverse direction

8. _euthanize_   the practice of intentionally ending a life to relieve pain and suffering

9. _murmur_   extra or unusual sound heard during a heartbeat, sometimes sounding like a whooshing or swishing noise

10. _dyspnea_   difficult or labored breathing; shortness of breath

11. _tachyrhythmia_   a rapid irregular heartbeat

12. _engorged_   swollen with blood, water, or another fluid

13. _echocardiography_ procedure that uses sound waves to create a moving picture of the heart

14. _pulmonary vein_ blood vessels that return blood from the lungs

15. _Atrium_   one of the upper chambers of the heart

16. ~~Atrium~~ _Morbidity_ in many cases, this term is used interchangeably with the following terms: disease, disorder, and illness

17. _edema_ swelling caused by a collection of fluid in the small spaces that surround the body tissues and organs

18. _Syncope_ fainting spells

19. _Congestive heart Failure_ condition in which the heart can no longer pump enough blood to the rest of the body; condition may affect only the right side or only the left side of the heart, but more often both sides of the heart are involved

20. _Necro_ a fatal outcome or, in one word, death

21. _Apex_ the pointed, bottom end of the heart

Check your answers at the end of the chapter, Answers to Exercises.

TABLE 7-3	Word Parts Associated with Cardiac Function		
Word Part	**Meaning**	**Example and Definition**	**Word Parts**
rhythm/o	rhythm, regularly occurring motion	**arrhythmia** abnormal rate of muscle contractions in the heart—the heartbeats may be too slow, too rapid, too irregular, or too early	a- = without, no, not rhythm/o = rhythm, regularly occurring motion -ia = pertaining to
tachy-	fast	**tachyrhythmia** an excessively or abnormally rapid heart rate; tachycardia *Sports cars have a tachymeter (also known as a tachometer) to measure engine speed.*	tachy- = fast rhythm/o = rhythm -ia = pertaining to
brady-	slow	**bradycardia** slow heart rate	brady- = slow cardi/o = heart -ia = pertaining to
electr/o	electricity	**electrocardiograph** instrument for recording electrical activity in the heart	electr/o = electricity cardi/o = heart -graph = instrument used to write or record

rhythm/o

tachy-

brady-

electr/o

TABLE 7-3	Word Parts Associated with Cardiac Function—cont'd		
Word Part	**Meaning**	**Example and Definition**	**Word Parts**
echo-	returned sound	**echocardiogram** image of the heart produced by ultrasound; a test that uses sound waves to create a moving picture of the heart	echo- = returned sound cardi/o = heart -gram = written record produced
steth/o	chest	**stethoscope** instrument to "view" the chest, to listen to thoracic sounds	steth/o = chest -scope = instrument for examining or viewing
sten/o	narrow	**arteriostenosis** abnormal condition of narrowing of the arteries *Think of the steno*grapher*, who writes in shorthand (narrow words).*	arteri/o = artery sten/o = narrow -osis = disease or abnormal condition
mega- megal/o	large or enlarged	**megagnathia** enlargement or elongation of the jaw	mega- = large or enlarged gnath/o = jaw -ia = pertaining to
		cardiomegaly enlargement of the heart *Visualize a cheerleader's mega*phone*, a cone-shaped device used to intensify, amplify, or direct the voice. Or think of a mega*lopolis*, a city of enormous size.*	cardi/o = heart megal/o = large or enlarged -y = made up of, characterized by
scler/o	hard	**arteriosclerosis** various disorders of arteries, particularly hardening due to fibrosis or calcium deposits	arteri/o = artery scler/o = hard -osis = disease or abnormal condition
-centesis	surgical puncture	**pericardiocentesis** procedure of removing fluid from the sac enclosing the heart by puncturing its wall and aspirating	peri- = around, surrounding cardi/o = heart -centesis = surgical puncture
edem/o	swelling	**dactyledema** swelling of a digit, finger, or toe	dactyl/o = digit, finger, toe edem/o = swelling -a = structure, thing
-philia phil/o	loving, or more than normal	**thermophilia** preferring a warm temperature; requiring high temperatures for normal development	therm/o = heat -philia = loving, or more than normal
		ergophilous a special love or desire for working, as in some breeds of dogs and horses *Have you ever heard of the city of Phil*adelphia *referred to as the "City of Brotherly Love"?*	erg/o = work phil/o = loving, or more than normal -ous = pertaining to
-phobia	intense or abnormal fear	**hydrophobia** extreme fear of water; a former name for rabies because hydrophobia is one of the later symptoms of the rabies virus infection	hydr/o = water -phobia = intense or abnormal fear

echo-

steth/o

sten/o

mega-

megal/o

scler/o

-centesis

edem/o

-philia

phil/o

-phobia

CIRCULATION AND THE HEARTBEAT

The circulation of blood in its loop through the body takes place in two parts. **Pulmonary circulation** occurs when deoxygenated blood leaves the heart via the **pulmonary artery,** flows through the lungs for oxygenation, and flows back into the heart via the **pulmonary vein. Systemic circulation** occurs when oxygenated blood leaves the heart via the **aorta,** is distributed throughout the body (except the lungs), where oxygen and other nutrients are exchanged for waste materials (mostly carbon dioxide), and then returns to the heart via the **vena cava.**

The flow of blood through the heart is not as complicated as it may seem at first glance. Figure 7-7 illustrates the two-part path that blood takes as it goes through the heart. It may help you to envision that blood is bright red in color when it is carrying oxygen, and that it takes on a darker, more-bluish cast when it is deoxygenated (and contains more carbon dioxide).

Another way to think of the path of circulation is to think of the shape of a figure eight (Figure 7-8).

Circulation starts with the beating heart that propels blood out of its ventricles when the ventricular walls (myocardium) contract. Sounds simple? It is really quite complicated, but the nice thing about circulation is that an animal does not have to think about it. The heart regulates itself in such a way that different areas of the heart contract in a coordinated rhythm—the heartbeat. In the animal, the heartbeat starts in one place and spreads throughout the heart. That starting place is a group of specialized cardiac muscle cells called the **sinoatrial (S-A) node,** located in the wall of the right atrium.

The Cardiac Cycle

Go back to Figure 7-7 and review the path of blood flow through the heart. At the beginning of one **cardiac cycle,** blood from the body enters the heart into the right atrium and from the lungs into the left atrium. It leaves the heart to circulate through the body out of the left ventricle, and to circulate through the lungs out of the right ventricle (Table 7-3).

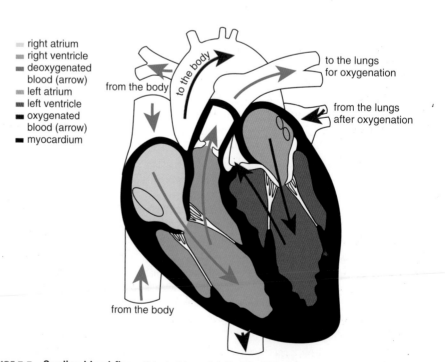

- right atrium
- right ventricle
- deoxygenated blood (arrow)
- left atrium
- left ventricle
- oxygenated blood (arrow)
- myocardium

to the body

from the body

to the lungs for oxygenation

from the lungs after oxygenation

from the body

FIGURE 7-7 **Cardiac blood flow.** (Adapted from Colville TP: *Clinical Anatomy and Physiology Laboratory Manual for Veterinary Technicians,* ed 2, St Louis, 2009, Mosby.)

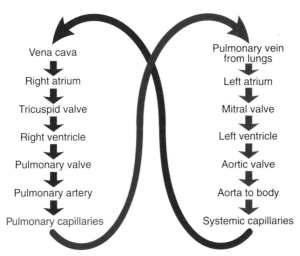

FIGURE 7-8 Schematic of blood circulation.

The S-A node initiates a wave of contractions that travels through the atrial walls causing them to contract at the beginning of the cardiac cycle. As the atria contract, they force blood into their respective ventricles: through the tricuspid (right side) and mitral (left side) valves. When the ventricles are full, the valves snap shut, so blood does not flow back into the atria. Remember the chordae tendineae and their function?

After the wave of contractions has passed through the walls of the atria, the atrial muscles relax and the atria start to fill again. The waves from the walls of the atria are then gathered by the **atrioventricular (A-V) node,** which is another group of specialized cardiac muscle cells that is located in the septum between the atria and the ventricles. The A-V node sends the contraction impulse down the **interventricular septum** to the apex of the heart. The wave of contraction then turns around and spreads up the ventricular walls, causing them to contract from the bottom up, "milking" the blood out through the two semilunar valves into the aorta and the pulmonary artery. When the ventricles are empty, the semilunar valves snap shut to prevent backflow of blood into the ventricles. Then the tricuspid and mitral valves open to allow blood from the atria to enter the ventricles. This completes one cardiac cycle.

The S-A node is the natural pacemaker for the heart. It sends out signals so that the atria and ventricles contract and relax at a coordinated rhythmical rate. This is the animal's heart rate or **pulse rate.** A normal resting heart rate has been established for most animals. If the S-A node is sending signals at a rate normal for an animal, the heart is in **sinus rhythm.** An animal's heart rate will vary throughout the day, depending on its level of activity and the related need for oxygen. **Tachycardia** is a fast heart rate with a normal rhythm. **Bradycardia** is a slow heart rate with a normal rhythm.

Any abnormality in the heart rate or rhythm is an **arrhythmia. Sinus arrhythmia** is a normal mild variation in heart rate associated with breathing in and out. An arrhythmia is detected or measured by *electro*cardiography **(ECG)** with the use of an **electrocardiograph** instrument. Electrocardiography follows electrical impulses as they travel through the myocardium.

The record of the electrocardiography is an **electrocardiogram.** Electrical leads (electrodes) are placed on the external surface of the animal's body at specified locations. When the electrocardiograph is turned on, electrical impulses generated in the heart muscle are picked up at various locations on the body surface and are recorded. A series of heartbeats are followed for a specified period, and they are recorded at a standardized rate on a strip of graph paper moving through the instrument (Figure 7-9).

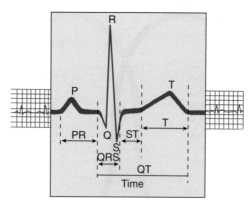

FIGURE 7-9 **The electrocardiogram (ECG) of normal heartbeats.** (From Koeppen BM and Stanton BA: *Berne & Levy Physiology,* ed 6, Philadelphia, 2010, Mosby.)

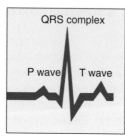

FIGURE 7-10 **One cardiac cycle or heartbeat.** (Adapted from Thibodeau D: *Structure and Function of the Body,* ed 12, St Louis, 2004, Mosby.)

Figure 7-10 is an illustration of the electrical record of one cardiac cycle (or one heartbeat). An explanation of the various components in Figure 7-9 follows:

- P wave
  - measures the time it takes the wave of **contractions** to travel from the S-A node through the atria **(depolarization)**
  - corresponds to the mechanical activity of atrial contractions in a normal animal
- QRS complex
  - measures ventricular **depolarization (contraction)**
  - corresponds to the mechanical activity of ventricular contraction
  - is composed of three different waves
- T wave
  - measures ventricular relaxation (repolarization)
  - corresponds to the time the ventricles are getting ready for the next contraction by refilling with blood from the atria

Another way to evaluate the heart is through **echocardiography** (ECHO or cardiac ultrasound). This procedure uses ultrasound (sound frequencies above the range of human hearing) to bounce sound waves off parts of the heart to watch the heartbeat. It is a **transthoracic** procedure; a probe that emits ultrasound waves is moved over the chest in the area of the heart. This is the same type of procedure that is used to take ultrasound pictures of unborn babies in pregnant mothers.

If you have had the opportunity to listen to a heart through a **stethoscope,** you have heard the sounds that are made when the heart valves snap shut. Even though there are four valves, there are only two sounds. Remember how the four valves are located close to each other? The two A-V valves close at the same time, and just a fraction of a second later, the two semilunar valves also close simultaneously. These sounds are translated into *LUBB-dubb.* The *LUBB* part of the heartbeat, or the first heart sound (S1), is caused by the two A-V valves closing. This means that the ventricles are full and are beginning to contract. The quiet time between the two heart

The letters P, Q, R, S, and T used in an ECG are not abbreviations for actual words but were chosen for their position in the middle of the alphabet.

sounds is known as **systole** and represents ventricular contraction and emptying. When the ventricles are empty, the semilunar valves shut, creating the *dubb* part of the heartbeat, or the second heart sound (S2). Between the *dubb* of one heartbeat and the *LUBB* of the next heartbeat, the ventricles are relaxing and filling with blood again. This time between one heartbeat and the next is known as **diastole.** Simply stated, systole is the working phase of the heart and diastole is the resting phase.

Blood Pressure

When the elastic in the walls of the arteries expands and contracts in response to the heartbeat, the change in diameter is felt as the pulse. Blood pressure is an evaluation of the amount of force exerted by the blood on the walls of the arteries. In dogs and cats, high blood pressure is rarely a primary disease; instead it most often develops secondary to another disease. Blood pressure is difficult to measure in animals, so it is not done on a routine basis.

In dogs and cats, the **central venous pressure (CVP)** can be measured instead of blood pressure. To measure CVP, a catheter attached to a pressure gauge is placed in the jugular vein in the neck and is advanced to the right atrium through the vena cava. The pressure in the right atrium and vena cava raises when the amount of circulating blood coming to the heart increases, or when the amount of blood leaving the heart decreases.

Box 7-1 lists words that are associated with cardiac function but cannot be evaluated by our word analysis method.

BOX 7-1   **Terms That Defy Word Analysis**

- aorta—large artery that directly leaves the heart to deliver blood to the body; largest artery in the body
- ascites—accumulation of fluid in the abdominal cavity; also known as *dropsy*
- auscultate—to evaluate by listening, usually with the aid of a stethoscope
- edema—excess fluid accumulation around the cells of connective tissue
- fibrillation—rapid, irregular myocardial contractions resulting in loss of a simultaneous heartbeat and pulse
- infarct—a localized area of tissue that is dying or dead because of lack of blood supply
- lavage—washing out a hollow organ by rinsing with fluid that is introduced into the organ and suctioned out
- murmur—an atypical heart sound associated with a functional or structural valve abnormality

---

EXERCISE 7-5 *Recall It!*

Repetitive use of terms that defy word analysis will help you commit them to memory. Circle the correct words to complete each definition. You will find some terms here that were introduced in previous chapters.

1. A localized area of tissue that is dying or dead because of lack of blood supply is an (infarct), (inflammation), or (ilium).

2. The large artery that leaves the heart is the (apex), (aorta), or (auricle).

3. An acute involuntary muscle contraction is a (spasm), (septum), or (stenosis).

4. Ascites and dropsy are also referred to as a form of (avian), (edema), or (infarct).

5. You might hear a (murmur), (systole), or (echo) in the quiet time between two heartbeats.

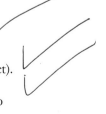

6. To auscultate, you will (examine the PQRST waves), (listen with a stethoscope), or (cull an animal from the herd).

7. Plaque is (what plugs arteries), (a joint dislocation), or (blood leaking from a ruptured blood vessel).

8. To treat palliatively, you would (treat symptoms to effect a cure), (treat symptoms, but not cure the cause), or (prepare the patient for euthanasia).

9. Idiopathic is (a disease of unknown origin) (the worsening severity of a disease), or (the cause of a disease).

10. Chordae tendineae are (part of the vocal cords), (found in the heart), or (cords that attach a muscle to a bone).

Check your answers at the end of the chapter, Answers to Exercises.

EXERCISE 7-6 *Case It!*

Using medical abbreviations can certainly increase your speed in recording the veterinarian's comments about your patient. Rewrite the following sample examination in your own words, without the abbreviations.

Miss Kitty, an M/C K-9, arrived at the Frisbee SA Hospital. His owners insisted that he be seen stat. Miss Kitty was DDN c̄ so many lacerations about his face we thought he was an HBC victim. Miss Kitty's HR was measured at 200 bpm, and he displayed a 105° F FUO. Upon further questioning of the owners, the dx was that Miss Kitty had a run-in with an F/S DLH. IV antibiotics and an overnight stay at the hospital returned Miss Kitty's TPR to normal, and he was released BAR.

_____

_____

_____

_____

_____

_____

_____

_____

_____

_____

_____

Check your answers at the end of the chapter, Answers to Exercises.

BOX 7-2   Cardiovascular System Abnormalities

- **Arteritis** is an inflammation of an artery.
- **Phlebitis** is an inflammation of a vein.
- **Venostasis** is an abnormally slow or completely stopped blood flow through a vein.
- **Insufficiency** is a condition that results when valves do not completely close, allowing some blood to flow back. This also can cause a **murmur.**
- **Stenosis** is an abnormal narrowing of a passageway, a vessel, or a valve.
- **Aortic stenosis** and **mitral stenosis** occur in the heart. The aortic and mitral valves do not open completely and consequently impede the flow of blood through them. Either case would produce a heart murmur.
- **Ventricular fibrillation (Vfib)** is a condition in which there is uncoordinated contraction of the muscle cells of the ventricle. It is a form of arrhythmia. Instead of one smooth contraction to empty the ventricle, the muscles tremble, and normal blood flow through the heart stops. Causes can include electrical shock (puppy chewing an electrical cord), electrolyte imbalance (calcium, potassium), and some poisonings (foxglove [digitalis] plants). This is a life-threatening condition.
- **Atrial fibrillation (Afib)** is a cardiac arrhythmia involving the two atria. It is often seen in older animals and is not as life threatening as ventricular fibrillation.
- **Hypertension** is an increase in arterial blood pressure. The clinical significance of high blood pressure is that it may result in a buildup of fluid in tissue **(edema)** or in the abdominal cavity **(ascites).** In these cases, the fluid leaks out of blood vessels as a result of high pressure in the arteries. Many causes of edema and ascites are known, not just high blood pressure.
- **Congestive heart failure (CHF)** is a condition that results from impaired pumping ability of the heart. The most common complication of CHF is fluid retention. Where the fluid accumulates is dependent on which part of the heart is not pumping adequately.
- **Left-sided CHF** results if the left ventricle does not completely contract, so it does not get rid of all the blood it contains. This prevents it from filling adequately with blood returning from the lungs. The pulmonary veins become distended or **engorged.** Eventually, fluid seeps out of the pulmonary veins because of increased pressure in the veins and collects in the pleural cavity, producing **pulmonary edema** and **pleural effusion.**
- **Right-sided CHF** occurs when the right ventricle does not empty completely. It cannot accept the blood returning from the body, so these veins engorge and lose fluid under increased pressure. Eventually, systemic edema, distended systemic veins, and ascites develop.
- **Effusion** is an abnormal buildup of fluid within a space. It can be **idiopathic** or can result from inflammation, infection, or hemorrhage. Ascites is a specific form of effusion.
- **Pericardial effusion** is a buildup of fluid between the fibrous layer of the pericardial sac and the epicardium. The fluid can be removed by **pericardiocentesis** in a procedure where a needle is inserted into the pericardial sac and the fluid is removed through aspiration with a syringe.
- **Cardiac tamponade** happens when the pericardial sac is so full of fluid that the heart is no longer able to beat. The outer fibrous layer of the pericardial sac is not elastic. As pericardial effusion builds up, the heart becomes unable to fully fill with blood because the heart chambers cannot expand.

TABLE 7-4	Abbreviations	
Abbreviation	**Meaning**	**Example**
bpm	beats (or breaths) per minute	If you see 120 bpm on Rocky's physical exam sheet, you should think heart rate, not breaths, even if he is panting.
HR	heart rate	Dudley's HR is 100 bpm, which is just a little slower than the reference range of 120 to 140 bpm.
CVP	central venous pressure	Instead of Sparky's blood pressure, his CVP was measured.
Afib	atrial fibrillation	Lotus Blossom was diagnosed with three cardiac problems often seen together in dogs: a mitral valve endocardiosis, an enlarged heart, and Afib.
Vfib	ventricular fibrillation	Rosebud chewed through an electrical cord, which caused her heart ventricles to go into uncontrolled and uncoordinated contractions typical of Vfib.
CHF	congestive heart failure	Daisy developed edema in her legs as a result of right-sided CHF.
ECG	electrocardiography, electrocardiograph, and electrocardiogram	To detect a cardiac arrhythmia, Tuliptoes's ECG was recorded immediately after vigorous exercise.
$\bar{c}$ or c $\bar{s}$ or s	with without *Sometimes you will see the letters c and s written without a line above them.*	Sparky will receive antibiotics $\bar{c}$ a painkiller but $\bar{s}$ narcotics.

Here is the completed Case Study 7-1 from the beginning of the chapter.

CASE STUDY 7-1 COW RFID TAG #985120008191595

Signalment and History: A 1675-lb 4-year-old Holstein **cow** with an **acute** history of **brisket edema** was examined at the Frisbee LA Hospital. At the time of evaluation, the cow was 6 months into her **gestation** period. The owner reported that the brisket edema had progressed to **ventral abdominal edema** the day before. The cow was not eating and was listless.

Physical Examination: At the time of examination, Dr. Murdoch noted the following abnormalities: **tachycardia** (100 to 120 bpm), muffled **heart sounds, ventral abdominal and limb edema,** and **jugular vein distention.** The cow had a mild fever (103.5° F). **Electrocardiography** (ECG) revealed **sinus tachycardia. Echocardiography** revealed a large volume of **pericardial fluid** and moderate **bilateral pleural effusion. Right atrium** and **right ventricle** collapse during **diastole** was also detected on echocardiography. The cow was admitted to the hospital.

Diagnosis: Idiopathic cardiac tamponade.

Treatment: Pericardiocentesis was performed through the left fifth **intercostal** space with the use of a **thoracic** catheter. An **ECG** monitor was run during the entire procedure. Two liters of blood-tinged fluid was drained from the pericardial space, and the cow's heart rate immediately decreased to 90 bpm. Pericardial sac **lavage** was performed, after which the drainage tube was sutured in place. The cow was administered antibiotics **SQ q12h.**

Laboratory Findings: **Cytological** evaluation of the **pericardial fluid** showed a **chronic inflammatory effusion** with blood contamination. In addition to normal blood cells, large **binucleate** cells with multiple large nucleoli and deeply **basophilic cytoplasm** were present. At this point, **neoplasia** could not be ruled out. Cytological examination of the **pleural fluid** revealed chronic inflammation with **hemorrhage,** similar to the pericardial fluid, indicating a concurrent **pleuritis.**

Outcome: Overnight, the cow developed a mild **hyperthermia** and was treated with an **anti-inflammatory, analgesic,** and **antipyretic** drug **IV.** Four days after admission, the cow's laboratory results had returned to within the normal reference range. On the seventh day, the cow's **venous** distention and edema were greatly reduced. **Inflammation** at the pericardiocentesis site was treated with **topical** medication. The cow appeared clinically normal with a normal **TPR** and was discharged from the hospital on the eighth day after admission.

Outcome: Follow-up checks confirmed that the cow **calved** successfully this time and once more before being **culled** from the herd years later.

EXERCISE 7-7 *Case It!*

Just by recalling word parts, what you have learned will help you to understand many of the details reported in Case Study 7-1 of the cow with idiopathic pericarditis and cardiac tamponade. The meaning of each underlined word part will help you to complete the sentences. You will have retold the story!

1. idio<u>path</u>ic — This is a case of a ___disease___ of unknown origin.

2. <u>cardi</u>ac — The ___heart___ is the organ involved.

3. <u>peri</u>carditis — The inflammation is found ___around the heart___

4. Holstein <u>cow</u> — This patient is a ___bovine Intact Female___

5. <u>LA</u> Hospital — The patient was seen at a ___large animal___ hospital.

6. <u>ventral abdominal</u> <u>edem</u>a — You would look on the ventral surface of the abdomen for ___a swelling___.

7. <u>tachy</u>cardia — The cow's heartbeat is ___fast___.

8. <u>bpm</u> — The heart rate is measured in ___beats per minute___

9. <u>electro</u>cardiography — One procedure involved ___electricity___.

10. <u>echo</u>cardiography — Another procedure involved ___returned sound___.

11. <u>bi</u><u>later</u>al — The cow's condition appeared on two ___sides___.

12. pericardio<u>centesis</u>   The surgical procedure performed was a
      Surgical puncture

13. inter<u>costal</u>   The surgery was performed between the
      Ribs .

14. <u>thoracic</u>   The body area involved in treatment was the
      thorax .

15. <u>SQ q12h</u>   The antibiotics were administered _subcuy 12 hrs_

16. <u>cyto</u>logical   _Cells_ in the fluid were examined.

17. <u>bi</u>nucleate   The large cells had _two_ nuclei.

18. <u>neo</u>plasia   _New_ growth could not be ruled out.

19. <u>hem</u>orrhage   _blood_ was found in the fluids examined.

20. <u>hyper</u>thermia   The cow's temperature was _high_ .

21. <u>an</u>algesic   The cow received this drug that _without_ pain.

22. anti<u>pyr</u>etic   This drug worked against _pus_ .

23. <u>IV</u>   The antipyretic drug was introduced _within a vein_ .

24. <u>ven</u>ous   When the edema was minimal, _veins_ had returned to normal size.

25. <u>TPR</u>   Before discharge, the tests performed on the cow were
      Temp, pulse, respiration

Check your answers at the end of the chapter, Answers to Exercises.

ANSWERS TO EXERCISES

Exercise 7-1
1. blood
2. force and energy in pumping blood
3. pain
4. paralysis; cold
5. white
6. inflamed
7. work
8. instrument for measuring
9. heart muscle
10. all the structures
11. on the right side of the body

Exercise 7-2
1. T
2. F—Heart valves ensure that blood passes through a healthy heart in one direction only.
3. T
4. F—A ventricle is refilling with blood when it relaxes.
5. F—Blood from the right ventricle is pumped to the lungs.
6. T
7. F—Blood travels through the lungs to exchange the carbon dioxide in the blood for oxygen in the air.
8. T
9. T
10. T

Exercise 7-3
There are no right answers; the following terms are examples.
1. cardialgia
2. cardiosis
3. cardiorrhexis
4. lithocardia
5. acardia
6. cardiothermia
7. cardiopathy
8. cardiorhythmia
9. cryocardia
10. hemicardia
11. pyrexocardia
12. pancardia
13. cardioid
14. trichocardia
15. melanocardia
16. cardiorooster
17. catacardiosis
18. purpurocardia
19. cardioparesis
20. cardiole
21. cardiostasis
22. cardiotomy
23. cardiosclerosis
24. metacarpocardia

Exercise 7-4
1. cardiomyopathy
2. cardiomegaly
3. chronic
4. ventricle
5. signalment
6. mitral
7. insufficiency
8. euthanize
9. murmur
10. dyspnea
11. tachyarrhythmia
12. engorged
13. echocardiography
14. pulmonary veins
15. atrium
16. morbidity
17. edema
18. syncope
19. congestive heart failure
20. mortality
21. apex

Exercise 7-5
1. infarct
2. aorta
3. spasm
4. edema
5. murmur
6. listen with a stethoscope
7. what plugs arteries
8. treat symptoms but do not cure the cause
9. a disease of unknown origin
10. found in the heart

Exercise 7-6
Miss Kitty, a male castrated canine, arrived at the Frisbee Small Animal Hospital. His owners insisted that he be seen immediately (if not sooner). Miss Kitty was dull, depressed, and nonresponsive with so many lacerations about his face that we thought he was hit by a car. Miss Kitty's heart rate was measured at 200 beats per minute, and he displayed a 105° Fahrenheit fever of unknown origin. Upon further questioning of the owners, the differential diagnosis was that Miss Kitty had a run-in with a female spayed domestic longhair cat. Intravenous antibiotics and an overnight stay at the hospital returned Miss Kitty's temperature, pulse, and respiration to normal, and he was released bright, alert, and responsive.

Exercise 7-7

1. disease
2. heart
3. around the heart
4. intact female that can go through pregnancy and give birth
5. large animal
6. a swelling
7. fast
8. beats per minute
9. electricity
10. returned sound
11. sides
12. surgical puncture
13. ribs
14. thorax
15. subcutaneous every 12 hours
16. cells
17. two
18. new
19. blood
20. elevated, above normal
21. takes away (*an-* = without, no, not)
22. pus
23. within a vein
24. veins
25. temperature, pulse, and respiration

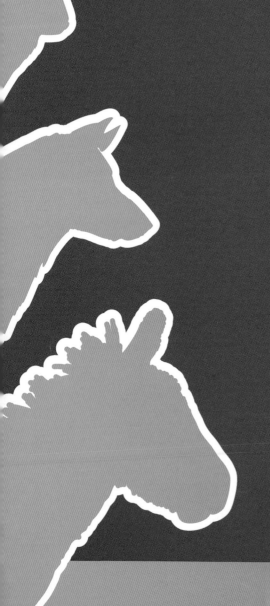

Chapter 8
Blood and Lymph

Real blood is for suckers.

Vampira

WORD PARTS

OUTLINE

LEARNING OBJECTIVES

When you have completed this chapter, you will be able to:

1. Understand the components and functions of blood and lymph.

2. Identify and recognize the meanings of word parts related to blood and lymph, using them to build or analyze words.

3. Apply your new knowledge and understanding of clinical veterinary language in the context of medical reports.

CASE STUDY 8-1 **#2011-2309 BUSTIFER JONES**

Signalment and History: A 6-month-old 2.5-**kg M(C) DSH** cat named Bustifer Jones was brought to the Frisbee **SA** Clinic because of an episode of **hematemesis** (emesis = vomiting) and subsequent **lethargy** that occurred in the morning. Bustifer had appeared healthy before his episode of hematemesis. He was kept indoors or outdoors on a leash. His vaccination status was current. He was being fed a commercial growth diet.

Physical Examination: On examination, Dr. Frisbee confirmed veterinary technician Jess Nelson's initial findings: Bustifer had very pale mucous membranes, a normal heart rate of 120 **bpm**, a weak pulse, a fast respiratory rate of 52 **bpm**, and a low rectal temperature of 96.8° F. No signs of external bleeding, skin **petechiae**, or **ecchymoses** were observed. Other findings of the physical examination were unremarkable.

 Hematology lab results showed a severe **normochromic normocytic** nonregenerative **anemia**, along with a marked **thrombocytopenia. WBC**s were adequate, and a differential count of the WBCs showed that the percentage of each was within the expected reference range. On a stained blood smear, the **erythrocytes**, platelets, and WBCs had normal **morphological** features. Results of serum **biochemical** tests and measures of **coagulation** function were within the expected reference ranges.

 (See the rest of the story at the end of this chapter.)

BLOOD

Without this essential fluid, your prototype animal's body would be like a country that was completely shut off from its supply of food and water, with no means to rid itself of its waste materials, and without oxygen to breathe. That is not compatible with life, and neither is an animal without blood. In Chapter 7, you were introduced to the cardiovascular system, which carries blood. The animal you are building system by system could have a heart and all the arteries and veins it needs, but without blood running through them, the heart and vessels are useless.

Function of Blood

Blood is a fluid connective tissue that travels within the cardiovascular system to all parts of the body. It is capable of multitasking via three general functions:

- transportation
  - Blood acts as a transport system for gases, nutrients, waste products, hormones, blood cells, and platelets. All of these components are essential for life.
- regulation
  - The temperature of blood can affect and can be affected by the temperature of the body.
  - The fluid content of blood can affect the fluid content of tissues outside of the cardiovascular system.
  - Blood helps to regulate body pH (acidity or alkalinity).
- protection
  - Some white blood cells can destroy microorganisms.
  - Some white blood cells are involved with immunity.
  - Blood clots help prevent blood loss.

Composition of Blood

Blood is not colored water. It is a fluid that contains formed elements and dissolved substances (Table 8-1). The formed elements are the blood cells. The fluid portion of blood is **plasma**, in which are dissolved nutrients, hormones, enzymes, proteins,

TABLE 8-1	Word Parts to Describe the Composition and Morphology of Blood		
Word Part	**Meaning**	**Example and Definition**	**Word Parts**
hem/o hemat/o sanguin/o	blood	**electrohemostasis** the stopping of bleeding by means of an electrical device, as in cauterizing	electr/o = electricity hem/o = blood -stasis = stopping, slowing, or a stable state
		hematology the study of the function and diseases of the blood and of blood-forming organs	hemat/o = blood -logy = to study, or to have knowledge of
		exsanguination extensive loss of blood resulting from bleeding	ex- = out, outside, outer, away from sanguin/o = blood -ation = state, condition, action, process, or result
-emia	blood condition (usually abnormal)	**anemia** not a disease itself but a symptom of disease that occurs when the amount of hemoglobin is less than normal	an- = without, no, not -emia = blood condition (usually abnormal)
plasm/o	plasma or related to plasma	**plasmacytoma** any abnormal new growth of plasma cells (plasmocytes)	plasma = plasma cyt/o = cell -oma = a tumor or an abnormal new growth; a swelling
		⚠ A plasmacytoma is a **neoplasm!** The combining form for plasma could be easily confused with the suffix -plasm, *meaning formed material (as of a cell or tissue).*	neo- = new -plasm = formed material (as of a cell or tissue)
		⚠ *Now add to the mix the combining form of* plas/o, *meaning growth, development, or formation. Sometimes you might need to use a word like* **plasmodysplasia.**	plasm/o = plasma dys- = bad, defective, painful, or difficult plas/o = growth, development, or formation -ia = pertaining to
ser/o	serum; the liquid portion of blood after it has clotted and the clot is removed	**serosanguineous** containing or related to both blood and serous fluid (fluid that resembles serum)	ser/o = serum sanguin/o = blood -(e)ous = pertaining to
morph/o	structure, shape	**morphology** (in biology) the study of the form or shape of an organism or its parts	morph/o = structure, shape -logy = to study, or to have knowledge of
-esis	process of an action	**morphogenesis** the biological process that causes an organism to develop its shape	morph/o = structure, shape gen/o = formation or beginning -esis = process of an action

hem/o

hemat/o

sanguin/o

-emia

plasm/o

-plasm

plas/o

ser/o

morph/o

-esis

Continued

cyt/o

-cyte

kary/o

clast/o

-clast

erythr/o

erythemat/o

eosin/o

rubr/o

rubri-

leuk/o

leuc/o

granul/o

		Word Parts to Describe the Composition and Morphology of Blood—cont'd	
Word Part	**Meaning**	**Example and Definition**	**Word Parts**
cyt/o -cyte	cell	**polycythemia** pertaining to a condition involving many cells in the blood	poly- = much or many cyt/o = cell hem/o = blood -ia = pertaining to
		plasmocyte a plasma cell, also known as a plasmacyte	plasm/o = plasma -cyte = cell
kary/o	nucleus	**karyorrhexis** rupture of a nucleus (the nuclear membrane)	kary/o = nucleus -rrhexis = rupture, bursting
clast/o -clast	to break	**karyoclastic** the breaking up of a cell nucleus or its nuclear membrane	kary/o = nucleus clast/o = break into pieces, crush -ic = pertaining to
		chondroclast a cell that breaks down cartilage	chondr/o = cartilage -clast = to break
erythr/o erythemat/o eosin/o rubr/o rubri-	red	**erythrocyte** a red blood cell (RBC)	erythr/o = red -cyte = cell
		erythematous redness of the skin, often a sign of inflammation or infection	erythemat/o = red -ous = pertaining to
		eosinophil a blood cell seen with red granules in its cytoplasm when it is stained and viewed under the microscope	eosin/o = red phil/o = loving, or more than normal
		rubric red; specifically pertaining to the red blood cell nucleus during development	rubr/o = red -ic = pertaining to
		rubricyte an (immature) red blood cell *Rubeola is another name for measles, a disease best known for its typical red rash.*	rubri- = red -cyte = cell
leuk/o leuc/o	white	**leukocyte** a white blood cell (WBC)	leuk/o = white -cyte = cell
		leucocytometer instrument for counting white blood cells *Use of either combining form is acceptable. Words beginning with leuk/o or leuc/o are normally spelled with leuc/o in Britain; in the United States, the leuk/o spelling tends to dominate.*	leuc/o = white cyt/o = cell -meter = measure, a device to measure
granul/o	granule, small grain	**agranulocyte** a type of blood cell that has no colored granules seen in its cytoplasm when it is stained and viewed under the microscope	a- = without, no, not granul/o = granule, small grain -cyte = cell

TABLE 8-1	Word Parts to Describe the Composition and Morphology of Blood—cont'd		
Word Part	**Meaning**	**Example and Definition**	**Word Parts**
phil/o -philia	loving, or more than normal	**hydrophilic** a substance that is water-loving	hydr/o = water phil/o = loving, or more than normal -ic = pertaining to
		hematophilia a hereditary disorder characterized by a strong tendency to bleed; also known as *hemophilia*	hemat/o = blood -philia = loving, or more than normal
baso-	chemically basic (blue)	**basophil** a blood cell seen with blue granules in its cytoplasm when it is stained and viewed under the microscope	baso- = chemically basic (blue) phil/o = loving, or more than normal
neutr/o	neutral	**neutrophil** a blood cell that has both pale red and blue granules visible in its cytoplasm when it is stained and viewed under the microscope—it is neutral!	neutr/o = neutral phil/o = loving, or more than normal
lymph/o	lymph, a transparent fluid that comes from body tissue and is conveyed back to the bloodstream by the lymphatic vessels	**lymphangitis** inflammation of lymph vessels	lymph/o = lymph ang/o = vessel, often a blood vessel, but not this time! -itis = inflammation
immun/o	immunity; immune; inherited, acquired, or induced resistance to infection by pathogens	**immunocyte** a cell involved in immunity; a transformed lymphocyte	immun/o = immunity, immune -cyte = cell
coagul/o	process of clotting	**coagulation** complex process by which blood forms clots	coagul/o- = process of clotting -ation = state, condition, action, process, or result
anti-	against, opposed to	**anticoagulant** an agent that prevents or retards the clotting of blood *Do not confuse this* **anti-** *with the* **ante-** *that means "before, in front of, prior to." Examples of words using* **ante-** *are* anterior, antechamber, *and* antedate.	anti- = against, opposed to coagul/o = process of clotting -ant = a person or a thing that does something specific
thromb/o	thrombus, clot	**thrombectomy** surgical procedure to remove a blood clot still attached to its place of origin within a blood vessel	thromb/o = thrombus -ectomy = surgical removal

phil/o

-philia

baso-

neutr/o

lymph/o

immun/o

coagul/o

anti-

ante-

thromb/o

Continued

fibrin/o

fibr/o

heter/o

is/o

macro-

phag/o

vacu/o

TABLE 8-1	Word Parts to Describe the Composition and Morphology of Blood—cont'd		
Word Part	Meaning	Example and Definition	Word Parts
fibrin/o	fibrin, an insoluble protein that is an essential part of the clotting process	**fibrinolysis** the breakdown of fibrin; the clot-dissolving part of the coagulation process	fibrin/o = fibrin lys/o = destruction, dissolution, dissolving, breakage -is = structure, thing
		⚠ *The combining form* fibrin/o *is not to be confused with* fibr/o *(fiber, which is composed of tissue).*	
		diacutaneous fibrolysis a physical therapy technique in which metallic instruments called "hooks" are used to reposition various connective tissue structures close to the skin (e.g., better positioning of the patella in relationship to the femur)	dia- = across, through cutane/o = skin -ous = pertaining to fibr/o = fiber lys/o = destruction, dissolution, dissolving, breakage -is = structure, thing
heter/o	different, other, unlike	**heterophil** a blood cell in birds and reptiles that is functionally similar to a neutrophil, characterized by granules that have variable sizes and staining characteristics	heter/o = different, other, unlike phil/o = loving, or more than normal
is/o	equal	**anisocytosis** extensive variation in the size of cells that are normally uniform, especially with reference to red blood cells	an- = without is/o = equal cyt/o = cell -osis = disease or abnormal condition
		💡 *Something that is* iso*metric has equal dimensions. When you do your isometric exercises, you use the same muscles on both sides of your body.* **Isotonic saline** *used intravenously has the same osmotic pressure or tension as plasma, so that it will not destroy red blood cells suspended in the plasma.*	is/o = equal ton/o = pressure, tension -ic = pertaining to saline = a solution of salt; when sterile it can be injected intravenously in patients who cannot take fluids orally
macro-	large, enlarged	**macrobiotic** having a long life span; long-lived	macro- = large, enlarged bi/o = life -(t)ic = pertaining to
phag/o	eat	**dysphagia** any difficulty in eating; a sensation of food sticking in the throat; difficulty swallowing	dys- = bad, defective, painful, or difficult phag/o = eat -ia = pertaining to
vacu/o	to empty, emptiness	**vacuole** one of the tiny spaces in cell cytoplasm containing air, water, sap, partially digested food, or other materials	vacu/o = to empty, emptiness -ole = indicating something small

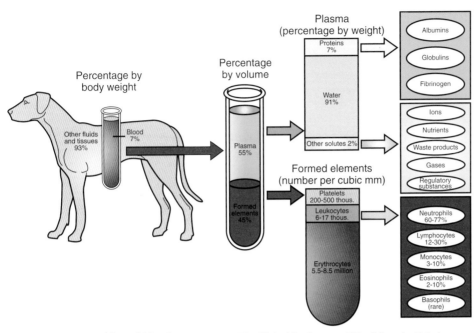

FIGURE 8-1 **Composition of blood.** (From Colville TP: *Clinical Anatomy and Physiology for Veterinary Technicians,* ed 2, St Louis, 2009, Mosby.)

and electrolytes. Because plasma is more than 90% water, if you took all the formed elements out of plasma and tasted it, you would find that it tastes like sea water (Figure 8-1).

"Drawing blood" is a common expression for collecting a blood sample. Veterinarians analyze the results of blood tests to determine changes in the amounts of an assortment of substances in plasma, and in the numbers of the different blood cells. Through these tests, they can study the function of almost every tissue and organ in the body.

When blood is removed from the body and is put into a clean tube, it will thicken and congeal naturally. This thick mass or lump of blood is referred to as a **clot.** After sitting in the tube for a while, the clot will get more compact and will decrease in size, and a clear, yellowish fluid will be left around the clot. This is **serum,** which is plasma with its clotting proteins removed.

Plasma and serum are interchangeable for many laboratory tests. However, if an analysis calls for plasma specifically, you must put a chemical into the blood collection tube to prevent the blood from clotting after it is removed from the body. This chemical is called an **anticoagulant.** If an anticoagulant is added to a blood sample and the sample is centrifuged, the fluid that is left is plasma because the clotting proteins have not been removed. Many different anticoagulants are available. All prevent clotting, but they may use different mechanisms to do so. For example, ethylenediaminetetraacetic acid (EDTA) is a commonly used anticoagulant that prevents clotting by irreversibly binding with the blood calcium necessary for clotting to take place.

Formed Elements

Suspended in plasma are the formed elements, which are the blood cells and platelets. Blood cells are classified into two main categories: red blood cells **(RBCs)** and white blood cells **(WBCs)** (Figure 8-2).

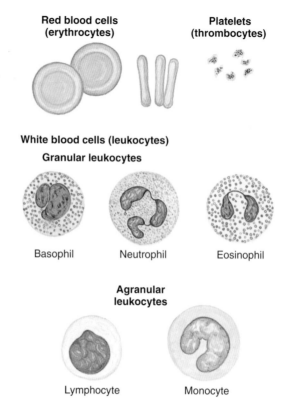

Red blood cells (erythrocytes)

Platelets (thrombocytes)

White blood cells (leukocytes)
Granular leukocytes

Basophil   Neutrophil   Eosinophil

Agranular leukocytes

Lymphocyte   Monocyte

FIGURE 8-2 **The formed elements in blood.** Blood cells as they would appear on a stained blood smear. (From Thibodeau GA, Patton KT: *Anatomy & Physiology,* ed 5, St Louis, 2003, Mosby.)

Red blood cells are also known as **erythrocytes.** They are the smallest and most numerous of the blood cells. The number of erythrocytes in a blood sample is measured as a counted number $\times 10^6$/microliter (μL). For example, the reference range for an RBC count in a cat is 5 to $10 \times 10^6/\mu$L. A mature mammalian red blood cell is **anucleate,** meaning that it does not have a nucleus. In birds and reptiles, the mature red blood cells retain a nucleus.

It is the red blood cell's responsibility to carry oxygen to body tissues. Red blood cells produce the protein **hemoglobin,** to which oxygen directly binds. The erythrocytes must contain their full complement of hemoglobin for them to carry sufficient oxygen to body cells. Iron is one of the essential ingredients of hemoglobin. Insufficient amounts of iron will lead to less hemoglobin being produced and therefore reduced oxygen-carrying capacity of the RBC. Hemoglobin gives blood its red color. If hemoglobin in the RBCs is insufficient, they appear pale when stained and are classified as **hypochromic.** Hemoglobin is measured as grams/deciliter (dL). For example, the reference range for hemoglobin in sheep is 9 to 15 g/dL.

White blood cells are also known as **leukocytes.** Unlike erythrocytes, they do not contain hemoglobin. Leukocytes are grouped into two categories: **granulocytes** and **agranulocytes** (sometimes called *nongranulocytes*). No matter into which category a leukocyte is placed, its function is to provide some form of protection for the animal. The total number of leukocytes in a blood sample is measured as a counted number $\times 10^3$/microliter (μL). For example, the reference range for WBCs in a pig is 11 to $22 \times 10^3/\mu$L.

The granulocytes are **basophils, eosinophils,** and **neutrophils.** All mature granulocytes have granules in their cytoplasm that can be stained and viewed under the microscope. The granulocytes are named for how their granules pick up specific colors using particular hematological stains. Look at Figure 8-2. The basophil contains blue granules, and the eosinophil contains red granules. The neutrophil's granules can stain light blue or light pink, or a combination of both. So to make identification easy, early **hematologists** decided that the neutrophil's granules would be considered neutral. Notice also that the mature granulocytes have nuclei with distinct lobes. Neutrophils are also known as **PMNs** or **polymorphonuclear cells** because their nuclei can take on many shapes and may segment into as many as five distinct lobes. Birds and reptiles have cells called **heterophils** that have the same function as mammalian neutrophils but a different morphology.

The most common granulocyte in animal blood is the neutrophil; in small animals, it is also the most abundant WBC. In **ruminants** (cattle, sheep, goats so named because of characteristics of their digestive system [see Chapter 10]), the neutrophil is also the most abundant *granulocyte*, but it is the lymphocyte (an agranulocyte) that is the most abundant *WBC*. In horses and pigs, the number of neutrophils varies widely in apparently healthy animals. Neutrophils play a major role in an **inflammatory** response. They phagocytize microorganisms, kill them, and spit out debris that may become pus.

Eosinophils are the next most common granulocyte. Their granules contain substances that attack parasites in the body. They also **phagocytize** some products of an immune response. The basophil is the least common granulocyte in a healthy animal. Its granules contain substances that take part in a **hypersensitivity** or allergic reaction.

The agranulocytes, so named because they do not have distinct granules in their cytoplasm, are the **monocytes** and **lymphocytes.** The monocyte is a master of disguise. Its cytoplasm ranges from lightly **basophilic** to deeply basophilic and contains many holes or **vacuoles,** or no vacuoles at all. It also changes its size and nucleus shape depending on its level of activity. Monocytes become **macrophages** when they migrate into body tissues, where they are capable of ingesting particles that are too large for other **phagocytes.** The term *monocyte* literally means "one cell"; however, the definition really refers to the fact that a monocyte nucleus never segments into distinct lobes but remains one continuous nucleus.

Lymphocytes are nice round cells with nice round nuclei and basophilic cytoplasm. Some lymphocytes will be found in circulating blood. However, lymphocytes are the predominant cell found in **lymph,** the clear to white fluid of the **lymphatic system.**

CASE STUDY 8-2 #2007-1459 STARFIRE'S WISH

Signalment and History: A 6-year-old 960-lb mare named Starfire's Wish was brought to the Frisbee **LA** Clinic at the end of May because of an **acute** onset of anorexia and signs of depression and lethargy. She was one of a pair of horses that had been fed wilted red maple leaves picked by the owners 10 days ago. Five days ago, both horses became sick. No other animals were on the property. The horses were offered a large quantity of clippings, but the amount ingested by each horse was unknown.

Physical Examination: At the time of evaluation, Starfire's Wish had a **tachycardia** of 92 **bpm** and an elevated respiratory rate of 20 **bpm.** Her blood was chocolate brown, and she was passing dark red **discolored** urine. Further physical examination findings included pale brown mucous membranes. Abnormalities of the **CBC** showed a marked **hemolysis,** with **packed cell volume (PCV)** of 18% and serum total protein concentration of 5.9 **g/dL.** Other abnormalities of the CBC included **leukocytosis** characterized by absolute **neutrophilia** and **monocytosis.** The RBC evaluation revealed a low hemoglobin concentration and a slight **polychromasia** and moderate **anisocytosis.** Nucleated **RBCs** were observed, and marked denatured hemoglobin Heinz body formation was noticed via staining with new methylene blue stain.

Diagnosis: The **ddx** at this point was nitrate-nitrite **toxicosis,** copper toxicosis, **hypophosphatemia,** or some other toxic insult such as ingestion of onions, canola, kale, or other plants. Initial supportive care included maintenance **IV** fluid therapy.

The following morning, the PCV had fallen to 9%. **Biochemical** analysis of the blood suggested a possible secondary **hemoglobinemic nephropathy.** After further treatment, Starfire's Wish remained moderately **tachycardic** and tachypneic with a marked increase in respiratory effort. A transfusion with 2 units of whole blood was performed. After the transfusion was complete, the PCV had increased to 18%. Starfire's Wish appeared more comfortable, and her vital signs stabilized.

Outcome: Supportive care was continued during the next 5 days. After that period, Starfire's Wish thrived with a daily increase in appetite and activity level. By day 6, the PCV had stabilized at 20%. All other clinical parameters, including the WBC count, had returned to normal reference ranges. Starfire's Wish remained in the hospital as a companion to the other affected horse and was discharged 24 days after admission.

EXERCISE 8-1 *Case It!*

Read Case Study 8-2. Decide whether each of the following statements is True or False. Rewrite to correct the false statements on the lines below.

(T) F   1. The reference range describes the variations of a measurement or value in healthy individuals. It provides a basis from which a set of results for a particular patient can be interpreted.

T **(F)**   2. The mare is a member of the family of murines.

(T) F   3. The monocytosis is diagnosed because of the increase in the number of WBCs with vacuoles in the cytoplasm.

T **(F)**   4. The presence of nucleated RBCs was mentioned in the CBC report because this is one of the normal parameters of a CBC.

T **(F)**   5. Starfire's Wish had an irregular heartbeat.

(T) F   6. <u>Poly</u>chromasia refers to a condition wherein colors in addition to red are found in the RBCs.

(T) F   7. Hemolysis tells you that the mare's blood cells were breaking down.

(T) F   8. Biochemical analysis consists of testing for dissolved nutrients, hormones, enzymes, proteins, and electrolytes found in blood.

T **(F)**   9. One of the combining forms meaning kidney is *nephr/o*, as found in *nephr*opathy. The mare's kidneys were affected by too much hemoglobin being released from the white blood cells.

(T) F   10. The acute onset that prompted the visit to the LA Clinic means that this medical situation developed rapidly.

_____

_____

_____

_____

Check your answers at the end of the chapter, Answers to Exercises.

The Lymphatic System

The exchange of oxygen and carbon dioxide takes place in the capillaries. But because of the high pressure in the circulatory system, water, proteins, and other materials seep out through the capillary walls into the intercellular tissues, where there is less pressure. It is this fluid that bathes and nourishes each cell in the body. If there was no way for the fluid to return to the blood, tissues eventually would become very water-logged and swollen **(edema).** Most of this fluid seeps back through the capillary wall. The rest of the fluid (now called **lymph**) returns to the blood by way of the **lymphatic system.** The lymphatic system is composed of lymph vessels, lymph nodes, and lymph organs (spleen, thymus, tonsils). The lymph vessels are a series of tubes that run closely beside veins. Their function is to pick up excess tissue fluid and return it to the blood. Lymph vessels start small and converge to form larger vessels, until they form one **thoracic duct.** The thoracic duct enters the vena cava in the thoracic cavity near the heart.

Along the way, each lymph vessel passes through a **lymph node** that acts as a biological filter to remove microorganisms and other foreign substances such as viruses and toxins to prevent these particles from traveling around in the body. The lymphatic system also plays a major role in the animal's immune system. Lymphocytes in the lymph node proliferate and transform to produce antibodies in response to foreign substances **(antigens)** in or on the body. An **antibody** (also known as an **immunoglobulin**) is a protein substance produced in the blood or tissues by lymphocytes in response to a particular antigen. A specific antibody is produced to attack each antigen. The antibody destroys and weakens or neutralizes the antigen. This is the basis of immunity in a nutshell.

Lymph nodes that drain a certain area may swell up and become painful. The swelling indicates that macrophages and lymphocytes are busy working to keep the infection from spreading. Such swellings are often called "swollen glands," but it is actually the lymph nodes that are swollen.

Platelets

Another type of formed element found in blood is platelets or **thrombocytes.** They are not complete cells but are pieces of cytoplasm that have broken off from a **megakaryocyte,** a large multinucleated cell, in the red bone marrow. The primary function of platelets is to prevent bleeding. Any break in the endothelium will attract platelets like a magnet. When the platelets arrive at the break, they stick together to form a plug in an attempt to stop the bleeding. Platelets also participate in the **coagulation** (clotting) process by providing some of the initial substances needed to start clot formation. The number of platelets in a blood sample is measured as a counted number $\times 10^5$/microliter. For example, the normal reference range for platelets in a cat is 3 to 7×10^5/μL.

-blast

-poiesis

-penia

norm/o

plur/i

lys/o

-lytic

splen/o

-phobia

TABLE 8-2	Word Parts Associated with Blood Formation and Analysis		
Word Part	**Meaning**	**Example and Definition**	**Word Parts**
-blast	bud, seed, formative cell	**hematoblast** a primitive blood cell	hemat/o = blood -blast = bud, seed, formative cell
-poiesis	making, producing	**hematopoiesis** the formation of blood or blood cells in the living body; also called **hematogenesis** *Spelling tip! It is easy to forget the first i in -poiesis because it is not distinctly pronounced. If you look at a keyboard, you will notice that the p, o, and i are all placed in a row. If you remember to use all three keys in order, you will not forget the i.*	hemat/o = blood -poiesis = making, producing hemat/o = blood gen/o = formation or beginning -esis = process of an action
-penia	lack, deficiency	**leukopenia** abnormally low number of white blood cells in the circulating blood	leuk/o = white -penia = lack, deficiency
norm/o	normal	**normocytic** a descriptive term applied to a red blood cell of normal size	norm/o = normal cyt/o = cell -ic = pertaining to
plur/i	several, more than one	**pluripotent** referring to a cell that has the capacity to develop into various tissues and organs of the body *A plural number is a quantity of more than one.*	plur/i = several, more than one potent = powerful, or able to do something
lys/o -lytic	destruction, dissolution, dissolving, breakage	**hemolysis** the destruction or dissolution of red blood cell membranes, with release of hemoglobin	hem/o = blood lys/o = destruction, dissolution, dissolving, breakage -is = structure, thing
		cellulolytic the destruction or dissolution of cells	cellul/o = cell -lytic = destruction, dissolution, dissolving, breakage
splen/o	spleen	**splenomyelomalacia** pathologic softening of the spleen and bone marrow	splen/o = spleen myel/o = bone marrow malac/o = soft, softening -ia = pertaining to
-phobia	intense or abnormal fear	**hippopotomonstro- sesquipedaliophobia** fear of long words (similar to some clinical veterinary words?)	hippopot/o = large monstr/o = monstrous sesquipedali/o = long word -phobia = intense or abnormal fear

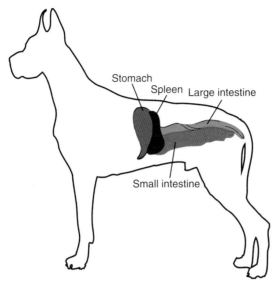

FIGURE 8-3 The location of the spleen in relation to the stomach and intestines.

BLOOD FORMATION AND ANALYSIS

Most blood cells, with the exception of some lymphocytes, are produced and mature in red bone marrow. (Lymph nodes can act as maturation centers for some lymphocytes that migrated to them from the bone marrow.) All blood cells that are produced in the bone marrow are formed from one undeveloped **pluripotent** stem cell that can mature into any of the blood cells, depending on what type of stimulus it receives from the body. The process of making blood cells is **hematopoiesis.** If the pluripotent stem cell is stimulated to make red blood cells, it goes through the stages of **erythropoiesis.** The same is true for **leukopoiesis** concerning production of all white blood cells. If you want to specify the production of a specific white blood cell, you use the cell's name (e.g., **lymphopoiesis**).

When you are studying hematology, you will find when you know the word parts that the stages of development of the blood cells follow a logical pattern. For example, the stages of development of a neutrophil are as follows:

pluripotent stem cell → myelo**blast** → **pro**myelocyte → **myelo**cyte →
metamyelocyte → band cell → mature neutrophil

Look at the highlighted word parts. By deconstructing the words, you can recognize that (1) the myeloblast is an immature bone marrow cell; (2) the promyelocyte is the bone marrow cell stage before it develops into the myelocyte (literally, the bone marrow cell stage); and (3) the metamyelocyte is the stage right after the myelocyte stage. See how it all makes sense?

Erythropoiesis can also take place in the spleen if the bone marrow cannot keep up with the body's need for red blood cells. This may happen when the animal is losing blood, or when blood is being destroyed at a rapid rate. The **spleen** is a large, tongue-shaped organ found on the left side of the abdominal cavity near the stomach (Figure 8-3). In addition to hematopoiesis, the spleen has other hematological functions:
- storage of blood
  - The spleen contains sinuses where it stores blood. Think of a sponge soaking up liquid and being squeezed to push out the liquid. When the body needs blood, muscles in the spleen contract and squeeze out the blood. In racing animals, the spleen contracts when a sudden burst of energy requires a sudden large increased demand for oxygen. The red blood cells produced and stored in the spleen provide the extra transportation needed to carry the increased amount of oxygen.

- filtering of foreign materials
  - The spleen contains numerous macrophages that clean the blood of foreign materials as the blood passes through the spleen or is stored there. The macrophages line the sinuses where the blood is stored.
- removal of dead and dying red blood cells
  - All blood cells have a finite life span. They go from an immature cell to a mature cell, to an old cell, and to a dead cell. When red blood cells get old, they become functionally less effective and need to be retired. The splenic macrophages will remove these dead and dying red blood cells, as well as any abnormal red blood cells. The red blood cells are hemolyzed by the macrophages. Some of the proteins and iron molecules are recycled to make new red blood cells.
- participation in the immune response
  - The spleen contains localized areas of lymphoid tissue, called *white pulp*, which contain many lymphocytes. During an immune response, the lymphocytes in the white pulp can clone themselves and take part in the immune response.

Animals can live without their spleens. A splenectomy may be performed if the spleen has a large rupture, if a hemangiosarcoma is present, or if the spleen is necrotic. The red bone marrow will then take over the hematopoietic duties of the spleen. Tissue macrophages and monocytes will fill in for lost phagocytic functions, and other lymphoid tissues will take over for the white pulp.

CASE STUDY 8-3 #2008-3024 CHASE

Signalment and History: Chase, a 9-year-old F(S) Golden Retriever, was examined at the Frisbee SA Clinic because of weakness, depression, mild weight loss, and on-again, off-again **pyrexia**. The **signs** had been getting progressively worse for the past 2 weeks. Chase had bouts of diarrhea and one seizure during that period. Chase was admitted to the hospital.

Physical Examination: Chase was depressed and was mildly **ataxic** when she was brought into the examination room. Jess reported to Dr. Frisbee that Chase currently was **pyrexic** with a fever of 104.5° F, was panting, and had tachycardia, and her mucous membranes were a pale yellow. Chase also had an extended **abdomen**. On palpation, Dr. Frisbee felt fluid in the **abdominal cavity,** so she performed an **abdominocentesis.** A total of 200 **mL** of clear orange fluid was removed. Palpating the abdomen again, Dr. Frisbee felt an enlarged spleen. Chase was prepped for an abdominal **ultrasound,** which showed numerous diffuse, irregular structures in the spleen. Dr. Frisbee did a **bx** of some of the structures and sent the material to the lab for analysis. Blood for a CBC was drawn.

The CBC results showed a **pancytopenia.** Histological results of the spleen bx showed both **extramedullary hematopoiesis** and areas of **infarct** and **necrosis.** With a pancytopenia present, Dr. Frisbee decided that the next course of action would be a bone marrow bx. The material from the bone marrow of the **ilial crest** was analyzed and showed **hypercellularity** caused by the presence of numerous **macrophages** that had **phagocytized** mature blood cells and their precursor cells.

Diagnosis and Treatment: At this point, Dr. Frisbee had a **ddx** of immune-mediated **hemolytic anemia, neoplasm,** massive infection, or **hemophagocytic** syndrome. Tests were run that eliminated immune disease, neoplasm, and infection. A diagnosis of **idiopathic** hemophagocytic syndrome was reached. The prognosis for Chase's survival was poor. An IV blood transfusion and palliative therapy were begun.

Outcome: Despite the best efforts of the entire veterinary team over the next 24 hours, Chase died. The owners did not want a **necropsy** performed and took Chase to the local pet cemetery to be cremated.

EXERCISE 8-2 *Case It!*

Read Case Study 8-3. Circle the correct word or phrase that makes each statement true.

1. Idiopathic refers to a disease that (has an unknown cause), (is passed from animals to humans), or (affects the lymphatic system).

2. Cytopenia is a general term for an abnormally (increased number of abnormal cells), (increased number of cells), or (decreased number of cells).

3. Bone marrow was aspirated from the (breastbone), (hip), or (spleen).

4. Chase was ataxic. She was (uncoordinated), (dehydrated), or (feverish).

5. Within hypercellular bone marrow, you will find (an abnormally low number of cells), (an abnormally high number of cells), or (abnormally overactive cells).

6. A macrophage was a (monocyte), (neutrophil), or (red blood cell) before it migrated into the body tissues.

7. The term for a localized area of dead tissue is (infarct), (ataxia), or (necropsy).

8. A mL is a unit of (length), (volume), or (weight).

9. The abbreviation bx means (blood cell), (bilateral examination), or (biopsy).

10. The clinical veterinary word for production of red blood cells is (erythro-trichia), (catabiosis), or (hematopoiesis).

Check your answers at the end of the chapter, Answers to Exercises.

The words listed in Box 8-1 are words pertaining to blood and the cardiovascular system. These words cannot be evaluated using the word analysis method.

BOX 8-1 **Terms That Defy Word Analysis**

- embolism—abnormal material circulating in blood that could become lodged in a vessel and block blood flow; could be composed of a blood clot, parasites, fat, gas bubbles, or clumps of bacteria
- globin—protein; the protein portion of hemoglobin and myoglobin
- globulin—a class of simple proteins that are insoluble in water
- goblin—a mischievous, malicious wandering sprite; an elf
- lethargic—drowsy, dull, listless, unenergetic
- occlude—to close off or shut
  - You will occlude a vein before you draw a blood sample from it.
  - When you close your mouth, you often also occlude your teeth.
- pH—potential hydrogen; a scale from 0 to 14 that measures the acidity or alkalinity of a substance
  - acidic—a pH less than 7
  - alkaline—a pH greater than 7
  - neutral—a pH of 7
- thrombus—a blood clot that forms and adheres to the wall of a blood vessel at its site of formation (it becomes an embolus when it breaks away from the endothelium and circulates in blood)

EXERCISE 8-3 *Recall It!*

Repetitive use of terms that defy word analysis will help you commit them to memory. Write a word or a group of words in each blank to complete the following statements. You will find some terms here that were introduced in previous chapters.

1. A thrombus becomes an ___embolus___ when it breaks away and begins to circulate in the blood.

2. To ___ausculate___ is to listen to internal sounds in the body, usually with the aid of a stethoscope.

3. An ___immunoglobulin___ is a protein that takes part in the immune response.

4. To be drowsy, dull, listless, and unenergetic is to be ___lethargic___.

5. The M DSH parent of his offspring is called a ___sire___.

6. An acute tendon injury that occurs where the tendon is forcibly torn is called an ___avulsion___.

7. A detailed description that includes distinctive features of an animal is the ___signalment___.

8. The rounded proximal end of a bone that is also the end nearest the muscle origin is called the ___head___.

9. A topical substance is applied on the ___surface of the body___

10. Rigor mortis is a temporary stiffening of ___muscles after death___ resulting from lack of energy to allow the muscles to relax.

Check your answers at the end of the chapter, Answers to Exercises.

BLOOD DISORDERS

The analysis of a blood sample can be revealing. Not only can you identify abnormalities in all portions of the sample, but these abnormalities in turn can indicate the presence of other disease conditions somewhere else in the body. When analyzing blood cells, you will be most interested in their total numbers and the **morphology** of cell populations or individual cells. Many of the blood disorders commonly seen in veterinary medicine are named using word parts you already know. With red blood cells used as an example, these are some of the conditions that may develop:

- **anemia** = literally means "without blood"

For veterinary medical purposes, *anemia* means that a decreased number of red blood cells are available, or that the existing red blood cells do not contain enough hemoglobin to carry sufficient oxygen to the body. Once anemia has been diagnosed, it is classified by how the red blood cells appear when they are spread on a microscope slide, stained, and analyzed under the microscope:

  - **normocytic** anemia—red blood cells present appear normal in size
  - **hypochromic** anemia—red blood cells present are not staining as intensely as normal red blood cells
  - **macrocytic** anemia—red blood cells present are larger than normal; usually indicates immature red blood cells
  - **microcytic** anemia—red blood cells present are smaller than normal; may indicate lack of iron, which is necessary to make hemoglobin
  - **hemolytic** anemia—cell membranes of red blood cells are being ruptured; ruptured membranes may be observed on the stained blood smear
- **polychromasia**—pertaining to more than one color

In this condition, the red blood cells pick up both a red and a blue stain, resulting in a purple or lavender color of the cytoplasm. This usually indicates immaturity.

When white blood cells are analyzed, some of the conditions that may be seen to develop are:

- **leukemia**—literally means "white blood"

This term indicates that an overabundance of abnormal white blood cells is present in the blood sample, but it does not specify which white blood cell is responsible. Leukemia is blood cell cancer, an uncontrolled overproduction of one cell type. Leukemia is classified on the basis of the cell type involved, as determined from a stained blood smear or a bone marrow biopsy. For example, **acute lymphoblastic leukemia** is a leukemia of sudden onset that involves very immature lymphocytes.

- **leukocytosis**—disease or abnormal condition of more than the normal number of white blood cells in the blood

This term does not specify which cell is at fault. Leukocytosis is seen as a result of some other abnormal condition in the body (e.g., inflammation) and does not involve uncontrolled proliferation of a specific cell (leukemia). Analysis of a stained blood smear will reveal the cell involved.

- **neutropenia**—an abnormally low number of neutrophils in the blood
- **eosinophilia**—an abnormally high number of eosinophils in the blood
- **monocytosis**—an abnormally high number of monocytes in the blood
- **pancytopenia**—an abnormally low number of all blood cells

EXERCISE 8-4 *Blood!*

Fill in the squares by combining the various word parts and defining the terms related to blood and analysis of a blood sample. **Hydremia** is done as an example.

Structure or Disorder	Word Parts	Definition
hydremia	hydr/o -emia	an abnormally large amount of water in the blood
1. Neutropenia	neutr/o -penia	low number of neutropenias in blood
2. leyoto cytosis	leuk/o cyt/o -osis	Disease of too many blood cells
3. anerythro plasia	an- erythr/o plas/o -ia	No formation of new blood cells condition
4. Basophil	bas/o phil/o	Blood cell with Blue granules stained
5. hemato poresis	hemat/o -poiesis	making blood cells
6. hemo cytometer	hem/o cyt/o -meter	Instrum counting Blood cells
7. thrombo lysis	thromb/o -lysis	Destruction of blood clot
8. leukemia	leuk/o -emia	white blood acrobundn of white blood cells
9. Macrocyte	macro- -cyte	Abnormally large cell
10. leuko cytoid	leuk/o cyt/o -oid	Resembling white blood cell
11. thrombo cytosis	thromb/o cyt/o -osis	Disease of abnormally increased number of platelets.
12. exsanguination	ex- sanguin/o -ation	Condition massive loss of blood

Structure or Disorder	Word Parts	Definition
13. *monocyte*	mono- -cyte	A white blood
14. *hemato phobia*	hemat/o -phobia	Abnormal fear of sight of blood
15. *lympho blast*	lymph/o -blast	formative lymph cell

Check your answers at the end of the chapter, Answers to Exercises.

TABLE 8-3	Abbreviations	
Abbreviation	**Meaning**	**Example**
CBC	complete blood count, analysis of all of the cellular components of a sample of blood	Licorice's CBC revealed a previously undiagnosed anemia.
WBC	white blood cell	All WBCs provide some form of protection for the animal.
PMN	polymorphonuclear	Neutrophils are also called PMNs because their nuclei can take on many shapes. The monocyte nucleus also can take on many shapes, but it is not classified as a PMN.
diff	differential white blood cell count	The diff includes the percentage of each WBC per 100 total WBCs counted on a stained blood smear.
TNTC	too numerous to count	In some cases of leukemia, the number of WBCs on a blood smear is TNTC.
RBC	red blood cell	The size of a normal RBC varies with the species. Goats have the smallest RBCs. Dogs have the largest RBCs.
TP	total protein	Total protein measures two proteins in serum: globulin and albumin.
Hb Hgb	hemoglobin	Licorice's Hgb (Hb) value was low because he was anemic.
Hct	hematocrit	The Hct is a measure of the percent of red blood cells in a volume of blood. It is calculated by an automated hematology instrument.
PCV	packed cell volume	The PCV also measures the percent of RBCs in a volume of blood. It is measured on a blood sample that has been centrifuged.
EDTA	ethylenediamine-tetraacetic acid	The anticoagulant of choice for collecting blood samples for a CBC is EDTA.

CBC WBC PMN diff TNTC RBC TP Hb *or* Hgb Hct PCV EDTA

CASE STUDY 8-1   #2011-2309 BUSTIFER JONES

Signalment and History: A 6-month-old 2.5-**kg M(C) DSH** cat named Bustifer Jones was brought to the Frisbee **SA** Clinic because of an episode of **hematemesis** (emesis = vomiting) and subsequent **lethargy** that occurred in the morning. Bustifer had appeared healthy before his episode of hematemesis. He was kept indoors or outdoors on a leash. His vaccination status was current. He was being fed a commercial growth diet.

Physical Examination: On examination, Dr. Frisbee confirmed veterinary technician Jess Nelson's initial findings: Bustifer had very pale mucous membranes, a normal heart rate of 120 **bpm,** a weak pulse, a fast respiratory rate of 52 **bpm,** and a low rectal temperature of 96.8° F. No signs of external bleeding, skin **petechiae,** or **ecchymoses** were observed. Other findings of the physical examination were unremarkable.

    Hematology lab results showed a severe **normochromic normocytic** nonregenerative **anemia,** along with a marked **thrombocytopenia. WBCs** were adequate, and a differential count of the WBCs showed that the percentage of each was within the expected reference range. On a stained blood smear, the **erythrocytes,** platelets, and WBCs had normal **morphological** features. Results of serum **biochemical** tests and measures of **coagulation** function were within the expected reference ranges.

Treatment and Outcome: Bustifer was immediately put into an oxygen cage to boost his oxygen intake. Blood typing and major cross matching with the clinic donor cat were performed to permit immediate transfusion of fresh whole blood (25 **mL** [4 **mL/kg/qh**]). After transfusion, Bustifer's clinical **signs** improved. **Thoracic** radiography and **abdominal ultrasonography** were performed. Even though Bustifer had an episode of hematemesis, gastric bleeding was considered an improbable cause for the severe anemia. The gastric bleeding was thought to be a consequence of severe thrombocytopenia and only a potential contributing factor to anemia. **Chronic** causes of anemia were thus more likely, and important **ddx** were infectious causes or a primary bone marrow disorder. The severe thrombocytopenia was suspected to be secondary to the same condition that caused anemia.

    A bone marrow **bx** specimen was collected. **Cytological** examination revealed massive **hypercellularity** attributable to a large number of small **lymphocytes** with normal morphological features. An adequate number of intermediate-sized lymphocytes and **lymphoblasts** with normal cytological features were observed. After scanning of multiple stained bone marrow bx slides, no **megakaryocytes** and only rare **erythroblasts** were found. More mature cell stages were absent, suggesting arrested development in both **erythrocyte** and **thrombocyte** cell lines. **Dysplastic** changes were not evident in the **myeloid** precursors. Disorders of the bone marrow including **myelodysplasia, fibrosis,** and **necrosis** were ruled out cytologically.

    Because other causes were excluded, an immune-mediated disease was suspected, and treatment was begun and lasted 10 days. At that time, on the basis of results of blood analyses, the initial treatment was not effective for improving the **hematological** disorder. Human **immunoglobulins** were then administered **IV** at a dose of 1.21 **g/kg** over 6 hours without signs of adverse effects.

    After 3 additional days, erythrocyte and thrombocyte counts had improved. Examination of a second bone marrow bx showed normal numbers of erythroblasts and small lymphocytes. The number of megakaryocytes was adequate. An increase in young cells (i.e., **megakaryoblasts**) relative to the mature stage was observed. Erythrocyte and thrombocyte counts returned to normal reference ranges 40 days after the initial **diagnosis.** Treatment was slowly tapered over 5 months to reach 1.5 mg/kg **q48h.** This dosage was administered for 8 weeks. At 38 weeks from diagnosis, Bustifer was still in good health, and the hematological disorder seemed to be controlled.

EXERCISE 8-5 *Case It!*

Several words used in Case Study 8-1 are highlighted with bold type. With practice, most words should be getting easier to dissect to comprehend their definitions. Match the words listed in the right column to their definitions.

1. _Thrombocyte_ platelet

2. _bpm_ beats per minute or breaths per minute

3. _hematemesis_ vomiting blood

4. _q 48h_ every 2 days

5. _hypercellularity_ abnormally large increase in number of cells

6. _megakaryoblast_ primitive cell with more than one nucleus

7. _myelodysplasia_ defective growth or development of bone marrow

8. _coagulation_ process of clotting of blood

9. _fibrosis_ disease or abnormal condition of fibers

10. _Necrosis_ death of body tissue

11. _lymphocyte_ predominant cell found in lymph

12. _petechiae_ tiny ecchymoses

13. _erythrocyte_ a red blood cell

14. _normochromic_ normal color

15. _cytological_ refers to the study or knowledge of cells

16. _immunoglobulins_ antibodies

bpm	
coagulation	
~~cytological~~	
erythrocyte	
fibrosis	
~~hematemesis~~	
hypercellularity	
~~immunoglobulins~~	
lymphocyte	
~~megakaryoblast~~	
~~myelodysplasia~~	
~~necrosis~~	
normochromic	
petechiae	
q48h	
~~thrombocyte~~	

Check your answers at the end of the chapter, Answers to Exercises.

SWERS TO EXERCISES

Exercise 8-1

1. T
2. F—The mare is a member of the family of equines.
3. T
4. F—Mention of the presence of nucleated RBCs was included in the CBC report because this is not an expected occurrence.
5. F—Starfire's Wish had a fast heart rate.
6. T
7. T
8. T
9. F—The mare's kidneys were affected by too much hemoglobin being released from the red blood cells.
10. T

Exercise 8-2

1. has an unknown cause
2. decreased number of cells
3. hip
4. uncoordinated
5. an abnormally high number of cells
6. monocyte
7. infarct
8. volume
9. biopsy
10. hematopoiesis

Exercise 8-3

1. embolus
2. auscultate
3. immunoglobulin
4. lethargic
5. sire
6. avulsion
7. signalment
8. head
9. surface of the body
10. muscles after death

Exercise 8-4

1. neutropenia = abnormally low number of neutrophils in the blood
2. leukocytosis = disease or abnormal condition of too many white blood cells
3. anerythroplasia = condition where there is no formation of red blood cells
4. basophil = a blood cell seen with blue granules in its cytoplasm when it is stained and viewed under the microscope
5. hematopoiesis = formation of blood cells in the body
6. hemocytometer = instrument for counting blood cells
7. thrombolysis = destruction of a blood clot
8. leukemia = "white blood"; an overabundance of white blood cells in blood
9. macrocyte = abnormally large cell
10. leukocytoid = resembling a white blood cell
11. thrombocytosis = disease or abnormally increased number of platelets
12. exsanguination = condition in which a massive loss of blood occurs
13. monocyte = a white blood cell with only one (unsegmented) nucleus
14. hematophobia = abnormal fear of the sight of blood
15. lymphoblast = formative lymph cell

Exercise 8-5

1. thrombocyte
2. bpm
3. hematemesis
4. q48h
5. hypercellularity
6. megakaryoblast
7. myelodysplasia
8. coagulation
9. fibrosis
10. necrosis
11. lymphocyte
12. petechiae
13. erythrocyte
14. normochromic
15. cytological
16. immunoglobulins

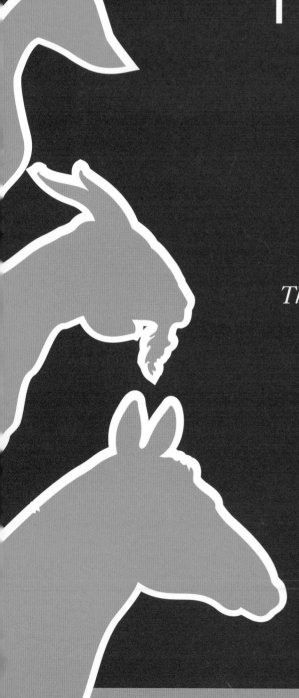

Chapter 9

The Respiratory System

The clever cat eats cheese and breathes down rat holes with baited breath.

W.C. Fields

WORD PARTS

aer/o	**ehr**-rō	hal/o	**hah**-lō	ox/o	**ohck**-sō	rhin/o	
alveol/o	ahl-**vē**-ō-lō	home/o	**hō**-mē-ō	pharyng/o	fah-**rihng**-gō	spir/o	
atel/o	aht-**ehl**-ō	iatr/o	**ī**-aht-rō	pleur/o	**ploor**-ō	spirat/o	
bronch/o	**brohng**-kō	laryng/o	lah-**rihng**-gō	pne/o	**nē**-ō *or* pah-**nē**-ō	-staxis	**stahck**-sihs
capn/o	**kahp**-nō	mediastin/o	mē-dē-ah-**stī**-nō	-pnea	pah-**nē**-ah	trache/o	**trā**-kē-ō
dynam/o	**dī**-nah-mō	muc/o	**myoo**-kō	pneum/o	**nū**-mō	tuss/o	**tuhs**-sō
-ectasis	**ehck**-tah-sihs	nas/o	**nā**-zō	pneumon/o	**nū**-mohn-ō	vestibul/o	veh-**stihb**-ū-lō
glott/o	**gloh**-tō	olfact/o	ohl-**fahck**-tō	re-	rē		

OUTLINE

THE RESPIRATORY SYSTEM

FUNCTION OF THE RESPIRATORY SYSTEM

ANATOMY OF THE RESPIRATORY SYSTEM
    Upper Respiratory System
    Lower Respiratory System

LUNGS

RESPIRATION

LEARNING OBJECTIVES

When you have completed this chapter, you will be able to:

1 Understand the components and functions of the respiratory system.

2 Identify and recognize the meanings of word parts related to respiration, using them to build or analyze words.

3 Apply your new knowledge and understanding of clinical veterinary language in the context of medical reports.

CASE STUDY 9-1 #1997-1488 FOOLISH RISK

Signalment and History: A 3-year-old Thoroughbred **gelding** named Foolish Risk was brought to the Frisbee LA Clinic because of an **acute** cough and **pyrexia** of 24 hours' duration. Two days ago, he had returned from a show where he had been stabled for 2 days. The owner had started treatment with an **antibiotic** injection (2.2 **mg/kg IM q12h**) as instructed over the phone by Dr. Murdoch and had administered an NSAID (nonsteroidal **anti-inflammatory** drug) (2.2 mg/kg **PO** once), but the pyrexia remained.

Physical Examination and Diagnosis: Foolish Risk was examined by Dr. Murdoch and veterinary technician, Pat Grouper, approximately 24 hours after the onset of clinical **signs.** At this time, Foolish Risk was **lethargic** but responsive and had pitting **edema** of the prepuce and **thoracic** and **pelvic** limbs. He had profuse **bilateral** blood-tinged seromucoid **nasal** discharge and a deep cough. There was **hyperemia** of the gingival mucous membranes, with numerous **petechiae.** Respiratory rate (44 **bpm**) and effort were increased, as were rectal temperature (103.5° F) and heart rate (64 **bpm**). **Auscultation** of the **thorax** revealed harsh respiratory sounds; cardiac rhythm was normal. Blood was collected for a **CBC.** A **nasal** swab specimen was collected and was sent to the lab along with the blood sample. **Petechiation** of the oral mucous membranes in conjunction with pitting edema of the prepuce and limbs was considered suggestive of **vasculitis.** IV antibiotics and anti-inflammatory drugs were started. Leg wraps were applied to help control the edema.

(See the rest of the story at the end of this chapter.)

THE RESPIRATORY SYSTEM

Your prototype animal is developing nicely. It now has a transport system (the cardiovascular system) to move blood around. It has blood to carry oxygen, nutrients, and waste materials. So now it needs to acquire oxygen and discard carbon dioxide. Animal bodies do not have the capability to exchange all the necessary oxygen and carbon dioxide on the surface area of their skin. That job now becomes the responsibility of the respiratory system—an internal surface through which this exchange of oxygen and carbon dioxide can readily take place. But that is not the only job of the respiratory system. Here is another system that is great at multitasking.

TABLE 9-1	Word Parts Associated with Respiratory System Functions		
Word Part	**Meaning**	**Example and Definition**	**Word Parts**
spir/o spirat/o	breathing	**spirograph** an instrument for measuring and recording breathing movements *Do not confuse this* spir/o *with another* spir/o, *which means a coil or a spiral. A* Spirograph® *is a geometric drawing toy that produces intricate mathematical curves.*	spir/o = breathing -graph = instrument used to write or record
		inspiration the act of breathing air into the lungs	in- = in, within, inward, into, not spirat/o = breathing -ion = state, condition, action, process, or result

spir/o

spirat/o

TABLE 9-1	Word Parts Associated with Respiratory System Functions—cont'd		
Word Part	**Meaning**	**Example and Definition**	**Word Parts**
re-	again, back	**respirator** a device for giving artificial breathing or to assist in breathing (to help breathe again—and again)	re- = again spirat/o = breathing -or = a person or a thing that does something specified
		review to look back on, like to study for a final exam	re- = back view = look
home/o	similar	**homeostasis** staying the same or remaining stable	home/o = similar -stasis = stopping, slowing, or a stable state
hal/o	breathing	**exhalation** the process of breathing out	ex- = out, outside, outer, away from hal/o = breathing -ation = state, condition, action, process, or result
		inhalant something, usually medicinal, that is inhaled	in- = in, within, inward, into, not hal/o = breathing -ant = a person who, things which
		Look for hal/o *in* hal*itosis, offensive and foul-smelling breath—an "abnormal condition" that you do not want to encounter often.*	
ox/o	oxygen, O_2	**hypoxia** a pathological condition in which the body, or a portion of it, is deprived of oxygen	hyp(o)- = under, beneath, below ox/o = oxygen -ia = pertaining to
capn/o	carbon dioxide, CO_2	**hypercapnia** an increased amount of carbon dioxide in the blood	hyper- = above, over, or excess capn/o = carbon dioxide -ia = pertaining to
olfact/o	smell	**olfaction** pertaining to the sense of smell	olfact/o = smell -ion = state, condition, action, process, or result
aer/o	air, gas	**aerobic** requiring air (oxygen) to live *An* aer*ial sticks up in the air to receive radio signals. You use an* aer*osol bomb to kill insects. And you strengthen your lungs by doing your* aer*obic exercises!*	aer/o = air, gas bi/o = life -ic = pertaining to
dynam/o	force, energy	**dynamogenesis** the generation of power, force, or energy, especially muscular or nervous energy	dynam/o = force, energy gen/o = formation or beginning -esis = process of an action

re-

home/o

hal/o

ox/o

capn/o

olfact/o

aer/o

dynam/o

EXERCISE 9-1 Analyze It!

This exercise will give you a chance to dissect "new-to-you" clinical veterinary language containing word parts introduced in this chapter. Complete the definitions by writing in the blank the word or words that correspond to the underlined word parts.

1. An<u>aer</u>obic describes any organism that does not require _____oxygen_____ for growth.

2. <u>In</u>halation is the act of breathing _____within or_____.

3. A <u>retr</u>actor is a surgical instrument by which the edges of a surgical incision or underlying organs can be held _____apart_____.

4. <u>Spiro</u>graphy is a method of measuring _____breathing_____ movements and capacity.

5. <u>Hyper</u>oxia is a condition characterized by _____more_____ levels of oxygen in the blood and tissues.

6. Hypo<u>capn</u>ia is a condition in which the level of _____carbon dioxide_____ in the blood is lower than normal.

7. <u>Neuro</u>dynamics has to do with energy from _____nerves_____.

8. An<u>ox</u>ia is a lack of _____oxygen_____.

9. <u>Re</u><u>sten</u>osis usually refers to an artery or other large blood vessel that has become _____, received treatment, and subsequently become _____ again.

10. <u>Olfacto</u>logy is the study of the sense of _____smell_____.

Check your answers at the end of the chapter, Answers to Exercises.

Inspiration and inhalation are used interchangeably. The same goes for expiration and exhalation.

FUNCTION OF THE RESPIRATORY SYSTEM

The function of the respiratory system is **respiration** (Table 9-1). However, respiration is more than just **inspiration** and **expiration**. Through **inhalation** and **exhalation,** the following functions are accomplished:

- air distribution
  - The airways in the lungs are responsible for distributing inhaled air to the small air sacs where gas exchange takes place.
- gas exchange
  - The body's cells require oxygen to run the cellular machinery.
  - This is a **dynamic** process that produces **energy** so the cell can use the nutrients that it requires to function.
  - The body also needs to get rid of the waste carbon dioxide that is produced during energy production.
  - external respiration
    - Air that an animal inhales contains **oxygen** that is absorbed by blood in the lungs.
    - Oxygenated blood will carry the oxygen throughout the body.

- Carbon dioxide in blood returning to the lungs is diffused back to the air.
  - internal respiration
    - At the cellular level in the body, the oxygen is exchanged for the waste carbon dioxide.
    - This is cellular gas exchange and is not considered part of the respiratory system.
- air modification
  - An animal does not inhale pure, warm air.
  - Passing through the respiratory tract, the inhaled air is filtered, warmed, and humidified.
- body temperature regulation
  - This helps prevent hyperthermia and hypothermia.
  - Most animals, except the horse, do not sweat through their skin or feet sufficiently to cool their overheated bodies. They have to rely on respiration, specifically, panting. As the animal pants, fluid from the lining of the respiratory passages (and mouth) evaporates. Evaporation cools the blood circulating just beneath the epithelium. The cool blood then continues to circulate through the body, cooling the body as it goes.
  - In very cold weather, these same superficial blood vessels warm the cold air as it passes down the respiratory tract. The warmed air does not cool the blood, so the blood does not cool the body.
- acid-base balance
  - Keeping the body at the right balance of acidity and alkalinity (pH) is crucial to an animal's **homeostasis.**
  - Carbon dioxide in the blood acts as an acidifier. If too much carbon dioxide is present in the blood, the animal's blood will become too acidic and the pH will fall beneath the safety zone.
  - In healthy animals, the amount of carbon dioxide in blood is controlled by how much is taken in and blown out, and how fast respiration takes place.
  - Normally, an animal's blood is kept slightly alkaline with a pH of around 7.4. If the pH goes below 7.35 or above 7.45, the animal's health is in danger.
- voice production
  - The **vocal cords** or **vocal folds** are two fibrous connective tissue bands attached to cartilage in the voice box (larynx).
  - The cords vibrate when exhaled air passes over them. The vibrations produce sound.
- olfaction
  - Many animals rely on their **olfactory** sense for survival.
  - As in humans, the smell receptors for olfaction are located in the nasal passages.

> Horses cannot breathe through the mouth, so they are not able to pant to cool their body temperature. Do you suppose that this is why they can sweat so profusely?

TABLE 9-2	Word Parts Associated with Respiratory System Anatomy		
Word Part	**Meaning**	**Example and Definition**	**Word Parts**
nas/o rhin/o	nose	**nasology** a scientific study of the nose, done by a nasologist	nas/o = nose -logy = to study, or to have knowledge of
		rhinoplasty surgical repair of the nose *A rhinoceros has a nose you can hardly forget, with a horn growing out of it. If you had a nose like a rhinoceros, you would need rhinoplasty.*	rhin/o = nose -plasty = surgical repair

nas/o

rhin/o

Continued

	TABLE 9-2	Word Parts Associated with Respiratory System Anatomy—cont'd		
	Word Part	**Meaning**	**Example and Definition**	**Word Parts**
pharyng/o	pharyng/o	pharynx, throat	**pharyngostomy** surgical creation of a new permanent opening in the pharynx; can be used to insert a tube for feeding *Many people want to call a pharynx the "fairnix." Note that the spelling is **not** phar**nyx**.*	pharyng/o = pharynx, throat -stomy = surgical creation of a new permanent opening
laryng/o	laryng/o	larynx, voice box	**laryngospasm** an uncontrolled/involuntary muscular contraction of the vocal cords that temporarily interrupts breathing; sometimes referred to as "the throat closes up" *Many people want to call a larynx the "lairnix." Note that the spelling is **not** lar**nyx**.*	laryng/o = larynx, voice box -spasm = intermittent involuntary abnormal muscle contraction
glott/o	glott/o	glottis; the vocal cords and the space between them	**glottitis** inflammation of the glottis portion of the larynx *Laryngitis would be a more general term for glottitis.*	glott/o = glottis -itis = inflammation
vestibul/o	vestibul/o	entrance, cavity, or channel that is an entrance to another cavity	**vestibular** pertaining to the entrance to a canal in the nose, mouth, larynx, ear, vagina, etc. *You are familiar with the vestibule that is a lobby, entrance hall, or passage between the entrance and the interior of a building. It is the same thing for the body.*	vestibul/o = entrance, cavity, or channel that is an entrance to another cavity -ar = pertaining to
trache/o	trache/o	trachea, windpipe	**tracheotomy** a surgical procedure performed in emergency situations when air cannot get to the lungs; a surgical incision into the trachea	trache/o = trachea, windpipe -tomy = surgical incision
			Tracheostomy *is sometimes used interchangeably with tracheotomy. Strictly speaking, tracheostomy usually refers to the permanent opening itself, but a tracheotomy is the initial incision into the trachea.*	trache/o = trachea, windpipe -stomy = surgical creation of a new permanent opening
bronch/o	bronch/o	bronchus, a branch from the trachea (*plural =* bronchi)	**bronchospasm** an uncontrolled/involuntary muscular contraction of the smooth muscle of the bronchi, as that which occurs in asthma	bronch/o = bronchus, a branch from the trachea -spasm = intermittent involuntary abnormal muscle contraction

TABLE 9-2	Word Parts Associated with Respiratory System Anatomy—cont'd		
Word Part	**Meaning**	**Example and Definition**	**Word Parts**
alveol/o	alveolus, air sac, small sac or cavity (*plural* = alveoli)	**alveolar dysplasia** pertaining to the abnormal development of the air sacs of the lung	alveol/o = alveolus, air sac, small sac or cavity -ar = pertaining to dys- = bad, defective, painful, difficult plas/o = growth, development, or formation -ia = pertaining to
pleur/o	pleura; thin membrane with two layers that lines the chest cavity and covers the lungs	**pleurisy** *or* **pleuritis** inflammation of the membrane that lines the chest and covers the lungs; condition leads to chest pain when an animal takes a breath or coughs	pleur/o = pleura -itis = inflammation
pne/o -pnea	breath or respiration	**pneopneic** breathing	pne/o = breath or respiration pne/o = breath or respiration -ic = pertaining to
		apnea absence of breathing *When a word begins with the letters* pne, *the "p" is silent; but when* pne *occurs later in a word, the "p" is pronounced. So the above words would be pronounced* nē-ō-pah-nē-ihk *and* ahp-nē-ah.	a- = without, no, not -pnea = breath or respiration
pneum/o	air, and sometimes the lung	**pneumothorax** a collection of air in the chest from a wound or tear in the lung itself, or it may result from a **thoracoplasty** that introduced air to collapse a lung to let it rest and heal faster	pneum/o = air, and sometimes the lung thorax = thorax thorac/o = thorax -plasty = surgical repair
		pneumocentesis surgical puncture of the lung	pneum/o = air, and sometimes the lung -centesis = surgical puncture
pneumon/o	lung	**pneumonoultramicroscopic-silicovolcanoconiosis** disease or abnormal condition of the lung; an obscure term sometimes cited as one of the longest words in the English language, referring to a disease of the lungs caused by the inhalation of very fine silica dust, and occurring especially in the lungs of miners—"miner's lung disease"	pneumon/o = lung ultra- = beyond, excess, on the other side of micr/o = small, very small scop/o = examine, view -ic = pertaining to silic/o = silicate or quartz volcan/o = fire, burn coni/o = dust -osis = disease or abnormal condition *Now, was that so hard? But can you pronounce it?*

Continued

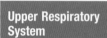

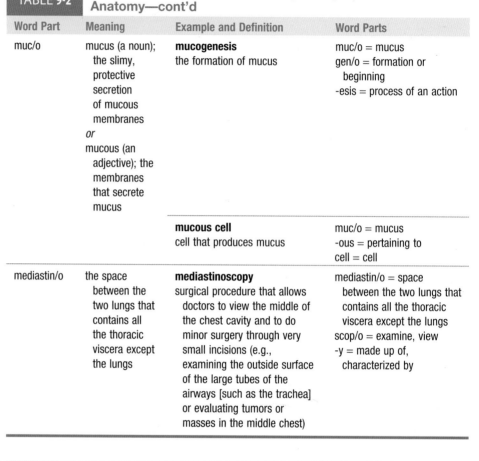

TABLE 9-2	Word Parts Associated with Respiratory System Anatomy—cont'd		
Word Part	**Meaning**	**Example and Definition**	**Word Parts**
muc/o	mucus (a noun); the slimy, protective secretion of mucous membranes *or* mucous (an adjective); the membranes that secrete mucus	**mucogenesis** the formation of mucus	muc/o = mucus gen/o = formation or beginning -esis = process of an action
		mucous cell cell that produces mucus	muc/o = mucus -ous = pertaining to cell = cell
mediastin/o	the space between the two lungs that contains all the thoracic viscera except the lungs	**mediastinoscopy** surgical procedure that allows doctors to view the middle of the chest cavity and to do minor surgery through very small incisions (e.g., examining the outside surface of the large tubes of the airways [such as the trachea] or evaluating tumors or masses in the middle chest)	mediastin/o = space between the two lungs that contains all the thoracic viscera except the lungs scop/o = examine, view -y = made up of, characterized by

ANATOMY OF THE RESPIRATORY SYSTEM

The structures of the respiratory system belong to the upper or the lower respiratory system, depending on their location in the body (Table 9-2).

Upper Respiratory System

The upper respiratory system includes the following respiratory structures: nostrils, nasal passages and sinuses, pharynx, larynx, and trachea (Figure 9-1).
- nostrils
  - These are the two external openings of the nose.
  - They are also called **nares** (*singular* = naris or nare).
  - They are the first respiratory system structures through which inspired air passes on its way to the lungs.
- nasal passages
  - They begin at the nostrils.
  - One extends back from each nostril, separated by a **nasal septum.** (Remember the interventricular septum in the heart? It separates the right and left ventricles. The nasal septum does the same thing, only in the nose; it separates the right and left nasal passages.)
  - Protruding into the lumen of the nasal passages are **nasal turbinates.** These thin, scrolled bones are covered with nasal epithelium and superficial blood vessels. The purpose of the turbinates is to increase the surface area of the nasal passages so more area is available to warm air and catch debris as the air passes through.
  - The epithelium of the nasal passages is a **ciliated mucous membrane** (Figure 9-2). The mucous cells in the epithelium produce **mucus,** which

Upper Respiratory System

nostrils
nasal passages
sinuses
pharynx
larynx
trachea

BOX 9-1   Terms That Defy Word Analysis

- agonal breathing, or agonal breaths—pertains to the last breaths taken near or at death, or after cardiac arrest; breathing is gasping and labored
- asthma—a chronic disease that often causes bronchoconstriction, making breathing difficult; sometimes caused by an allergic response
- cilia (*singular* = cilium)—small, hair-like structures on the surface of the epithelium that beat rhythmically; originates from the Latin word for "eyelash" (This must be related to batting one's eyelashes.)
- cough—reflex stimulated by irritation or foreign matter in the trachea or bronchi
- diaphragm—a thin, dome-shaped sheet of muscle that separates the thorax from the abdomen; also called the *midriff* in humans
- emphysema—overexpansion of alveolar walls causing the walls to break down and block other airways, resulting in less oxygen/carbon dioxide exchange in the lungs
- friable—crumbly, easily crumbled
- furcation—divided, branched
- hiccups—spasms of the diaphragm accompanied by sudden closing of the glottis; may be caused by nerve irritation, indigestion, or central nervous system damage; most often temporary and harmless
- paranasal sinus—a hollow cavity in the skull connected to the nasal passages; usually just called a *sinus*
- sigh—a deep breath through the nose that usually is taken in response to a slightly low blood oxygen level or a slightly high blood carbon dioxide level
- sinus—a cavity, recess, or passage in any organ or tissue
- sneeze—similar to a cough, but the irritation is in the nasal passages
- turbinate—scroll-shaped bone on the wall of a nasal passage; also known as a *nasal concha* (shell-shaped)
- ventilate/ventilator—breathing in and out, or a machine that artificially moves air into and out of the lungs
- yawn—a slow, deep breath taken through the wide open mouth; can be caused by mildly low blood oxygen levels, fatigue, boredom, or drowsiness

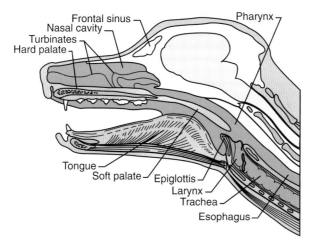

FIGURE 9-1 **Longitudinal section of canine upper respiratory tract.** (From Colville TP: *Clinical Anatomy and Physiology for Veterinary Technicians,* ed 2, St Louis, 2009, Mosby.)

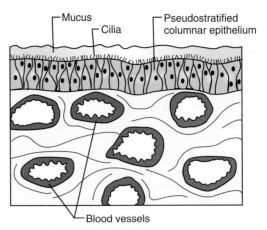

FIGURE 9-2 **Lining of nasal cavity.** Note cilia protruding up into overlying mucous layer and numerous large blood vessels immediately below the epithelium. (From Colville TP: *Clinical Anatomy and Physiology for Veterinary Technicians,* ed 2, St Louis, 2009, Mosby.)

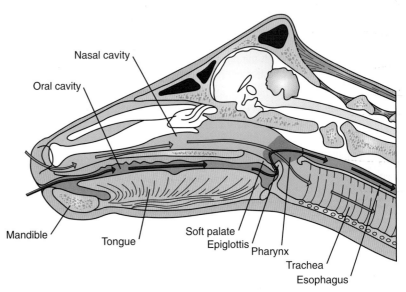

FIGURE 9-3 **The upper respiratory tract of a cow.** The blue arrows follow the path of air that is breathed in through the nostrils. The red arrows follow the route of food after it is taken into the mouth. Note that at the pharynx, the two paths cross. (From Colville TP: *Clinical Anatomy and Physiology Laboratory Manual for Veterinary Technicians*, St Louis, 2009, Mosby.)

captures foreign materials such as bacteria, insects, dust, and pollen. The **cilia** on the epithelium beat rhythmically to move the contaminated mucus to the throat, where it is swallowed.

- **paranasal sinuses** (usually just called *sinuses*)
  - These are the pouches of the nasal passages that fit into spaces inside the skull.
  - Most animals have four (two pairs of) sinuses. Some animals, including humans, have two additional sinuses.
  - The epithelial mucous membranes lining the sinuses produce mucus that is carried into the nasal passages by the action of the cilia on the epithelium. This action prevents debris caught on the mucus from clogging the sinuses and possibly the nasal passages.
- pharynx
  - This is the throat (Figure 9-3).
  - Both the respiratory system and the digestive system use this passageway.

- At the caudal end of the pharynx, the opening into the larynx lies ventrally and the opening into the esophagus (of the digestive system) lies dorsally. If you think about the position of the nose and the mouth in animals, you realize that the nose is dorsal to the mouth. This means that in the pharynx, the two systems cross over and invert their relationship to each other. Have you ever choked when your food went "down the wrong tube"?

- larynx
  - This is the voice box.
  - The larynx connects the pharynx to the trachea.
  - The opening into the larynx is the **glottis.**
  - Instead of one solid structure, the larynx is made up of segments of cartilage held together by muscles. The most rostral of these cartilages is the triangle-shaped flap called the **epiglottis.** It can cover the glottis when an animal swallows, thereby acting as the traffic director for the trachea and the esophagus. When an animal is taking a breath, the epiglottis is in its normal open position, allowing air to enter the glottis. Of course, nothing is ever as simple as it sounds. The entire process is a finely tuned reflex action, which sometimes does not work perfectly, and choking results.
  - The larynx also prevents foreign material from entering the trachea and the lower respiratory tract by means of the action of the epiglottis.
  - **Vocal cords,** or **vocal folds,** in the larynx are responsible for voice production. Two vocal cords act as a sort of curtain that closes over the laryngeal lumen. When exhaled air passes between the cords, they vibrate much like a string when it is plucked to produce a sound. The muscles attached to the cartilage that hold the vocal cords can adjust the tension of the vocal cords and affect the pitch of the sound.

- trachea
  - This is the windpipe, the end of the upper respiratory system.
  - It runs from the larynx, down the neck, and into the thoracic cavity, where it **bifurcates** into two branches.
  - The walls of the trachea contain incomplete cartilage rings that are spaced along the length of the trachea. They keep the trachea open and prevent it from collapsing when an animal inhales (Figure 9-4).
  - The **tracheal** epithelium is also a ciliated mucous membrane, similar to that in the nasal passages. It too produces mucus, to which foreign material sticks. The cilia beat in one direction only. This action takes the foreign material up the trachea, through the larynx, and into the pharynx, where it is eventually swallowed.

One of the cartilages that make up the larynx is what is known as the *Adam's apple* in humans.

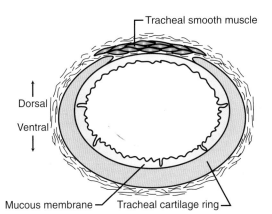

FIGURE 9-4 Cross section of canine trachea. Note that the tracheal cartilage ring is incomplete dorsally. (From Colville TP: *Clinical Anatomy and Physiology for Veterinary Technicians,* ed 2, St Louis, 2009, Mosby.)

Lower Respiratory System

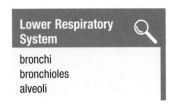

The lungs make up the lower respiratory system, which includes all the respiratory structures subsequent to the bifurcation of the trachea: bronchi (*singular* = bronchus), bronchioles, and alveoli (*singular* = alveolus) (Figure 9-5).

The **right and left bronchi** are the first branches of the trachea. The right bronchus goes to the right lung, and the left bronchus goes to the left lung (see Figure 9-5). Each bronchus branches into secondary bronchi, then into tertiary bronchi, and finally times into **bronchioles.** The area from the bifurcation of the trachea to the branching of the bronchioles is called the **bronchial tree.** The bronchioles get smaller and their lumens get narrower with each successive branching, until the very smallest bronchioles branch into **alveolar ducts.** Each alveolar duct terminates in a cluster of microscopic blind sacs called the **alveolar sac,** which contains many alveoli. Think of a bunch of grapes. The alveolar duct is the main stem and the alveoli are the grapes (Figure 9-6). Each alveolus has a wall that is only one cell thick and is surrounded by capillaries with walls that are also one cell thick.

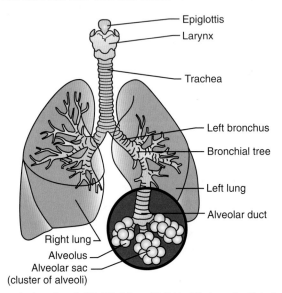

FIGURE 9-5 Lower respiratory tract. (Modified from McBride DF: *Learning Veterinary Terminology,* St Louis, 1996, Mosby. In Colville TP: *Clinical Anatomy and Physiology for Veterinary Technicians,* ed 2, St Louis, 2009, Mosby.)

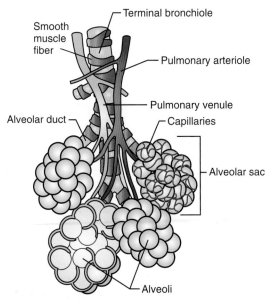

FIGURE 9-6 Alveoli and alveolar sacs. Smallest terminal bronchioles divide into alveolar ducts that lead to clusters of alveoli called *alveolar sacs.* (From Colville TP: *Clinical Anatomy and Physiology for Veterinary Technicians,* ed 2, St Louis, 2009, Mosby.)

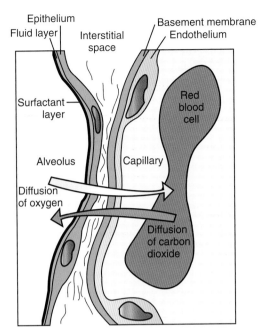

FIGURE 9-7 **Diffusion of gases between alveolus and capillary.** (From Cunningham J, Klein B: *Textbook of Veterinary Physiology,* ed 4, St Louis, 2008, Saunders.)

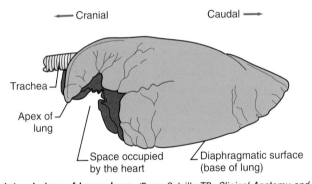

FIGURE 9-8 **Left lateral view of horse lung.** (From Colville TP: *Clinical Anatomy and Physiology for Veterinary Technicians,* ed 2, St Louis, 2009, Mosby.)

External respiration uses air containing oxygen that an animal inhales to exchange for carbon dioxide to exhale. This takes place in the alveoli. When inhaled air enters an alveolus, it is high in oxygen and low in carbon dioxide, but the capillaries surrounding the alveoli are carrying blood that is high in carbon dioxide and low in oxygen. At this microscopic level, where only a two-cell-wall thickness separates the air in the alveoli from the blood in the capillaries, oxygen diffuses into the blood and carbon dioxide diffuses into the air that will be exhaled (Figure 9-7).

LUNGS

Put together all the bronchi, all the bronchiole branches, all the alveolar ducts, and all the alveoli sacs, along with a good blood supply, some nerves, and interstitial tissue—and you have a lung. Animals have two lungs that are divided into varying numbers of **lobes,** depending on the species (Figure 9-8). The base of the caudal lobe of each lung rests on the **diaphragm.** The apex of each lung is the cranial aspect of the cranial lobe. The lungs fill the thoracic cavity except for a space between the two lungs called the **mediastinum,** where the heart, large blood vessels, nerves, trachea, esophagus, lymphatic vessels, and lymph nodes are located.

All of the thoracic organs and structures are covered with a thin membrane called the **visceral pleura,** which folds back on itself to line the thoracic cavity and become the **parietal pleura.** The pleural membrane is not continuous on the right and left sides of the thorax. Each side has its own membrane. Between the visceral pleura and the parietal pleura is a potential space that contains a small amount of lubricating fluid to allow the lungs to move smoothly along the chest wall when the animal breathes.

EXERCISE 9-2 *Label It!*

Label each blank in the diagram below with the name of the structure in the respiratory system. Labels on the diagram will provide answers for the definitions that follow.

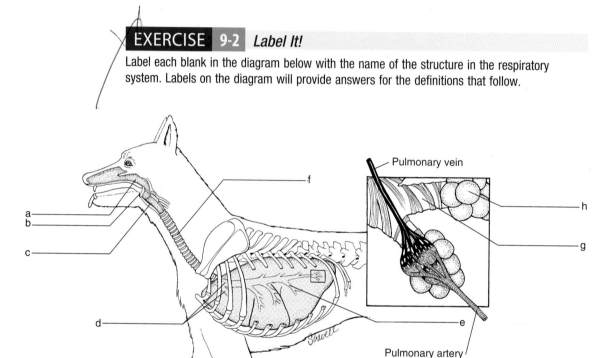

Canine respiratory system. (Adapted from Wanamaker BP: *Applied Pharmacology for Veterinary Technicians,* ed 4, St Louis, 2009, Saunders.)

1. The _____ is commonly referred to as the windpipe.

2. The _____ is used by both the respiratory system and the digestive system.

3. The opening of the _____ is covered by the epiglottis.

4. The _____ is where the vocal cords are found.

5. The _____ bifurcates into two branches.

6. The _____ is commonly called the throat.

7. The _____ are the first branches of the trachea.

8. The _____ is only one cell thick and is surrounded by capillaries with walls that are also one cell thick.

9. The _____ is the vessel that carries oxygenated blood back to the heart.

10. The _____ connects the pharynx to the trachea.

Check your answers at the end of the chapter, Answers to Exercises.

CASE STUDY 9-2 #2010-1974 HOLDEN

Signalment and History: A 7-year-old **M(N)** Golden Retriever dog named Holden was referred to the Frisbee **SA** Clinic for evaluation of an acute increased respiratory noise **(inspiratory stridor)** and snoring **(stertorous** breathing), which the referring veterinarian, Dr. Kaftan, suspected to be secondary to a **laryngeal** mass or laryngeal **paralysis.** Dr. Kaftan had evaluated Holden on the day before referral because of inspiratory stridor and stertorous breathing detected by the owner.

Physical Examination and Diagnosis: Physical examination revealed that Holden was **panting,** appeared anxious, and was obviously having trouble breathing. **Thoracic auscultation** revealed typical lung sounds in all lung fields; auscultation of the heart also revealed typical sounds with a slight tachycardia of 125 **bpm.** His temperature was 100.5° F—within the expected reference range. Results for the remainder of the physical examination were unremarkable. Blood was drawn and was sent to the lab, where a **CBC** was requested. All the results were within their respective reference ranges. Because of the difficulty Holden was having breathing, he was anesthetized and **intubated.** A temporary cuffed **tracheotomy tube** was inserted **transversely** between **tracheal rings** on the midline in the **midcervical** region of the trachea. A mass compressing the left side of the **larynx** was found. Holden recovered from anesthesia without complication and was administered another dose of anti-inflammatory drug given **IV.** The next day, Holden was sedated for examination, which revealed that the mass was noticeably smaller. Laryngeal **paralysis** was suspected.

The initial **diagnostic** plan included **serum** biochemical analysis and urinalysis. Thoracic and **cervical** radiographs were taken and revealed mild **alveolar** infiltrates in the **cranial** lung lobes. The cause of this pattern was unknown, but it was consistent with **inhalation** of **hemorrhage** from the previously placed tracheotomy tube.

For further examination of the larynx, a short-term anesthetic was administered (5 **mg/kg** IV). A 2 × 2-**cm nodular** mass was visible on the **lateral** aspect of the **epiglottis.** A **bx** specimen of the mass was obtained, and impressions were made for **cytological** evaluation. **Septic suppurative inflammation** was diagnosed from the cytological specimen; small **intracellular** rod-shaped bacteria were observed. **Histological** examination of the **biopsy** specimen confirmed the cytological diagnosis. No evidence of **neoplasia** was noted.

Treatment: The temporary tracheotomy tube was replaced with a cuffed tracheotomy tube. A large blood **clot** was found on the **distal** end of the temporary tracheotomy tube when it was removed. It had obstructed approximately 90% of the tube lumen. An **anti-inflammatory** drug was again administered to decrease **inflammation. Antimicrobial** treatment was started.

Examination of new lateral radiographic views the following morning revealed an **intraluminal** soft tissue opacity in the distal portion of the trachea. The cuffed tracheotomy tube appeared to be in an appropriate position and was visible **proximal** to the soft tissue opacity.

On the basis of the severity of clinical signs and radiographic evidence of a mass or foreign body in the trachea, Holden was again anesthetized for immediate **tracheoscopy.** A mass that appeared to be obstructing most of the tracheal lumen was identified. The mass was dark red, and hair was incorporated within the structure of the mass. Small forceps were advanced through the bx port to remove the mass. Unfortunately, the mass was **friable,** and only small pieces could be removed with the forceps. A catheter was then introduced through the tracheal **stoma** and was advanced past the mass. A balloon was inflated and was retracted **retrograde** in the trachea to dislodge the mass. Biopsy forceps were then used to remove the mass. The trachea was subsequently examined, and no remaining mass or foreign material was detected.

The mass was submitted for histological examination, which revealed an organized thrombus that contained hair and plant material. The following morning, results of physical examination were unremarkable. Air movement through the tracheotomy tube was appropriate, and auscultation revealed adequate sounds in all lung fields. Later that day (approximately 28 hours after the initial thrombus was removed from Holden's trachea), the patient had another episode of **dyspnea,** became **cyanotic,** and vomited and urinated in his cage. It was apparent that the tracheotomy tube was obstructed, so it was removed, and a suction catheter was advanced through the tracheotomy site in an attempt to dislodge or remove the obstruction. When the suction tube was removed, there was blood on it. Holden regained air movement through the trachea, and the cyanosis resolved. Lateral cervical and thoracic X-rays revealed another soft tissue opacity in the distal portion of the trachea at approximately the same location as the previous soft tissue opacity.

Holden was immediately anesthetized to allow examination of the suspected thrombus. Grasping forceps were introduced, and the thrombus was removed. Dr. Frisbee assumed that the continued **hemorrhage** was a complication at the tracheotomy tube site. Because the laryngeal mass was greatly reduced in size, she decided to not replace the tracheotomy tube.

Coagulation tests were performed. An **arterial** blood sample was obtained while Holden was breathing room air during recovery from anesthesia. Holden recovered well from anesthesia and had no additional respiratory complications.

The following morning, Holden appeared to be resting comfortably and the results of physical examination were unremarkable. Thoracic X-rays showed a mild **pneumomediastinum,** which Dr. Frisbee assumed to be a result of the previous tracheotomy site.

Outcome: Holden was discharged with instructions to continue oral administration of antimicrobials until they were finished. Holden's owner reported 12 days later that Holden was doing fine and was breathing normally.

EXERCISE 9-3 *Case It!*

Several words used in Case Study 9-2 are highlighted with bold type. With practice, most of these words should be getting easier to dissect in order to comprehend their definitions. Match the words listed in the right column to their definitions.

1. _____	air is present in the space in the middle of the chest, between the lungs	antimicrobial
2. *tracheotomy*	incision into the trachea	auscultation
3. *CBC*	diagnostic test performed to examine cells in the blood	biopsy
4. *coagulation*	complex process by which blood forms clots	CBC
5. *cyanotic*	bluish coloration of the skin or mucous membranes	coagulation
6. *dyspnea*	difficulty breathing	cyanotic
7. *stoma*	a surgically created permanent opening	dyspnea
8. *transversely*	lying across, or extending across	inhalation
9. *auscultation*	listening to the sounds of internal organs	pneumomediastinum
10. *serum*	liquid portion of blood after clotting has occurred	serum
11. *inhalation*	breathing in	stoma
12. *antimicrobial*	substance that kills or inhibits the growth of microorganisms such as bacteria, fungi, or protozoans	tracheotomy
13. *biopsy*	medical procedure that involves obtaining a sample of cells or tissues for examination	transversely

Check your answers at the end of the chapter, Answers to Exercises.

RESPIRATION

So what causes an animal to inhale and exhale? Ultimately, all these many structures of the respiratory system from the nostrils through the alveoli must work together to effectively move air in sufficient volume to do their part to maintain homeostasis.

A couple of factors play an important role in respiration. Within the thoracic cavity is a partial vacuum, which makes the pressure in the thorax less than atmospheric pressure. And because the lungs are sufficiently soft and flexible, the partial vacuum allows the lungs to pretty much fill up the thoracic cavity from the diaphragm and all along the ribs and the thoracic vertebrae. As the thoracic cavity expands and contracts, the lungs passively follow along.

Inspiration is the process of drawing air into the lungs. It is also called *inhalation*. Because the lungs do not contain muscles, they cannot expand or contract on their own. They must rely on **intercostal** muscles between the ribs and the muscular diaphragm.

The muscles of inspiration are the **external intercostal** muscles and the diaphragm. When these muscles contract, the size of the thoracic cavity is increased. The flexible lungs expand along with the cavity size, and air is sucked into the lungs. Of course, all of this is possible only if the partial vacuum in the thoracic cavity is maintained.

Expiration is the process of pushing air out of the lungs. It is also called *exhalation*. The muscles of expiration are the **internal intercostal** muscles and the abdominal muscles. When these muscles contract, the size of the thoracic cavity is decreased. This causes the lungs to compress, and the air within them is pushed out.

EXERCISE 9-4 *Recall It!*

Repetitive use of terms that defy word analysis will help you commit them to memory. You will find some terms below that were introduced in previous chapters. Circle the correct word or phrase that makes each statement true.

1. Tetany is intermittent, painful, sustained muscle contractions related to (toxins released from the *Clostridium tetani* bacteria), (alternating spasms and muscle relaxations), or (defective calcium metabolism).

2. A cavity, recess, or passage in any organ or tissue is a (furcation), (turbinate), or (sinus).

3. Something friable is (easily crumbled), (diseased), or (cancerous).

4. Hiccups are spasms of the (larynx), (vocal cords), or (diaphragm).

5. Small, hair-like structures on the surface of the epithelium that beat rhythmically are (cilia), (melanotrichia), or (bradyrhythmia).

6. Emphysema is overexpansion of the walls of the (bronchioles), (alveoli), or (arterioles).

7. Suppurate means to produce or discharge (blood), (pus), or (water).

8. A suture is the (line of junction of two bones forming an immovable joint), (the smooth end of a bone that forms part of a joint), or (a depression, trench, or hollow area).

9. Breathing in and out is (inspiration), (expiration), or (ventilation).

10. Accumulation of fluid in the abdominal cavity is (aorta), (ascites), or (auscultation).

Check your answers at the end of the chapter, Answers to Exercises.

Table 9-3 lists some of the more common respiratory diseases seen in large and small animals.

TABLE 9-3   **Word Parts Associated with Respiratory System Diseases**

Word Part	Meaning	Example and Definition	Word Parts	
-staxis	bleeding, escape of blood from the vessels	**epistaxis** nosebleed *Have you ever noticed how sometimes word analysis can paint a picture in your mind? Epistaxis is one such word; you can visualize bleeding from the nose.*	epi- = on or upon -staxis = bleeding, escape of blood from the vessels	-staxis
-ectasis	expansion, dilation, distention	**cardiectasis** dilation of the heart, which could be a physiological, pathological, or artificial enlargement of a cavity, blood vessel, or opening in the heart	cardi/o = heart -ectasis = expansion, dilation, distention	-ectasis
atel/o	incomplete, imperfect	**atelectasis** incomplete expansion of the lungs at birth or as a result of bronchial obstruction	atel/o = incomplete, imperfect -ectasis = expansion, dilation, distention	atel/o
iatr/o	physician, medicine	**iatrogenic** caused by medical personnel, or by treatment or diagnostic procedures	iatr/o = physician, medicine gen/o = formation or beginning -ic = pertaining to	iatr/o
tuss/o	cough	**tussiculation** a short, dry hacking cough as seen in kennel cough	tuss/o = cough -ic = pertaining to -ule = indicating something small -ation = state, condition, action, process, or result	tuss/o
		antitussive a cough suppressant	anti- = against, opposed to tuss/o = cough -ive = pertaining to	

BOX 9-2   **Diseases of the Respiratory System**

- laryngeal hemiplegia—**"roaring"** in horses; a high-pitched wheezing sound made when the horse is breathing deeply (e.g., during a cantor or gallop)
  - Roaring is caused by damage to the nerve supply to one of the cartilages on the (most often) left cartilages of the larynx.
  - The result is that the larynx cannot open all the way, and less air (oxygen) is reaching the lungs.
- aspiration pneumonia—an inflammatory reaction resulting from inhaled foreign material
  - This may occur when oral liquids are administered too rapidly, not allowing the epiglottis to close off the larynx.
- RAO (recurrent airway obstruction)—**"heaves"** in horses
  - The former name was chronic obstructive pulmonary disease (COPD).
  - This allergic, obstructive inflammatory airway disease is similar to human asthma.
- URI (upper respiratory infection)
  - This is an infection of any of the structures of the upper respiratory tract.
  - In humans, URI is a head cold.
- LRI (lower respiratory infection)
  - This is an infection of any of the structures of the lower respiratory tract.
  - In humans, LRI is a chest cold.
- pneumonia—an acute or chronic infection of the lungs accompanied by inflammation
- bovine respiratory disease complex—**shipping fever pneumonia** in cattle
  - The origin involves many factors, including stress, decreased immunity, and an infectious agent.
  - Shipping fever is so named because it is frequently seen in animals that are being transported. Stress factors include dehydration, starvation, crowding, exhaustion, and inhalation of toxic fumes.
  - Morbidity can approach 35%; mortality is 5% to 10%.
- infectious canine tracheobronchitis—**kennel cough**
  - This highly contagious bacterial respiratory disease of dogs is characterized by inflammation of the trachea and bronchi.
  - Inflammation results in a dry hacking cough, retching, nasal discharge, pneumonia, fever, and lethargy.

CASE STUDY 9-1 #1997-1488 FOOLISH RISK

Signalment and History: A 3-year-old Thoroughbred **gelding** named Foolish Risk was brought to the Frisbee LA Clinic because of an **acute** cough and **pyrexia** of 24 hours' duration. Two days ago, he had returned from a show where he had been stabled for 2 days. The owner had started treatment with an **antibiotic** injection (2.2 **mg/kg IM q12h**) as instructed over the phone by Dr. Murdoch and had administered an NSAID (nonsteroidal **anti-inflammatory** drug) (2.2 mg/kg **PO** once), but the pyrexia remained.

Physical Examination and Diagnosis: Foolish Risk was examined by Dr. Murdoch and veterinary technician, Pat Grouper, approximately 24 hours after the onset of clinical **signs.** At this time, Foolish Risk was **lethargic** but responsive and had pitting **edema** of the prepuce and **thoracic** and **pelvic** limbs. He had profuse **bilateral** blood-tinged seromucoid **nasal** discharge and a deep cough. There was **hyperemia** of the gingival mucous membranes, with numerous **petechiae.** Respiratory rate (44 **bpm**) and effort were increased, as were rectal temperature (103.5°F) and heart rate (64 **bpm**). **Auscultation** of the **thorax** revealed harsh respiratory sounds; cardiac rhythm was normal. Blood was collected for a **CBC.** A **nasal** swab specimen was collected and was sent to the lab along with the blood sample. **Petechiation** of the oral mucous membranes in conjunction with pitting edema of the prepuce and limbs was considered suggestive of **vasculitis.** IV antibiotics and anti-inflammatory drugs were started. Leg wraps were applied to help control the edema.

Hematological abnormalities noted on the **CBC** results included mild **leukopenia, anemia,** and **thrombocytopenia.** Results of **serological** testing for **antibodies** against **equine** viral **arteritis** virus and other viruses were negative.

Treatment: Foolish Risk became increasingly lethargic and developed **anorexia** over the next 24 hours. The **distal** portions of his extremities became cool. His heart rate remained high and the nasal discharge became more **mucopurulent.** Thoracic auscultation revealed wheezes and end **inspiratory** crackles that were more prominent on the right side of the thorax. The brief use of a rebreathing bag elicited **dyspnea** and a **paroxysmal** deep **productive** cough.

On day 3, a **transtracheal** wash produced a **serosanguineous** fluid that was submitted for bacterial culture and **cytological** examination. **Microscopic** examination of the fluid showed cellular debris consisting of moderate numbers of **neutrophils;** moderate numbers of **erythrocytes;** small numbers of **macrophages, lymphocytes,** and plasma cells; and a few **eosinophils.** Numerous **intracellular** bacteria were also seen. Serum biochemical abnormalities included **hyperfibrinogenemia, hypoproteinemia,** and **acidosis.** Foolish Risk was started on antibiotics and fluid therapy.

During the next 12 hours, Foolish Risk developed right **thoracic limb** lameness. His wraps were removed, and multiple epithelial **vesicles** were seen in the **dorsal metacarpal region** of the right thoracic limb. The distal portion of the limb was swollen, and **signs** of pain were elicited on **palpation.** Epithelial vesicles were seen in the **caudal pastern regions** of the other three limbs. Approximately 50% of the skin over the dorsal right metacarpal area eventually came off. The areas of the distal portions of the limbs that lost their skin improved with **topical** antibacterial and zinc oxide treatment. The frequency of coughing was reduced, and the cough became **nonproductive.**

Thoracic ultrasonography through the sixth and seventh **intercostal** spaces revealed bilateral **ventral** lung consolidation and minimal **pleural** fluid accumulation. **Leukocytosis** and **thrombocytosis** were indicative of **chronic** inflammation.

Outcome: Thirty days after admission, results of a CBC and of serum biochemical tests were within expected reference ranges. Foolish Risk had normal lung sounds, and only a few coughs were induced by the examination. Foolish Risk was discharged from the hospital. Results of a CBC performed 10 days later were also within expected reference ranges.

EXERCISE 9-5 *Case It!*

Re-read Case Study 9-1. Complete the statements following the case study by writing the words in the blanks to complete the definitions.

1. Describe a gelding: _____

2. Pleural fluid was found in the _____.

3. Serosanguineous fluid contains _____

   and _____.

4. Edema can be demonstrated by depressing the skin of a swollen area. What would you expect to see in pitting edema? _____

5. A productive cough is one that produces _____.

6. Where would you look for the caudal pastern region? _____

7. If thrombocytosis is a high count of platelets, what do you call a high count of WBCs? _____

8. This disease was diagnosed as chronic because _____.

9. Topical treatment was administered _____.

10. Mucopurulent nasal discharge contains _____

    and _____.

11. In acidosis, the pH of the blood is _____.

12. Bilateral nasal discharge comes from _____.

Check your answers at the end of the chapter, Answers to Exercises.

TABLE 9-4	Abbreviations	
Abbreviation	**Meaning**	**Example**
URI	upper respiratory infection	Diagnosis: Because she was coughing, sneezing, had a runny nose and nasal ulcers, Midnight was diagnosed with URI.
LRI	lower respiratory infection	*Pasteurella pneumotropica* was the etiology of LRI in Shadow's litter of puppies.
RAO	recurrent airway obstruction	The tentative diagnosis for Slivers was RAO because he had a chronic cough and exercise intolerance that had been present for nearly 4 months.
CO_2	carbon dioxide	Midnight's vomiting is probably the cause of her higher than normal CO_2 blood level.
O_2	oxygen	O_2 therapy is often used in emergency and critical care medicine.
CPR	cardiopulmonary resuscitation	Misty lived because of the best efforts of our veterinary staff and the administration of CPR.
ETT	endotracheal tube	After Misty was anesthetized, an ETT was placed and she was hooked up to an anesthetic machine.
QNS	quantity not sufficient	The blood sample was QNS for a CBC on Oscar's blood.
xs	excessive	There was xs mucus dripping from Oscar's nose.

URI

LRI

RAO

CO_2

O_2

CPR

ETT

QNS

xs

ANSWERS TO EXERCISES

Exercise 9-1

1. air (oxygen)
2. in
3. back
4. breathing
5. abnormally high
6. carbon dioxide
7. nerves
8. oxygen
9. narrow; narrow
10. smell

Exercise 9-2

a. pharynx
b. epiglottis
c. larynx
d. bronchi
e. secondary bronchus
f. trachea
g. bronchus
h. alveolus

1. trachea
2. pharynx
3. larynx
4. larynx
5. trachea
6. pharynx
7. bronchi
8. alveolus
9. pulmonary vein
10. larynx

Exercise 9-3

1. pneumomediastinum
2. tracheotomy
3. CBC
4. coagulation
5. cyanotic
6. dyspnea
7. stoma
8. transversely
9. auscultation
10. serum
11. inhalation
12. antimicrobial
13. biopsy (bx)

Exercise 9-4

1. defective calcium metabolism
2. sinus
3. easily crumbled
4. diaphragm
5. cilia
6. alveoli
7. pus
8. line of junction of two bones forming an immovable joint
9. ventilation
10. ascites

Exercise 9-5

1. male, neutered/castrated equine
2. in the space between the membranes that line the chest and cover the lungs
3. serous fluid (fluid that resembles serum) and blood
4. an indentation remains for some time after release of the pressure
5. mucus
6. back of the leg, above the hoof; the joint between the proximal and middle phalanges
7. leukocytosis
8. onset was slow, and the condition persisted for a long time
9. on the surface areas of the body
10. mucus and pus
11. less than 7.35
12. both nostrils

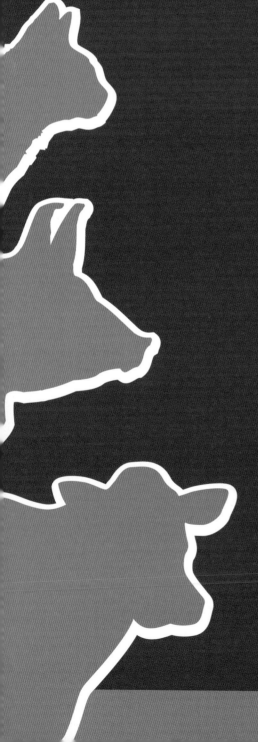

Chapter 10

The Digestive System

If toast always lands butter-side down, and cats always land on their feet, what happens if you strap toast on the back of a cat and drop it?

Steven Wright

WORD PARTS

abomas/o	ahb-ō-**mā**-sō	dips/o	**dihp**-sō	lapar/o	**lahp**-ah-rō	prandi/o	**prahn**-dē-ō
aliment/o	ahl-ih-**mehn**-tō	dont/o	**dohn**-tō	lingu/o	**lihng**-gwah-ō	pre-	prē
amyl/o	**ahm**-mehl-ō	duoden/o	**doo**-ō-**də**-nō	lip/o	**lī**-pō	proct/o	**prohck**-tō
an/o	**ā**-nō	enter/o	**ehn**-tehr-ō	-lith	lihth	-ptosis	pah-**tō**-sihs
-ase	ās	esophag/o	ē-**sohf**-ah-gō	lith/o	**lihth**-ō	ptyal/o	**tī**-uh-lō
brachy-	**brahk**-ē	gastr/o	**gahs**-trō	mal-	mahl	-ptysis	pah-**tuh**-sis
bucc/o	**būk**-ō	gingiv/o	**jihn**-jih-vō	odont/o	ō-**dohn**-tō	pylor/o	pī-**lohr**-ō
carni-	**kahr**-nē	gloss/o	**glohs**-ō	omas/o	ō-**mā**-sō	rect/o	**rehck**-tō
cec/o	sē-**cō**	gluc/o	**gloo**-cō	oment/o	ō-**mehn**-tō	reticul/o	reh-**tihck**-yoo-lō
-cele	sēl	glyc/o	**glī**-co	omni-	**ohm**-nē	-rrhea	**rē**-ah
cheil/o	**kī**-lō	hepat/o	heh-**paht**-ō	or/o	**ohr**-ō	rumen/o	**roo**-mehn-ō
chol/e	**kō**-lē	herbi-	**hərb**-ih	-orexia	ō-**rehck**-sē-ah	rumin/o	**roo**-mihn-ō
choledoch/o	**kō**-lē-dō-kō	herni/o	**hər**-nē-ō	palat/o	**pahl**-ah-tō	sacchar/o	**sahck**-ahr-ō
chyl/o	**kī**-lō	hyps/o	**hihps**-ō	pancre/o	**pahn**-krē-ō	sial/o	sī-**ahl**-ō
col/o	**kō**-lō	-iasis	**ī**-ah-sihs	pancreat/o	**pahn**-krē-aht-ō	steat/o	stē-**aht**-ō
colon/o	**kō**-lohn-ō	ile/o	**ihl**-ē-ō	peps/o	**pehp**-sō	stom/o	**stō**-mō
copr/o	**kohp**-rō	jejun/o	jeh-**joo**-nō	pept/o	**pehp**-tō	stomat/o	stō-**mah**-tō
dent/o	**dehn**-tō	labi/o	**lā**-bē-ō	phag/o	**fā**-gō	-vore	vohr

OUTLINE

THE DIGESTIVE SYSTEM

ANATOMY OF THE DIGESTIVE SYSTEM

FUNCTION OF THE DIGESTIVE SYSTEM
 Digestion
 Absorption
 Elimination

A FEW WORDS ABOUT THE LIVER AND PANCREAS

DISORDERS OF THE DIGESTIVE SYSTEM

LEARNING OBJECTIVES

When you have completed this chapter, you will be able to:

1 Understand the components and functions of the digestive system.

2 Identify and recognize the meanings of word parts related to digestion, using them to build or analyze words.

3 Apply your new knowledge and understanding of clinical veterinary language in the context of medical reports.

CASE STUDY 10-1 #2010-5832 SARGE

Signalment and History: An 8-year-old 145-lb **M(C)** Great Dane dog named Sarge was brought to the Frisbee SA Clinic because of a distended abdomen and an **acute** history of **regurgitation, retching, vomiting** of white foam, and excessive salivation. Sarge was whining continuously when he was brought into the clinic.

Physical Examination: Dr. Frisbee recognized an emergency situation coming on, so she quickly performed an initial physical examination with Jess's help. Notable findings included **lethargy,** pale mucous membranes, abdominal distention, **tachycardia** (210 beats/min), and a **palpably** large mass in the **mid-abdominal** region. **IV** fluids were started immediately and included 5 **L** of crystalloids to expand Sarge's blood volume. Fresh plasma was also administered because Dr. Frisbee was concerned about Sarge's cardiovascular condition and the possibility that he might develop a **coagulopathy,** or disseminated **intravascular coagulation.**

Blood was collected for serum biochemical analyses, a **CBC,** and coagulation tests. The serum biochemical results showed **hypoglycemia, hyperphosphatemia,** and **hyperproteinemia.** A **neutrophilia, lymphocytopenia,** and **macrocytic, normo-chromic RBCs** were seen on the **hemogram.** Results of coagulation tests were within expected reference limits.

Right lateral thoracic and **abdominal** X-rays showed indications of **gastric dilation** and **volvulus (GDV)** with secondary **megaesophagus.** With Sarge in right lateral recumbency, Dr. Frisbee inserted a 16-gauge needle through the abdominal wall lateral to the ventral midline and into the stomach to immediately relieve gas distention. After providing mild sedation, Dr. Frisbee tried to pass a stomach tube but was unsuccessful. A 16-gauge needle was again inserted into the stomach, and this time gas and approximately 475 **mL** of malodorous, dark brown fluid were removed. Sarge was then prepared for **sx.**

(See the rest of the story at the end of this chapter.)

THE DIGESTIVE SYSTEM

Back in Chapters 7 and 8, you learned that the functions of the cardiovascular system and of blood were to carry, among other substances, oxygen, carbon dioxide, and nutrients. The animal you are building system by system now has the respiratory system needed to exchange oxygen and carbon dioxide. It is time to learn about how this animal deals with the food it eats and what happens to turn the food into usable nutrients (Table 10-1). The digestive system does all of this.

Animals cannot absorb food or nutrients through their skin. Some other mechanism is needed by which food is taken into the body and is made available to the cells that need nutrients to function. When a horse eats alfalfa pellets, the pellets do not go directly to the body cells and say, "Here we are. Use us!" Why not? The pellets are not in a form that can be used by the body. They are too large to pass through the wall of the digestive tract into the body. So chemicals in the digestive system break down the pellets, convert them into a mushy consistency, and then break them down into much smaller compounds. It is these individual compounds that can pass through or be carried through the digestive tract wall, enter a capillary, and get distributed to the body's cells.

Therefore, the digestive system is responsible for all of the following processes:

- **prehension**—gathering food, grasping or seizing it
- **mastication**—mechanical digestion, chewing to break food into smaller particles
- **digestion**—chemical or microbial breakdown of food particles into simpler chemical compounds that can be absorbed and used by the body

TABLE 10-1   Word Parts Associated with Digestive System Functions

Word Part	Meaning	Example and Definition	Word Parts
omni-	all, every	**omnivision** seeing everything or perceiving all things	omni- = all, every vision = seeing, sight	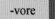
-vore	eat, devour, swallow	**omnivore** animal that eats all kinds of plants and animals	omni- = all, every -vore = eat, devour, swallow	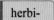
herbi-	plant, green crop	**herbivore** animal that subsists on a diet consisting of only plants	herbi- = plant, green crop -vore = eat, devour, swallow	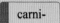
carni-	flesh, meat	**carnivore** animal that subsists on a diet consisting of only meat	carni- = flesh, meat -vore = eat, devour, swallow	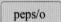
peps/o pept/o	digestion	**apepsia** lack of digestion	a- = without, no, not peps/o = digestion -ia = pertaining to	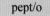
		bradypeptic pertaining to slow digestion *Is this where* Pepto-Bismol® *gets its name? It claims to help relieve the symptoms of indigestion. What about* Pepsi Cola®?	brady- = slow pept/o = digestion -ic = pertaining to	

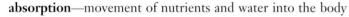

- **absorption**—movement of nutrients and water into the body
- **defecation**—getting rid of feces, the leftover waste material of the digestive system

Not all animals eat the same diet. **Herbivores** (horses, cows, sheep, and goats) eat only plant material, **carnivores** (cats and dogs) eat primarily meat, and **omnivores** (pigs and humans) eat both plants and meat. Over time, digestive tracts have adapted to these varied diets. For example, herbivore animals have developed additional specialized organs of digestion to efficiently break down the hard-to-digest cellulose that makes up much of plant material. Carnivore and omnivore species have not needed to develop these specialized organs of digestion; these species are called simple-stomach, or **monogastric** animals (Figure 10-1).

Much of the absorption of nutrients into the body occurs after the partially digested food has passed through the stomach into the intestines. Not every bit of the food that is taken in is used by the animal. Some waste material will always be left over after all the usable nutrients in food have been removed. The leftover material moves into the rectum. Here, most of the water is removed, and this material becomes **feces.** The amount of water left in the feces determines the consistency of the feces. Compare a soft cow pie with firm sheep fecal pellets.

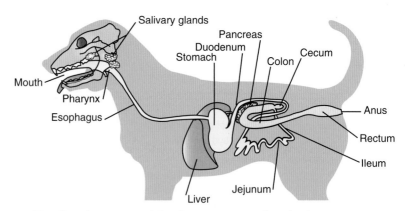

FIGURE 10-1 **The digestive system of the dog, a monogastric animal.** (Modified from Dyce KM, Sack WO, Wensing CJG: *Textbook of Veterinary Anatomy,* ed 3, Philadelphia, 2002, Saunders. In Colville TP: *Clinical Anatomy and Physiology for Veterinary Technicians,* ed 2, St Louis, 2009, Mosby.)

EXERCISE 10-1 *Opposites!*

Below is a list of word parts. For each one, there is a word part that means the opposite. Define the word part, and then write and define its opposite. The first one is done for you as an example.

Word Part	Definition	Opposite	Definition
1. dextr/o	right	sinistr/o	left
2. dors/o	toward top	ventro belly	
3. intra-	within	inside	outside
4. hydr/o	water	dry	
5. heter/o	Different	similar	
6. therm/o	heat	cold	
7. malac/o	soft	hard	
8. melan/o	black	white	
9. brady-	slow	fast	
10. ab-	away	toward	
11. ante-	before	after	
12. hypo-	under below	onton above	
13. -philia	loving	non loving	
14. macr/o	large	small	
15. pan-	all	without	

Check your answers at the end of the chapter, Answers to Exercises.

TABLE 10-2 Word Parts Associated with the Anatomy of the Digestive System

Word Part	Meaning	Example and Definition	Word Parts
or/o stom/o stomat/o	mouth	**oral** pertaining to the mouth	or/o = mouth -al = pertaining to
		anastomosis a surgical connection of two hollow organs, or a place where two hollow organs naturally join (such as branching blood vessels or bronchioles)	an- = without, no, not a- = without, no, not *(this second "no" makes it a "yes, there is a mouth")* stom/o = mouth -osis = disease or abnormal condition
		stomatomalacia pathological softening of any of the structures of the mouth *Remember the suffix -stomy? The permanent opening created is often referred to as a stoma, or a mouth.*	stomat/o = mouth malac/o = soft, softening -ia = pertaining to
phag/o	eat	**hyperphagia** overeating, gluttony *Sarcophagus literally means "eating flesh." You know a sarcophagus to be a funeral holder for a corpse.*	hyper- = above, over, excess phag/o = eat -ia = pertaining to
prandi/o	meal	**postprandial** happening after a meal	post- = after, behind, later prandi/o = meal -al = pertaining to
aliment/o	food	**alimentary canal** digestive tract; tube that runs from the mouth to the anus	aliment/o = food -ar = pertaining to -y = made up of, characterized by canal = a tubular passageway either in bone or formed by soft tissue
dips/o	thirst	**polydipsia** excessive or abnormal thirst	poly- = much or many dips/o = thirst -ia = pertaining to
cheil/o labi/o	lip	**cheilophagia** excessive biting of the lips	cheil/o = lip phag/o = eat -ia = pertaining to
		labionasal pertaining to the lips and the nose *Labia also refers to the lip-like structures that are part of the female genitalia.*	labi/o = lip nas/o = nose -al = pertaining to
gingiv/o	gums, gingiva	**gingivostomatitis** inflammation of the gums and mouth	gingiv/o = gums stomat/o = mouth -itis = inflammation

or/o

stom/o

stomat/o

phag/o

prandi/o

aliment/o

dips/o

cheil/o

labi/o

gingiv/o

Continued

palat/o

dent/o

dont/o

odont/o

brachy-

hyps/o

bucc/o

TABLE 10-2	Word Parts Associated with the Anatomy of the Digestive System—cont'd		
Word Part	**Meaning**	**Example and Definition**	**Word Parts**
palat/o	palate, roof of the mouth	**palatorrhaphy** surgical procedure of suturing a cleft palate, a birth defect affecting the roof of the mouth *You are familiar with the phrase "cleansing the palate," which is common in wine tasting or fine dining. It involves clearing your mouth of any previous taste before trying the next item. The palate was once considered the source of the sense of taste.*	palat/o = palate, roof of the mouth -rrhaphy = suture
dent/o dont/o odont/o	teeth	**dentist** doctor who diagnoses and treats problems with teeth and tissues in the mouth	dent/o = teeth -ist = a person or a thing that does something specified
		orthodontic pertaining to the branch of dentistry that deals with the prevention or correction of irregularities of teeth	orth/o = straight, normal, correct dont/o = teeth -ic = pertaining to
		odontopathy any disease of the teeth or their sockets	odont/o = teeth -pathy = disease
brachy-	short	**brachydactyly** general term referring to shorter than normal phalanges *The two prefixes,* brachy- *and* brady-, *can be easily confused if you are not paying attention.* bradydactyl = *slow phalanges (A slow typist?)*	brachy- = short dactyl/o = digit, a finger or toe -y = made up of, characterized by
hyps/o	height, altitude	**hypsography** procedure for measuring height (used to measure height above sea level)	hyps/o = height, altitude -graphy = method of recording
bucc/o	cheek	**buccal** oriented toward the side of the mouth (e.g., the buccal side of a tooth is next to the cheek)	bucc/o = cheek -al = pertaining to

TABLE 10-2	Word Parts Associated with the Anatomy of the Digestive System—cont'd		
Word Part	**Meaning**	**Example and Definition**	**Word Parts**
gloss/o lingu/o	tongue	**glossopalatolabial** pertaining to the tongue, the roof of the mouth, and the lips	gloss/o = tongue palat/o = palate labi/o = lips -al = pertaining to
		lingual oriented toward the tongue (e.g., the lingual side of a tooth is next to the tongue) *The combining form of* lingu/o *has also come to mean "speech and language." Lingu*istics *is the science of language, or the study of a particular language. You may have asked, "What is his native tongue?", meaning language. A linguist is someone who speaks many tongues (several languages).*	lingu/o = tongue -al = pertaining to
sial/o ptyal/o	saliva, salivary gland	**sialectasis** dilation of the ducts of the salivary glands, indicative of an infection	sial/o = saliva, salivary gland -ectasis = expansion, dilation, distention
		hypoptyalism abnormal decrease in the amount of saliva, leading to xerostomia	hypo- = under, beneath, below ptyal/o = saliva, salivary gland -ism = state, condition, action, process, or result
		xerostomia dry mouth which may or not be associated with a lack of saliva	xer/o = dry stom/o = mouth -ia = pertaining to
-ptysis	spitting	**hemoptysis** spitting up blood *Would* gingiptysis *mean spitting out your gum?*	hem/o = blood -ptysis = spitting
esophag/o	esophagus, gullet	**esophagoplegia** paralysis of the esophagus *Did you see* phag/o *in* esophag/o? *The esophagus is the "eating" tube, connecting the throat to the stomach.*	esophag/o = esophagus, gullet -plegia = paralysis

gloss/o

lingu/o

sial/o

ptyal/o

-ptysis

esophag/o

Continued

TABLE 10-2	Word Parts Associated with the Anatomy of the Digestive System—cont'd		
Word Part	**Meaning**	**Example and Definition**	**Word Parts**
rumen/o rumin/o	rumen, the first compartment of the forestomach	**rumenotomy** surgical incision into the rumen	rumen/o = rumen -tomy = surgical incision
		ruminant any mammal with a stomach that has multiple forestomach chambers, such as a cow, goat, camel, or giraffe *When you ruminate, you are thinking or pondering—or "chewing the cud." Ruminants will bring food back up out of their rumen into their mouths to chew it a second time (chew the cud).*	rumin/o = rumen -ant = a person or a thing that does something specified
reticul/o	reticulum, the second compartment of the forestomach	**reticulorumen** composed of the reticulum and the rumen	reticul/o = reticulum rumen = rumen
omas/o	omasum, the third compartment of the forestomach	**omasal stenosis** inability of food to move from the reticulum into the omasum because of a narrowed opening	omas/o = omasum -al = pertaining to sten/o = narrow -osis = disease or abnormal condition
gastr/o	stomach in simple-stomached animals	**gastropexy** surgical fixation of the stomach of a simple-stomached animal to the body wall	gastr/o = stomach in simple-stomached animals -pexy = surgical fixation
abomas/o	stomach in ruminants	**abomasopexy** surgical fixation of the stomach of a ruminant to the body wall *See? Same surgery as a gastropexy in different species!*	abomas/o = stomach in ruminants -pexy = surgical fixation
pylor/o	pylorus, the region of the stomach that connects to the small intestine	**pyloric sphincter** the ring-like muscle at the end of the stomach that normally remains closed but relaxes to allow the release of food into the small intestine	pylor/o = pylorus -ic = pertaining to sphincter = ring-like muscle
lapar/o	abdominal wall, flank	**laparosplenotomy** surgical incision into the abdominal wall to gain access to the spleen	lapar/o = flank, loin splen/o = spleen -tomy = surgical incision
enter/o	intestines in general; referring collectively to the small and large intestines	**enterokinesia** muscle contractions of the intestines by which their contents are moved onward; more commonly known as **peristalsis**	enter/o = intestines in general kinesi/o = movement -ia = pertaining to
duoden/o	duodenum, first segment of the small intestine	**esophagoduodenostomy** surgical creation of a new permanent opening between the esophagus and the duodenum; surgical procedure after a total gastrectomy	esophag/o = esophagus duoden/o = duodenum -stomy = surgical creation of a new permanent opening

rumen/o

rumin/o

reticul/o

omas/o

gastr/o

abomas/o

pylor/o

lapar/o

enter/o

duoden/o

TABLE 10-2	Word Parts Associated with the Anatomy of the Digestive System—cont'd		
Word Part	**Meaning**	**Example and Definition**	**Word Parts**
jejun/o	jejunum, second and middle segment of the small intestine	**esophagojejunoplasty** surgical repair of the esophagus using a segment of the jejunum	esophag/o = esophagus jejun/o = jejunum -plasty = surgical repair
ile/o	ileum, last segment of the small intestine	**ileopathy** disease of the ileum *This is just a reminder not to confuse this ile/o with the ili/o that means the ilium bone of the pelvis.*	ile/o = ileum -pathy = disease
col/o colon/o	colon, the major portion of the large intestine	**colocentesis** surgical puncture of the colon to relieve distention	col/o = colon -centesis = surgical puncture
		colonoscopy endoscopic examination of the colon	colon/o = colon -scop/o = examine, view -y = made up of, characterized by
cec/o	cecum, the blind pouch located at the junction of the ileum and colon	**cecorrhaphy** suturing of the cecum	cec/o = cecum -rrhaphy = suture
rect/o proct/o	rectum, the most caudal end of the large intestine	**rectalgia** pain in the rectum	rect/o = rectum -algia = pain
		proctologist a specialist in the branch of medicine that deals with the rectum and anus	proct/o = rectum -log/o = to study, or to have knowledge of -ist = a person or a thing that does something specified
an/o	anus, the caudal opening of the GI tract through which waste material is eliminated	**anospasm** intermittent involuntary abnormal muscle contractions of the anus	an/o = anus spasm = intermittent involuntary abnormal muscle contractions
copr/o	feces	**coprophagia** eating feces, normally done by dung beetles, rabbits, and chickens; abnormally done by other animals	copr/o = feces phag/o = eating -ia = pertaining to
hepat/o	liver	**hepatocyte** a liver cell	hepat/o = liver -cyte = cell
chol/e	bile, gall	**choleangitis** infection of the common bile duct, the tube that carries bile from the liver to the gall bladder and intestines *Note that the combining vowel e is used here.*	chol/e = bile, gall angi/o = vessel, not always a blood vessel -itis = inflammation

Continued

TABLE 10-2	Word Parts Associated with the Anatomy of the Digestive System—cont'd		
Word Part	**Meaning**	**Example and Definition**	**Word Parts**
choledoch/o	common bile duct, the tube that carries bile from the liver and gall bladder to the duodenum	**choledochohepatostomy** surgical procedure that creates a new permanent opening between the common bile duct and some part of the liver	choledoch/o = common bile duct hepat/o = liver -stomy = surgical creation of a new permanent opening
pancreat/o pancre/o	pancreas	**pancreatitis** inflammation of the pancreas	pancreat/o = pancreas -itis = inflammation
		pancreopathy disease of the pancreas	pancre/o = pancreas -pathy = disease
oment/o	omentum, membrane covering some of the abdominal organs (*plural* = omenta)	**omentopexy** surgical procedure in which omentum is fastened to some other tissue	oment/o = omentum -pexy = surgical fixation

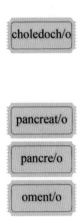

choledoch/o

pancreat/o

pancre/o

oment/o

ANATOMY OF THE DIGESTIVE SYSTEM

The digestive system, also known as the **digestive tract,** the **gastrointestinal (GI) tract,** the **alimentary canal,** or the **gut,** is very complex (Table 10-2). Think of the digestive system as a very long tube passing through an animal, from its front end to its rear end. Food enters one end of the tube, passes through the tube, and exits the other end of the tube completely changed. You might also think of an animal as a fancy-shaped donut whose digestive tube is the hole in the middle, where anything inside the digestive tube is still considered to be outside the body. To enter the body, nutrients must pass through the wall of the tube and into blood and lymph vessels, which will carry them off to the rest of the body. This process of passing through the digestive tube wall is called **absorption.**

If you were a piece of dog food passing through Sparky's digestive system tube, you would be processed by or would go through these structures in the following order:

mouth → pharynx → esophagus → stomach → duodenum → jejunum → ileum → colon → rectum → anus

If you were an equine alfalfa pellet passing through Foolish Risk's digestive tract, you would be processed by or would go through these structures in the following order:

mouth → pharynx → esophagus → stomach → duodenum → jejunum → ileum → cecum → colon → rectum → anus

If you were a mouthful of grass passing through Daisy the cow's digestive system tube, you would be processed by or would go through these structures in the following order:

mouth → pharynx → esophagus → reticulorumen → esophagus → pharynx → mouth → pharynx → esophagus → reticulorumen → omasum → abomasum → duodenum → jejunum → ileum → cecum → colon → rectum → anus

Along the way, accessory organs are available to help with digestion. These organs are not located in the digestive tube itself, but they play an important role in digestion. The **pancreas** provides enzymes that help to break down complex food into absorbable nutrients. The **liver** produces bile, which helps to break down fats. Bile is stored in the **gall bladder.**

BOX 10-1   **Terms That Defy Word Analysis**

- antrum—cavity within a structure
- borborygmus—a rumbling noise that gas makes as it moves through the stomach and intestines; your "stomach growling"
- bowel—another name for the intestines
- cachexia—generalized wasting of the body as a result of disease
- chyme—a semifluid mass of partially digested food that enters the small intestine from the stomach
- cud—the portion of partially digested food that a ruminant returns to the mouth for further mastication before sending it to the omasum
- deciduous—temporary teeth; also known as milk teeth or baby teeth
- enzyme—protein produced by living cells that initiates a chemical reaction (e.g., digestion) but is not affected by the reaction
- eructation—burp; the method by which ruminants continually get rid of fermentation gases
- flatus—intestinal gas produced by the action of bacteria
- ingest—to take into the body (e.g., food, liquids)
- ingesta—ingested material, especially food taken into the body via the mouth
- melena—passing dark, tarry feces containing blood that has been acted upon by bacteria in the intestines
- occlusion—the way the upper and lower teeth line up against each other
- paralumbar fossa—the dorsal area of the flank; the dorsal, soft, triangular portion of the flank
- peristalsis—a progressive wave of contraction and relaxation of the smooth muscles in the wall of the digestive tract that moves food through the digestive tract
- reflex—automatic, unthinking reaction or behavior
- relapse—to fall back into a disease state after an apparent recovery
- retrograde—inverted, reversed, backward, recede, deteriorate
- rumination—bringing ingesta from the reticulorumen back to the mouth, followed by remastication and reswallowing
  - This occurs predominantly when the animal is resting and is not eating.
- sphincter—a circular band of voluntary or involuntary muscle that encircles an opening of the body or one of its hollow organs
- viable—capable of living, workable, capable of being done

FUNCTION OF THE DIGESTIVE SYSTEM

Digestion

Every structure and organ of the digestive system has a specific task, starting with gathering the food and finishing with eliminating feces (Table 10-3).

The **mouth** contains many structures that are necessary to begin the digestive process. The **lips** form the opening to the digestive system and are used by many animals for **prehension** of their food because they do not have hands or silverware.

The **gums** consist of a mucous membrane with its supporting fibrous tissue that covers the surfaces of the mandible and the maxilla in the mouth. They surround the teeth and provide a seal around them.

Structures of the Mouth

lips
gums
teeth
cheeks
tongue
salivary glands

Teeth are used for grooming and defense; however, their primary function is **mechanical mastication,** which breaks down food into smaller particles. The teeth that are rooted in the upper jaw (maxillary and incisive bones) make up the **maxillary arcade** (*arch*) or the **upper arcade.** The teeth rooted in the lower jaw (mandible) constitute the **mandibular arcade** or the **lower arcade.** Dental formulas label each tooth by its type using a number related to its position within the arcade.

Mammals have two sets of teeth: **deciduous** teeth (milk teeth, baby teeth), which are temporary in young animals, and **permanent** teeth, which replace deciduous teeth as the animal ages. Four types of permanent teeth are present in an animal's mouth:
- **incisor teeth** (represented by the letter "I")
  - These are the most rostral teeth and are used for grasping food.
  - Most animals have two upper incisors and two lower incisors on either side of the midline of the jaw.
  - When counting teeth, you begin with an incisor and work caudally.
  - Ruminants do not have upper incisors. Instead they have a **dental pad.** Think of someone with his false teeth out.
- **canine teeth** (represented by the letter "C")
  - These are the teeth next to the incisors; they are used for tearing food.
  - Ruminants are also missing their upper canine teeth. In piglets, the deciduous third incisors and the canine teeth are called **needle teeth;** they are clipped to prevent damage to the sow's mammary glands while piglets are suckling.
  - The tusks of wild boars are overgrown canine teeth.
  - Vampires need canine teeth to suck blood.
- **premolar teeth** (represented by the letter "P")
  - These are next to the canine teeth and are used to tear and cut food.
  - The upper P4 in a dog is the fourth upper premolar tooth counting from rostral to caudal.
  - Horses have an extra premolar **(wolf tooth)** left over from its ancestors.
- **molar teeth** (represented by the letter "M")
  - These are the most caudal teeth in the mouth and are used for grinding food.
  - Molars and premolars are sometimes called the **cheek teeth.**
  - **Carnassial teeth** are large cheek teeth in dogs and cats that are used for shearing or cutting. In the dog, they are upper P4 and lower M1. In the cat, they are upper P3 and lower M1.

Two styles of permanent teeth are seen in animals. **Brachydont** teeth ("short teeth") consist of a **crown** encased in **enamel,** a **neck,** and a **root** permanently embedded in a jaw bone. This type of tooth is seen in carnivores and pigs. **Hypsodont** teeth ("high teeth") consist of a body encased in enamel and a root embedded in a jaw bone. These teeth continue to erupt (grow) throughout the animal's life and must be worn down naturally, or must be cut or filed down manually. This type of tooth is seen in horses and in the cheek teeth of ruminants.

Occlusion is the way the upper and lower teeth line up against each other. **Malocclusions** can be inherited (breed disposition) or acquired. In cases of inherited malocclusion, the shape and length of the muzzle play an important role. If the lower jaw (mandible) protrudes farther rostral than the upper jaw (maxilla), the condition is known as **prognathism.** If the upper jaw protrudes farther rostral than the lower jaw (parrot mouth, overbite), the condition is known as **brachygnathism.** Acquired malocclusions can result from malnutrition, environmental factors, or mechanical forces.

The **cheeks** form the side walls of the mouth or **buccal cavity.**

The **tongue** is a muscular organ under voluntary control that is used for prehension and to move food through the mouth to the throat for swallowing. The tongue also contains minor salivary glands and taste buds. All vertebrates have taste buds; the number and type depend on the animal's diet. Herbivores have the greatest number of taste buds, so they can differentiate good plants from toxic plants. Many species develop food preferences and aversions through their taste buds.

Salivary glands lie outside the mouth, but they add saliva to moisten and lubricate food via their ducts that open into the mouth. Saliva contains some digestive enzymes that start to break down food, especially carbohydrates (sugars and starches). Adult cattle take the prize for producing the most saliva. In one day, they can generate 100 to 150 liters. They need this much saliva to moisten all that dry plant material that they eat.

The **pharynx** or throat is caudal to the mouth. This is the same pharynx that is used by the respiratory system. Remember the epiglottis? When an animal swallows, the epiglottis is pulled shut by the muscles of the larynx. Try this. Put your finger lightly on your Adam's apple and swallow. Did you feel the larynx move up? With that action, the epiglottis closes and food goes down the esophagus—usually.

The **esophagus** is the muscular tube that connects the pharynx to the stomach in monogastric animals. It travels down the neck, through the thoracic cavity and diaphragm, and into the abdominal cavity. The esophagus is the transport tube that moves food along by waves of smooth muscle contractions known as **peristalsis.**

The remaining organs of the digestive system are located in the abdomen, where they are covered by a thin membrane called the **visceral peritoneum.** The visceral peritoneum of the stomach extends into a double-layered flat sheet called the **omentum,** which is positioned over the stomach and other organs. It has a lacy appearance because of the patches of fat that it contains. The visceral peritoneum is also continuous with another membrane **(parietal peritoneum)** that lines the abdominal and pelvic cavities. The potential space between these two membranes is called the **peritoneal cavity.** The digestive tract is suspended in the peritoneal cavity by fused double layers of parietal peritoneum called **mesentery.** The mesentery carries blood vessels, lymphatics, and nerves to and from the digestive tract.

Remember those special organs of digestion mentioned earlier in the chapter? **Ruminants** are a group of animals that have developed three large compartments at the caudal end of the esophagus, where the plants they eat can stay awhile to initiate the digestive process. These three extra compartments, called **forestomachs,** are located between the end of the esophagus and the stomach (Figure 10-2). The compartments are the **rumen,** the **reticulum,** and the **omasum.**

The first compartment, the rumen, is the largest compartment. After food arrives from the esophagus, the muscular rumen wall with its many folds and sacs contracts rhythmically to mix food with the large amounts of saliva that all ruminants produce. The rumen is also a large fermentation vat, containing many microbes (microorganisms) that break down cellulose into substances that ruminants are able to use. The action of microbes produces large amounts of gas that rise to the top of the rumen. Fermentation generates about 30 to 50 liters of gas per hour in adult cattle, and about 5 liters per hour in sheep or goats. Fortunately, ruminants belch a lot. All the gas that is produced has to go somewhere, or it would just continue to accumulate within the rumen. You will not hear loud burps, though, because the gas that comes up the esophagus makes a U-turn in the pharynx and is inhaled before it is exhaled. This entire process is called **eructation.**

The lighter, more recently eaten plant material floats within the rumen for further digestion. The heavier, denser material drops to the bottom of the rumen and into the reticulum (Figure 10-3).

The smallest and most cranial forestomach compartment, the reticulum, compresses food. Because the reticulum and the rumen are nearly continuous with each other, they are referred to as the **reticulorumen.** The reticulum part is sometimes referred to as the **honeycomb** because the mucous membrane lining has numerous small, six-sided folds that make it look like a honeycomb (Figure 10-4).

Have you ever heard the term "chewing her cud" in reference to someone chewing gum? In people, it is not that attractive. In ruminants, it is part of digestion and is something they do naturally. Plant cellulose is very difficult to digest. Once through the mouth does not allow enough time for ruminants to break down plant food. So they **regurgitate** partially digested food back into their mouths through reverse

Tripe is the main ingredient in the Mexican soup, menudo. The lining of any of the three forestomachs is used. Tripe can be eaten by itself. Tripe is also slang for something that is false or worthless.

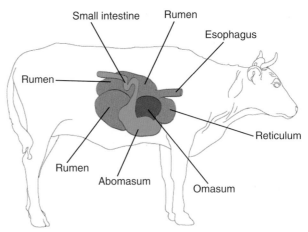

FIGURE 10-2 The forestomachs and abomasum of a cow. Location of the rumen, reticulum, omasum, and abomasum as seen from right side of cow.

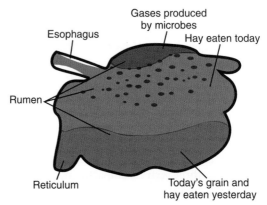

FIGURE 10-3 Layers of material in the rumen. Grain and yesterday's hay are the heaviest materials, so they have fallen to the bottom of the rumen and into the reticulum.

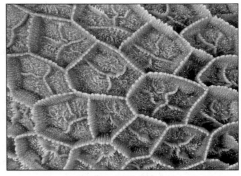

FIGURE 10-4 The mucous membrane lining of the reticulum. Note the honeycomb appearance. (From Dyce K, Sack W, Wensing CJG: *Textbook of Veterinary Anatomy,* ed 4, St Louis, 2010, Saunders.)

peristalsis via the esophagus. Back in the mouth, the animals will chew it some more (i.e., the cud) and then reswallow it. This breaks down the plant material into even smaller particles, providing a larger surface area upon which microbes can work. This entire process, called **rumination,** occurs most often when the animal has finished eating and is resting.

The entrance to the third compartment, the omasum, comes off the reticulum through the **reticulo-omasal orifice.** The omasum is sometimes referred to as the

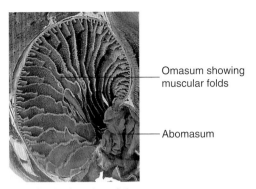

Omasum showing muscular folds

Abomasum

FIGURE 10-5 The many folds in the interior of the omasum. (Adapted from Dyce K, Sack W, Wensing CJG: *Textbook of Veterinary Anatomy*, ed 4, St Louis, 2010, Saunders.)

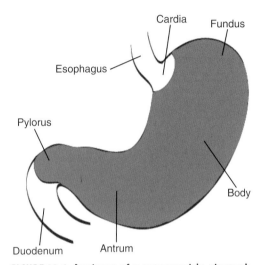

Cardia

Fundus

Esophagus

Pylorus

Body

Duodenum   Antrum

FIGURE 10-6 Anatomy of a monogastric stomach.

book or **manyplies** (*plies* = folds) because its interior contains many muscular folds that fill the lumen, making it look like the pages of a book (Figure 10-5). The function of the omasum is not well understood. Fluid rapidly passes through the omasum, leaving behind tiny food particles clinging to its folds. These particles drop off and enter the true stomach of the ruminant, the **abomasum.**

From this point on, the structures in the digestive tract of ruminants and of monogastric animals are the same. Some structures have become more developed in some species. For instance, the horse's cecum (in the large intestine) has adapted to its plant-based diet by becoming its main fermentation organ.

The **stomach** receives food from the esophagus (or the **abomasum** receives food from the omasum in ruminants) in an area called the *cardia*. The **cardiac sphincter** can close to prevent backup of food (Figure 10-6).

The body and fundus areas of the stomach distend when the food arrives. This area contains gastric glands that secrete hydrochloric acid, digestive enzymes, and mucus that partially digests the food. Food does not stay in one area of the stomach; it is further broken down as it is moved around by contractions of muscles within the stomach wall. In the **pyloric antrum** area, food is ground into even smaller particles by muscle contractions.

After all of this partial digestion and grinding, the food has become a semifluid material called **chyme.** Chyme slowly passes through the **pyloric sphincter** into the small intestines—the beginning of the intestinal tract. This sphincter closes to prevent food backup.

EXERCISE 10-2 *Position It!*

When reviewing the anatomy of the digestive tract, it is important to know the parts that make up the whole. It is also important to know the relative position of each part to the other parts. Below is a list of the parts of the digestive tract of a monogastric animal. Number the parts of the digestive tract in order from most caudal to most cranial/rostral.

___1___ anus

___10___ cardiac sphincter

___4___ cecum

___3___ colon

___7___ duodenum

___11___ esophagus

___5___ ileum

___16___ incisor

___6___ jejunem

___14___ molar

___12___ pharynx

___15___ premolar

___8___ pyloric sphincter

___2___ rectum

___9___ stomach

___13___ tongue

Check your answers at the end of the chapter, Answers to Exercises.

CASE STUDY 10-2 | 2004-1333 COW RFID TAG #230 123 500374

Signalment and History: A 4-year-old lactating Holstein **cow** was brought to the Frisbee LA Hospital because she had been "off feed" and her milk production had gone down over the past week and a half. She had **calved** 1 month previously. The owner noticed that the cow's left **flank** area was distended and reported that the cow was passing very little **feces.**

Physical Examination: Dr. Murdoch and veterinary technician Pat unloaded the cow from the trailer and performed an initial physical examination. The cow's **TPR** was normal. Her ears were cold and her eyes were dilated. A vaginal discharge suggested the presence of a metritis (**inflammation** of the uterus). Dr. Murdoch "flicked" and **auscultated** the cow's **abdomen** from her left **hook bone** to the point of her left elbow. In the upper third of the area between the 9th and 13th **intercostal** spaces, in the **paralumbar fossa,** he heard the diagnostic "ping" of a left displaced **abomasum.** On rectal palpation, Dr. Murdoch felt the right displaced **rumen** caused by the left displaced abomasum. He noted that the uterine horns were thick. Dr. Murdoch performed **ultrasonography** over the left abdominal area to confirm the **diagnosis.** Pat drew a blood sample and submitted it (along with a urine sample) to the lab for a **CBC** and **serum biochemical** testing. The **hemogram** was within expected reference ranges, but both serum analysis and urinalysis indicated inadequate carbohydrate metabolism (mild starvation) resulting in lipolysis for energy. A mild **hypocalcemia** was also present.

Diagnosis: Dr. Murdoch explained that an underlying condition, probably the metritis, had caused GI tract **atony**, which led to abomasal atony, with the abomasum filling with gas. The abomasum then floated dorsally and over the rumen to the left side of the cow. This resulted in a left displaced abomasum.

Treatment: Dr. Murdoch discussed treatment options with the owner, and together they decided that a combination of medical and surgical treatments offered the best course because the cow was one of the owner's top producers. Pat prepared the cow for a **right flank omentopexy** through a **laparotomy incision. Presurgical IV** fluids containing electrolytes and **antibiotics** were started. An antibiotic solution was placed in the uterus for treatment of the metritis.

Outcome: The surgery was uncomplicated and successfully returned the abomasum to its normal position, with its **omentum** fixed to the abdominal wall. The cow returned to her farm, where **IM** injections of antibiotics were administered by the owner for the next 3 days. The cow's milk production and appetite gradually returned to normal. A week after antibiotic injections ended, the cow was returned to her normal rotation in the milking line.

EXERCISE 10-3 *Case It!*

Read Case Study 10-2. Fill in the squares by identifying the word parts used in some of the clinical veterinary language of this case study. Then define each word. The first word is done as an example.

	Word Parts	**Word Definition**
presurgery	pre-, surgery	happening before surgery
1. laparotomy	tomy,	surgical incision into the flank
2. paralumbar	para, dr	near or beside the loin flank
3. atony	ton/y	without pressure or tension
4. diagnosis	Gnosis	through knowledge
5. lipolysis	lysis	breaking down of fat
6. hemogram	Gram	written record of blood
7. intercostal		Between the ribs
8. omentopexy	pexy, Surgery	fixation of the omentum.
	Surgical	

Check your answers at the end of the chapter, Answers to Exercises.

TABLE 10-3	Word Parts Associated with Digestion and the Digestive System		
Word Part	**Meaning**	**Example and Definition**	**Word Parts**
-orexia	appetite, desire	**anorexia** loss of appetite for food, especially when caused by disease	an- = without, no, not -orexia = appetite, desire
amyl/o	starch	**amylodyspepsia** unable to digest starchy foods	amyl/o = starch dys- = bad, defective, painful, or difficult peps/o = digestion -ia = pertaining to
sacchar/o glyc/o	sugar	**monosaccharide** a simple sugar, such as glucose or fructose, that cannot be broken down into simpler sugars	mono- = one sacchar/o = sugar -ide = pertaining to
		hypoglycemia abnormally low amount of sugar in the blood	hypo- = under, beneath, below glyc/o = sugar -emia = blood condition (usually abnormal)
gluc/o	glucose	**cytoglucopenia** a deficiency of glucose within the cells	cyt/o = cell gluc/o = glucose, sugar -penia = lack, deficiency
-rrhea	flow, flowing	**diarrhea** abnormally frequent discharge of semisolid or fluid fecal matter from the bowel ◆ *Dia*rrhea *literally means a "flow through." Do you agree?*	dia- = across, through -rrhea = flow, flowing
steat/o lip/o	fat	**steatorrhea** a large amount of fat is in the feces because of a failure to digest and absorb it	steat/o = fat -rrhea = flow, flowing
		lipolysis the breaking down of fat	lip/o = fat lys/o = destruction, dissolution, dissolving, breakage -is = structure, thing
-ase	enzyme	**lipase** an enzyme used to break down the fat in food so it can be absorbed in the intestines	lip/o = fat -ase = enzyme
pre-	before (in time and place)	**prefix** to attach or fasten something in front of	pre- = before (in time and place) fix = attach, fasten

TABLE 10-3	Word Parts Associated with Digestion and the Digestive System—cont'd		
Word Part	**Meaning**	**Example and Definition**	**Word Parts**
mal-	diseased, bad, abnormal, defective	**malodorous** smelly, stinky	mal- = diseased, bad, abnormal, defective odor = a scent -ous = pertaining to
-lith lith/o	stone	**cholelith** stone made of bile or gall; a gall stone	chol/e = bile, gall -lith = stone
		lithogenesis production or formation of stones *Even if you have not heard of a stone referred to as a* lith, *you are probably familiar with* lithographs, *the pictures made from specially prepared stones or flat plates that hold or repel the ink.*	lith/o = stone gen/o = formation, beginning -esis = process of an action
-iasis	pathological condition that results from	**lithiasis** pathological condition that results from a stone *Word parts that comprise the suffix* -iasis *will look familiar to you:* -ia = *pertaining to; and* -sis = *state, condition, action, process, or result.*	lith/o = stone -iasis = pathological condition that results
-ptosis	downward placement, drooping	**enteroptosis** abnormal downward placement of the intestines in the abdominal cavity	enter/o = intestines -ptosis = downward placement, drooping
herni/o	hernia, the protrusion of tissue or part of an organ through an opening in the surrounding walls	**herniorrhaphy** surgical repair by suturing closed an opening in the wall of a body cavity	herni/o = hernia -rrhaphy = suture
-cele	protrusion, hernia	**tracheoaerocele** a hernia in the mucous membrane of the trachea containing air	trache/o = trachea aer/o = air -cele = protrusion, hernia
chyl/o	chyle, a milky fluid consisting of fats and other products of digestion absorbed into lymph from the small intestine	**chylorrhea** flow or discharge of chyle	chyl/o = chyle -rrhea = flow, flowing

mal-

-lith

lith/o

-iasis

-ptosis

herni/o

-cele

chyl/o

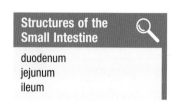

Structures of the Small Intestine

duodenum
jejunum
ileum

Absorption

The intestinal tract is divided into the **small intestine** and the **large intestine.** The **duodenum** is the first segment of the small intestine. Next is the **jejunum,** which is the longest segment. The **ileum** is the last segment.

Most of the absorption of nutrients takes place through the wall of the jejunum because it is the longest segment. Nutrients such as sodium, chloride, potassium, and vitamins are absorbed intact without further breakdown. Other more complex nutrients like carbohydrates, proteins, and fats must undergo further chemical breakdown before they can be absorbed. For this to occur, enzymes are needed. However, the intestines cannot produce sufficient quantities of the enzymes themselves. They rely on other abdominal organs to provide them.

Complex carbohydrates **(polysaccharides)** and starches are broken down by the enzyme **amylase,** which is produced by the **pancreas** and is secreted into the duodenum. Some species of animals have small amounts of amylase in their saliva; these species are able to start digesting sugars and starches in their mouths.

Proteins must be broken down into smaller segments (their component **amino acids**) before they can be absorbed. The enzyme **gastric pepsin** begins the breakdown process inside the stomach. Other enzymes called **proteases** help break down proteins. They are produced by the pancreas and are secreted into the small intestines.

When **fats** reach the stomach and encounter the water-based partially digested food, they ball up into large fat globules. (Remember—oil [fat] and water do not mix well.) These globules are broken down into smaller fat globules by the churning action within the pyloric antrum. When these smaller globules move into the small intestines, they are further broken down by **lipase** from the pancreas and by **bile,** which is produced by the **liver** and is stored in the **gall bladder** until it is needed. After an animal has eaten, the gall bladder empties by reflex action and sends bile into the duodenum via the bile duct. Horses, rats, and elephants do not have gall bladders, so bile produced within their livers is continuously secreted into the duodenum.

While the chyme is traveling through the small intestines, many nutrients are absorbed through the intestinal wall into capillaries. Blood vessels then carry the nutrient-rich blood to the liver via a system called the **hepatic portal system.** When blood reaches the liver, it enters hepatic sinusoids that are lined with phagocytes. These phagocytes remove bacteria, toxins, and other foreign material from the blood before it is distributed to the body.

The lymphatic system also picks up some of the nutrients (especially fats) from the chyme through tiny lymph vessels called **lacteals.** After absorption by the lacteals, the liquid that was chyme in the intestines is now called **chyle.** Eventually, the chyle will be carried to the thoracic duct, where it is dumped into the vena cava and enters the bloodstream.

The tiny fat droplets that make up chyle are called **chylomicrons;** they turn the lymph an opaque, milky white. Chylomicrons turn the plasma in the bloodstream the same opaque, milky white as they did in the lymph. The presence of chylomicrons in plasma after an animal eats is called **postprandial lipemia.** The number of chylomicrons present determines the degree of opacity of the plasma. This number is highest right after an animal has eaten and can make the plasma unsuitable for some biochemical analyses. Clear plasma is most desirable for analyses; therefore, most blood samples should be drawn before an animal eats.

Elimination

After most nutrients have been absorbed into the body, the "leftovers" pass into the large intestine. The **cecum, colon,** and **rectum** make up the large intestine.

At the place where the ileum joins the large intestine, a blind sac branches off the intestinal wall. This is the cecum, and it is found at the **ileocecal junction.** In carnivores and ruminants, the cecum is small and is poorly developed. However, in the horse (a nonruminant herbivore), the cecum is large and is very well developed. A

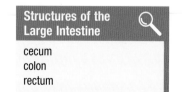

Structures of the Large Intestine

cecum
colon
rectum

horse's colon and cecum together are called the **hindgut.** It acts much like the fore-stomach (especially the reticulorumen in a ruminant) to serve as a fermentation vat for cellulose. Rats, rabbits, and guinea pigs also rely on hindgut fermentation to help them digest their food.

The colon in carnivores is merely a long tube that carries material from the small intestine directly to the rectum. The primary duty of the colon is to return fluid and electrolytes back into the body. What is left is eliminated from the body as **feces** (also known as **excrement** or **stercus**). The colon secretes mucus to help lubricate feces as they pass. Also, large numbers of microorganisms act on the feces. *Escherichia coli* and *Salmonella* spp. are two of the microorganisms you have probably heard about. Food contaminated by feces from one animal can cause disease in another animal. Animals do not get sick from their own microorganisms while they are still in the digestive tract because—remember—if they are still in the digestive tract, then these microorganisms are outside of the body!

The rectum is the most caudal segment of the large intestine. Its wall is capable of distending in the presence of feces. This allows the rectum to store feces until they are eliminated. The act of passing feces is called **defecation.**

The rectum terminates at the **anus,** which is surrounded by internal and external sphincter muscles. In some animals, the external sphincter is under voluntary control and will not open until the animal is ready to defecate. The internal sphincter, which works under involuntary control, opens reflexively when the rectum is distended with feces.

A FEW WORDS ABOUT THE LIVER AND PANCREAS

The **liver** is the largest gland and the second largest organ in an animal's body. (The skin is the largest organ.) The liver sits just caudal to the diaphragm in the cranial portion of the abdominal cavity and is grossly divided into several lobes. The stomach snuggles into its caudal surface. The many important functions of the liver include the following:

- production of bile
  - Bile contains acidic bile salts, cholesterol, and bilirubin (yellow pigment that comes from hemoglobin breakdown when red blood cells die or are destroyed).
  - The bile is stored until it is needed in the gall bladder, which is tucked in between the lobes of the liver.
  - After an animal eats, the gall bladder releases bile into the duodenum to aid in fat digestion.
  - Horses, rats, and elephants do not have gall bladders, so bile produced in their livers is continuously secreted into the duodenum.
- production and storage of glycogen
  - The liver takes glucose absorbed from the intestine, converts it to glycogen, and stores it.
  - When the body needs more glucose for energy, the liver converts the glycogen back to glucose.
- storage and metabolism
  - Nutrients such as amino acids, vitamins, and minerals are absorbed from the gastrointestinal tract.
- production of blood proteins
  - Three examples of blood proteins are those used to clot blood, the immunoglobulins, and albumin, which helps maintain fluid balance in the blood by preventing excessive movement of fluid into tissue through capillary walls.
- metabolism and neutralization of drugs, toxins, and alcohol
  - When an animal receives certain medications, they stay in the body only as long as it takes the liver to metabolize them.

- storage of iron from red blood cell (RBC) breakdown
- conversion of ammonia
  - Ammonia is a by-product of protein metabolism. It is converted to urea, which can be eliminated through the urine.

The **pancreas** lies along the walls of the pyloric antrum of the stomach and duodenum. It actually consists of two glands inside one organ. One of the glands produces digestive enzymes: amylase, protease, and lipase. The other gland produces hormones, in particular, **insulin** and **glucagon,** which help regulate blood glucose levels. Insulin is released after a meal when the blood glucose level rises. The function of insulin is to react to an elevated blood glucose level by facilitating movement of glucose from the blood into the cells, where it is used for energy production. This results in lowering of the blood glucose level. Glucagon is released in response to **hypoglycemia.** Glucagon is called an **insulin antagonist** because it encourages glucose release from the liver to raise the blood glucose level. The two hormones work together to maintain blood glucose homeostasis. **Diabetes mellitus** is a disease caused by lack of insulin, or by the inability of cells to react to insulin.

EXERCISE 10-4 *Build It!*

Using the word parts for the digestive tract and word parts you have learned in previous chapters, construct words with the following definitions. There may be more than one correct answer for a definition.

1. _____ not eating

2. _____ gall bladder stone

3. _____ inflammation of the pancreas

4. _____ suture of the stomach

5. _____ rupture of the middle segment of the small intestine

6. _____ tumor of the liver

7. _____ a blood-filled protrusion or hernia

8. _____ one who straightens teeth

9. _____ making an incision into the esophagus

10. _____ eating abnormally fast

11. _____ inflammation of the stomach and intestines

12. _____ removal of pieces of gum

13. _____ inflammation of the throat

14. _____ making a new opening into the rumen

15. _____ surgically fixing the abomasum to the body wall

16. _____ a disease of the rectum

Check your answers at the end of the chapter, Answers to Exercises.

BOX 10-2 **Terms That Defy Word Analysis**

- constipation—bowel movements that are infrequent or hard to pass
- displacement—movement of one segment of the digestive tract to an abnormal location
- distention—abnormal enlargement of a part of the digestive tract
- emesis—vomiting of food from the stomach (compare with regurgitation)
- emetic—a substance that causes vomiting
- enema—injection of a fluid into the rectum to stimulate a bowel movement
- gavage—tube-feeding through a stomach tube
- ileus—lack of neuromuscular control of the intestines, which prevents ingesta from moving through the intestines at a normal rate
- impaction—physical blockage of one part of the digestive tract by abnormal amounts of material
- intussusception—slipping or telescoping of one part of a tubular organ into a lower portion, causing obstruction; seen especially in the intestines
- laxative—a substance that induces bowel movements or loosens the stool; most often taken to relieve constipation
- lesion—localized pathological change in an organ or tissue; a wound or injury
- nosocomial—hospital-acquired
- regurgitation—bringing back to the mouth food that has not yet reached the stomach
- retch—involuntary spasms of ineffective vomiting; dry heaves
- ruminal tympany—overdistention of the reticulorumen as a result of rumen gas being trapped in the rumen when the ruminant is unable to eructate; also known as *bloat* or *hoven*
- torsion—twisting or rotating on a long axis
- ulcer—a depressed lesion on the skin or mucous membrane accompanied by inflammation, pus formation, and necrosis
- volvulus—abnormal twisting of the intestines, causing an obstruction

EXERCISE 10-5 *Ouch!*

Define the following conditions and in the blank before the word indicate whether it is (yes) or is not (no) considered a lesion. The first one is done for you as an example.

yes	**1.** abrasion	*a skin scrape*
	2. alopecia	
	3. gastric ulcer	
	4. pneumothorax	
	5. laceration	
	6. proud flesh	
	7. esophageal abscess	
	8. rhabdomyolysis	
	9. osteochondritis	
	10. papule	

Check your answers at the end of the chapter, Answers to Exercises.

DISORDERS OF THE DIGESTIVE SYSTEM

You have just learned that the digestive system is a complex system made up of many structures. Each of these structures is susceptible to injury, disease, and repair. You may witness everything from cheiloplasty to proctalgia, and you will be able to dissect the names of most of the disorders that you encounter. However, some gastrointestinal disorders have been given "common" names that people will use instead of the "medical" names. Examples of these common names include the following:

- colic in horses—a symptom, not a disease; a condition of abdominal pain often caused by an intestinal disorder or by infection elsewhere in the body
- bloat in ruminants—overdistention of the reticulorumen due to trapped rumen gas
- grain overload in ruminants—also known as **carbohydrate engorgement, rumen stasis,** and **lactic acidosis**
  - This results from eating too much grain (or other food), which in turn leads to indigestion, acidosis, and possibly death.
- hardware disease in ruminants—also known as **traumatic reticuloperitonitis**
  - This is most common in mature dairy cattle, which are indiscriminate eaters when it comes to ingesting foreign objects with their food.
  - Items such as nails and pieces of broken barbed wire are swallowed and get caught in the honeycomb folds of the reticulum. From there, they penetrate the reticular wall, causing an inflammatory reaction within the peritoneum. Sometimes the object will penetrate the diaphragm and pericardial sac, causing pericarditis.
- bloat in dogs—gastric dilation volvulus (GDV)
  - This life-threatening emergency situation is primarily seen in large, deep-chested dogs.
  - It involves a gastric obstruction that leads to gas buildup in the stomach, followed by torsion of the stomach clockwise at the distal esophagus.

- inflammatory bowel disease (IBD)—a group of gastrointestinal diseases of dogs and cats characterized by chronic inflammation of various areas of the GI tract
  - The cause is unknown.
  - Some of the diseases included in this group are chronic lymphocytic-plasmacytic colitis of dogs, lymphocytic-plasmacytic enteritis in cats, eosinophilic gastroenteritis and colitis, and suppurative colitis.

TABLE 10-4	Abbreviations	
Abbreviation	**Meaning**	**Example**
GI	gastrointestinal	The GI tract is a complex organ.
TPN	total parenteral nutrition	Analyzing to find the word parts in **parenteral,** you will discover: par- = other than, abnormal enter/o = intestines in general -al = pertaining to This means that nutrition must be administered by means other than the mouth (i.e., usually by IV administration).
PRN	as often as necessary, as needed	Many times analgesics are prescribed PRN. You give the medication at the prescribed dose as often as necessary. PRN *is not the same as* ad lib. *There is no prescribed amount to give when a medication is* ad lib; *you just give as much as you have to for the desired result.*
ASAP	as soon as possible	Maybe not a **right-now** emergency, but you should attend to the matter ASAP.
NA *or* N/A	not applicable	You can use NA or N/A on a form when the question does not apply to the animal in question, like How many pregnancies has the M(C) dog gone through?
>	greater than	Notice that in >, the open, wide part comes at the beginning and is larger than the closed ending.
<	less than	Owners of dogs that received >0.8 mg of diazepam/kg (0.36 mg/lb) were more likely to report increased activity as an adverse effect than were owners of dogs that received <0.8 mg/kg. Based on this, would you say the higher or the lower dose was more favorable?
PD	polydipsia	Use PD when Sparky's owner tells you that Sparky has been drinking a lot of water lately.
ICU	intensive care unit	An animal that is very ill will be put in the ICU, where it can receive special individual care.
MM mm	mucous membrane *or* millimeter *or* muscles	Apply a 3-mm strip of ointment to the mm of the mouth, or rub a 6-mm strip into the mm of the rump.
DA	displaced abomasum	The abomasum that is loosely suspended by the omentum so it moves around could become a DA.
LDA	left displaced abomasum	If the abomasum is displaced to the left, it becomes an LDA.
RDA	right displaced abomasum	If the abomasum is displaced to the right, it becomes an RDA.
BM	bowel movement	Some dogs are trained to have a BM on command. Try that with a cow.

CASE STUDY 10-1 #2010-5832 SARGE

Signalment and History: An 8-year-old 145-pound male (castrated) Great Dane canine named Sarge was brought to the Frisbee Small Animal Clinic because of a distended abdomen and an **acute** history of **regurgitation, retching, vomiting** of white foam, and excessive salivation. Sarge was whining continuously when he was brought into the clinic.

Physical Examination: Dr. Frisbee recognized an emergency situation coming on, so she quickly performed an initial physical examination with Jess's help. Notable findings included **lethargy**, pale mucous membranes, abdominal distention, **tachycardia** (210 beats per minute), and a **palpably** large mass in the **mid-abdominal** region. Intravenous fluids were started immediately and included 5 liters of crystalloids to expand Sarge's blood volume. Fresh plasma was also administered because Dr. Frisbee was concerned about Sarge's cardiovascular status and the possibility that he might develop a **coagulopathy**, or disseminated **intravascular coagulation.**

Blood was collected for serum biochemical analyses, a complete blood count, and coagulation tests. The serum biochemical results showed **hypoglycemia, hyperphosphatemia,** and **hyperproteinemia.** A **neutrophilia, lymphocytopenia,** and **macrocytic, normochromic** red blood cells were seen on the **hemogram.** Results of coagulation tests were within expected reference limits.

Right lateral thoracic and **abdominal** X-rays showed indications of **gastric dilation and volvulus** (GDV) with secondary **megaesophagus.** With Sarge in right lateral recumbency, Dr. Frisbee inserted a 16-gauge needle through the abdominal wall lateral to the ventral midline and into the stomach to immediately relieve gas distention. After providing mild sedation, Dr. Frisbee tried to pass a stomach tube but was unsuccessful. A 16-gauge needle was again inserted into the stomach, and this time gas and approximately 475 milliliters of malodorous, dark brown fluid were removed. Sarge was then prepared for surgery.

Treatment: After Sarge was anesthetized, his abdomen was opened via a **ventral midline incision.** Dr. Frisbee confirmed gastric dilation and volvulus. The large mass was the spleen, which was engorged but **viable** with adequate **venous** drainage. Dr. Frisbee repositioned the stomach. Jess passed an **orogastric** tube, and the stomach contents were removed. Dr. Frisbee was concerned about the viability of approximately 15% of the gastric wall, so she excised the area of discoloration and thinning, along with a margin of healthy tissue surrounding the area. Dr. Frisbee performed a **gastropexy** to fix the **pyloric end** of the stomach to the right abdominal wall, so hopefully it would twist again.

Outcome: Sarge recovered from anesthesia without complications. He received painkillers (0.05 milligrams per kilogram, intramuscular, as needed) for pain control and intravenous administration of a crystalloid solution (5 milligrams per kilogram every hour). Sarge was discharged 2 days after surgery; at that time, he had a good appetite, and his prescription had been discontinued.

CASE STUDY 10-3 #2010-5917 SARGE

History: Twenty-one days after surgery, Sarge was again admitted to the Frisbee Small Animal Clinic because of a 3-day history of listlessness, **anorexia,** and weakness. He had collapsed that morning. Sarge was admitted to the hospital.

Physical Examination: Jess performed an initial exam and found that Sarge was mildly depressed, pyrexic (**rectal** temperature, 103.5 degrees Fahrenheit), and tachycardic (120 beats per minute). His pulse quality was poor, and mucous membranes were pale and moist. Sarge had lost 6.82 pounds since his discharge 21 days before. A palpable mass was again detected in the mid-abdominal region. **Rectal palpation** revealed **melena.** Dr. Frisbee instructed Jess to draw blood for a complete blood count and serum biochemical testing. The results showed that Sarge was hypoproteinemic. The hemogram revealed **microcytic, hypochromic,** nonregenerative anemia. Additionally, mature neutrophilia and lymphocytopenia were detected. Results of a coagulation profile were within expected reference ranges. Transfusion of 2 units of packed red blood cells improved mucous membrane color and pulse quality.

Thoracic X-rays revealed a small volume of **pleural effusion.** Abdominal X-rays revealed a **peritoneal effusion** and possible **splenomegaly.** Dr. Frisbee performed an abdominal **ultrasonography,** which showed a splenic **infarct** secondary to a **thrombus** at the tip of the spleen, **edema** in the stomach consistent with the **gastric** surgery, and a peritoneal effusion.

Diagnosis: On the basis of diagnostic test findings, Dr. Frisbee thought gastric **ulceration** and splenic infarction was the primary differential diagnosis. The owner agreed to an exploratory **laparotomy.** Dr. Frisbee decided to perform an **endoscopy** of the upper portion of the gastrointestinal **tract** before performing the laparotomy, to identify any ulceration that might not be visible during surgery.

Treatment: Gastrointestinal endoscopy revealed a large focal area of gastric ulceration. Dr. Frisbee found a splenic **torsion** with a focal splenic infarct, so she performed a total **splenectomy.** A 5-centimeter **gastrotomy** incision was made along the ventral surface of the greater curvature of the stomach. A 5 × 3-centimeter gastric ulcer was located at the site of the previous surgery. The ulcerated area was **resected,** and the stomach was closed. Samples of splenic tissue and of the resected ulcerated gastric tissue were submitted for **histological** evaluation.

Outcome: Histology of the splenic tissue showed **necrotic changes** with marked congestion and **lymphocytolysis.** Dr. Frisbee thought this was most likely due to an **anoxia** that resulted from complete **occlusion** of the **arterial** supply to that area of the spleen.

Examination of the gastric biopsy specimen confirmed a gastric ulcer. The pathologist noted that some of the vessels contained fibrin thrombi and **necrotizing vasculitis.** No **neoplastic** tissue was identified.

Sarge was discharged from the hospital 4 days after surgery. He was still mildly anemic. Sarge's owner was instructed to administer two gastric protectants: one at 6.5 milligrams per kilogram by mouth every 8 hours; and one at 32 milligrams per kilogram by mouth every 6 hours for 14 days. Sarge was to be fed a bland diet of small, frequent meals for 3 weeks. On follow-up 1 month later, the owner reported that Sarge's activity level and behavior had returned to normal within 1 week after surgery, and that no subsequent medical problems had occurred.

EXERCISE 10-6 *Case It!*

Read Case Studies 10-1 and 10-3. You will find that some words have been underlined. All of these words could be replaced by abbreviations to which you have already been introduced. Write the abbreviation for each of the following sets of words.

1. _____ as needed

2. _____ beats per minute

3. _____ biopsy

4. _____ by mouth

5. _____ canine

6. _____ castrated

7. _____ centimeter

8. _____ complete blood count

9. _____ degrees Fahrenheit

10. _____ diagnosis

11. _____ differential diagnosis

12. _____ every hour

13. _____ every 6 hours

14. _____ every 8 hours

15. _____ gastrointestinal

16. _____ gastric dilation and volvulus

17. _____ history

18. _____ intramuscular

19. _____ intravenous

20. _____ kilogram

21. _____ liter

22. _____ male

23. _____ milligrams

24. _____ milliliters

25. _____ mucous membrane

26. _____ physical examination

27. _____ pound

28. _____ prescription

29. _____ red blood cells

30. _____ small animal

31. _____ surgery

32. _____ treatment

33. _____ with

34. _____ without

Check your answers at the end of the chapter, Answers to Exercises.

ANSWERS TO EXERCISES

Exercise 10-1

1. dextr/o; right; sinistr/o; left
2. dors/o; toward the top; ventr/o; belly
3. intra-; within, inside; extra- *or* ex- *or* exo-; outside
4. hydr/o; water; xer/o; dry
5. heter/o; different, other; home/o; similar (*or* is/o; equal)
6. therm/o; heat; cry/o; freezing, icy cold
7. malac/o; soft, softening; scler/o; hard
8. melan/o; black; leuk/o; white (*or* albin/o; no color)
9. brady-; slow; tachy-; fast
10. ab-; away from; ad- toward
11. ante-; before, in front, of, prior to; post-; after, behind, later
12. hypo-; under, beneath, below; hyper-; above, over, or excess
13. -philia; loving, or more than normal; -penia; lack, deficiency (*or* -phobia; intense or abnormal fear)
14. macr/o; large, enlarged; micr/o; very small
15. pan-; all; a- *or* an-; without, no, not

Exercise 10-2

1. anus
2. rectum
3. colon
4. cecum
5. ileum
6. jejunum
7. duodenum
8. pyloric sphincter
9. stomach
10. cardiac sphincter
11. esophagus
12. pharynx
13. tongue
14. molar
15. premolar
16. incisor

Exercise 10-3

1. lapar/o, -tomy; surgical incision into the flank (or loin)
2. para-, lumb/o, -ar; near or beside the loin or flank
3. a-, -ton/o, -y; without pressure or tension (i.e., lack of normal muscle tone)
4. dia-, -gnosis; through knowledge—the way to identify a disorder
5. lip/o, lys/o, -is; breaking down of fat
6. hem/o, -gram; a written record (of the cellular components) of blood
7. inter-, cost/o, -al; between the ribs
8. oment/o, -pexy; surgical fixation of the omentum

Exercise 10-4

1. aphagia
2. cholelith
3. pancreatitis
4. gastrorrhaphy
5. jejunorrhexis
6. hepatoma
7. hematocele
8. orthodontist
9. esophagotomy
10. tachyphagy *or* tachyphagia
11. gastroenteritis
12. gingivectomy
13. pharyngitis
14. rumenostomy
15. abomasopexy
16. rectopathy

Exercise 10-5

1. abrasion—yes; a skin scrape
2. alopecia—no; loss of hair
3. gastric ulcer—yes; a circumscribed depressed lesion on the mucous membrane of the stomach accompanied by inflammation, pus formation, and necrosis
4. pneumothorax—no; free air in the thoracic cavity
5. laceration—yes; a rough or jagged skin tear
6. proud flesh—yes; exuberant granulation tissue at the site of injury
7. esophageal abscess—yes; a localized collection of pus in the esophagus
8. rhabdomyolysis—no; destruction of skeletal muscle
9. osteochondritis—no; inflammation of bone and cartilage
10. papule—yes; an inflamed, small, solid, pointed elevation of the skin with no pus

Exercise 10-6

1. PRN
2. bpm
3. bx
4. PO
5. K-9
6. C
7. cm
8. CBC
9. °F
10. dx
11. ddx
12. qh
13. q6h
14. q8h
15. GI
16. GDV
17. hx
18. IM
19. IV
20. kg
21. L *or* l
22. M
23. mg
24. mL *or* ml
25. mm
26. PE
27. lb
28. Rx
29. RBCs
30. SA
31. sx
32. tx
33. $\bar{c}$ *or* c
34. $\bar{s}$ *or* s

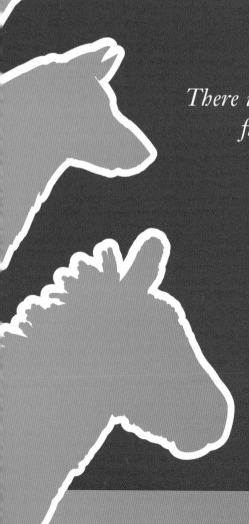

Chapter 11

The Nervous System

There is no way in which to understand the world without first detecting it through the radar-net of our senses.

Diane Ackerman, American poet

WORD PARTS

arachn/o	ah-**rahck**-nō	dendr/o	**dehn**-drō	gli/o	**glē**-ō	neur/o	**nər**-ō
astr/o	**ahs**-trō	em-	ehm	lept/o	**lehp**-tō	olig/o	**ohl**-ih-gō
cerebr/o	sehr-**ē**-brō	en-	ehn	mening/o	meh-**nihng**-ō	poli/o	**pohl**-ē-ō
corp/o	**kohr**-pō	encephal/o	ehn-**sehf**-ah-lō	myel/o	mī-**eh**-lō	tax/o	**tahck**-sō

OUTLINE

THE NERVOUS SYSTEM

THE ANATOMY AND FUNCTION OF THE NERVOUS SYSTEM
    The Central Nervous System (CNS)
    The Peripheral Nervous System (PNS)

LEARNING OBJECTIVES

When you have completed this chapter, you will be able to:

1. Understand the components and functions of the nervous system.

2. Identify and recognize the meanings of word parts related to the nervous system, using them to build or analyze words.

3. Apply your new knowledge and understanding of clinical veterinary language in the context of medical reports.

CASE STUDY 11-1 #2002-1296 BELLA

Signalment and History: A 9-year-old **F(S)** Golden Retriever named Bella was brought to the Frisbee SA Clinic because of a **chronic** history of progressive right **pelvic limb** lameness. The owner reported that occasionally, over the past 3 years, Bella would not bear weight on this leg. Within the past 4 months, Bella had episodes of **fecal** and urinary incontinence while asleep. About 4 weeks ago, Bella displayed **paresis** of the left pelvic limb, and the right pelvic limb had become progressively weaker. Bella was taken to another veterinarian, who prescribed an **anti-inflammatory** drug regime. Bella's owner had also been giving her glucosamine supplements **PO.**

Physical Examination: Jess performed a routine physical exam on Bella, and all parameters were within expected reference ranges. She also collected blood and urine samples from Bella. **Palpation** of both pelvic limbs revealed mild, diffuse **atrophy** of the musculature. Dr. Frisbee performed a complete **neurological** examination and discovered that Bella was **paraparetic** and had exaggerated **patellar** reflexes. She also detected mild **bilateral** atrophy of the **hamstring** muscles. Bella's **cranial nerve reflexes** were normal. Dr. Frisbee made a tentative diagnosis of right CCL (cranial cruciate ligament) rupture and a spinal cord abnormality involving the region from **T3 to L3.** The **ddx** for the spinal cord abnormality included **neoplasia, intervertebral** disk disease, **meningitis, myelitis,** and **diskospondylitis.** The **hemogram,** serum biochemical test findings, and urinalysis results were all within expected reference ranges.

(See the rest of the story at the end of this chapter.)

THE NERVOUS SYSTEM

The prototype animal that you are so carefully building has the potential for many functions. With the right stimulus, it can move, eat, digest, breathe, and pump blood throughout the body. It *could* do all this if something would just tell it to. Your animal is ready for its central processing unit (CPU) and an electrical-chemical wiring network that will relay messages back and forth between the brain and all parts of the body. It is ready for its nervous system.

THE ANATOMY AND FUNCTION OF THE NERVOUS SYSTEM

The nervous system is the boss of the animal. It is an animal's key homeostatic regulatory and coordinating system; it is what enables all parts of the body (including the internal organs) to work together and keep the animal alive. The nervous system is composed of two parts: the **central nervous system (CNS)** and the **peripheral nervous system (PNS)** (Table 11-1). Within each part are numerous subdivisions, each with a different role. In general, the nervous system responds to changes in the internal and external environment of an animal. For example,
- The spinal cord transmits a message to the brain.
- The brain analyzes the message and decides the appropriate response to the situation.
- The brain sends a message back to the body.
- The message initiates a response such as a muscle contraction, the release of a hormone from a gland, or breathing.

TABLE 11-1	Word Parts Associated with Nervous System Anatomy and Function		
Word Part	**Meaning**	**Example and Definition**	**Word Parts**
neur/o	nerve, nervous system	**neuropathy** disease of nerves	neur/o = nerve -path/o = disease -y = made up of, characterized by
dendr/o	tree, dendrite	**dendroid** something resembling a tree with many branches, e.g., the dendrites of nerves	dendr/o = tree, dendrite -oid = resembling
gli/o	glue, glial cells	**glioma** tumor that starts in the brain or spinal cord from glial cells	gli/o = glue, glial cells -oma = a tumor or abnormal new growth, a swelling
olig/o	little, few, small	**oligodendroglia** a small, branching glial cell	olig/o = little, few, small dendr/o = branching gli/o = glial cell -a = structure, thing
astr/o	star	**astrocyte** star-shaped glial cell found in certain structures of the nervous system *This combining form should be easy to remember. You will see a connection between astr/o and the "stars" in words such as astronaut and astrology.*	astr/o = star -cyte = cell
en- *or* em-	in, into, inward	**enchondroma** slow-growing tumor of cartilage growing into bone tissue *The prefix en- changes to em- before **b, p,** or **ph.** A few familiar words using these prefixes are enzootic, embolism, and emphysema.*	en- = in, into, inward chondr/o = cartilage -oma = a tumor or abnormal new growth, a swelling
cerebr/o encephal/o	brain	**cerebroatrophy** a wasting away of the brain tissue	cerebr/o = brain a- = without, no, not -trophy = growth
		electroencephalograph instrument used to record electrical activity in the brain; abbreviated EEG *How clever! The combining form of* encephal/o *is composed of the prefix en- meaning "in" and* cephal/o, *the combining form for "head or skull." The brain is IN the skull.*	electr/o = electricity encephal/o = brain -graph = instrument used to write or record
mening/o	meninges; the three membranes that enclose the brain and spinal cord	**meningocele** hernial protrusion of the meninges through a defect in the cranium or the vertebral column	mening/o = meninges -cele = protrusion, hernia

Continued

dendr/o

gli/o

olig/o

astr/o

en-

em-

cerebr/o

encephal/o

mening/o

TABLE 11-1	Word Parts Associated with Nervous System Anatomy and Function—cont'd		
Word Part	**Meaning**	**Example and Definition**	**Word Parts**
corp/o	body	**corpus** the trunk or main mass of a thing *A corporation is a body. A corpulent body is a large (fat) body. A corpse is a (dead) body.*	corp/o = body -(o)us = pertaining to
myel/o	spinal cord or bone marrow	**neuromyelitis** a neuritis combined with inflammation of the spinal cord (or bone marrow) *Did you remember that myel/o also refers to the bone marrow? Depending on the context in which this combining form is used, you should know whether myel/o refers to the spinal cord or to bone marrow. The term myelitis is a very general term; it does not tell the location of the inflammation. A neuromyelitis could also be called a myeloneuritis.*	neur/o = nerve myel/o = spinal cord or bone marrow -itis = inflammation
poli/o	gray	**poliomyelitis** a highly infectious viral disease that causes inflammation of the gray matter of the spinal cord and brainstem, leading to paralysis, muscular atrophy, and often deformity; commonly referred to as "polio" in humans	poli/o = gray myel/o = spinal cord or bone marrow -itis = inflammation
arachn/o	spider, spider web	**arachnoid** resembling a spider web	arachn/o = spider, spider web -oid = resembling
lept/o	thin, fine, slender, small	**leptocephaly** a head that is abnormally small and thin	lept/o = thin, fine, slender, small cephal/o = head, skull -y = made up of, characterized by
tax/o	order, coordinated movement	**ataxia** lack of coordination *Taxonomy is the ordered classification of animals and plants according to their natural relationships. Taxidermy is the art of mounting the skins of animals so that they have a life-like appearance.*	a- = without, no, not tax/o = order, coordinated movement -ia = pertaining to

corp/o

myel/o

poli/o

arachn/o

lept/o

tax/o

BOX 11-1   Terms That Defy Word Analysis

- aberrant—abnormal; deviating from the usual or ordinary
- afferent—to carry to or bring toward a place
- anomaly—a deviation from the average or norm
- axon—the long branch off a nerve cell (neuron) that carries impulses away from the cell
- blood–brain barrier—the separation of brain nervous tissue (which is bathed in a clear cerebrospinal fluid) from capillaries within the brain tissue
  - The walls of the capillaries and the glial cells near the capillaries selectively prevent various substances (such as some drugs and toxins) from entering the brain, while allowing other substances (such as barbiturates and other anesthetic drugs) to enter the brain.
- cerebellum—"little brain"; the second largest portion of the brain
- cerebrum—the largest portion of the brain
- corpus callosum—"tough body"; the bundle of nerve fibers that connect the right and left hemispheres of the cerebrum
- cortex—"outer shell"; the outer layer of nervous tissue in the brain
- dura mater—"tough mother"; the thick, fibrous outer membrane covering the brain
- efferent—to carry out or take away from a place
- ganglia (*singular* = ganglion)—cell bodies in the peripheral nervous system that cluster together in groups
- geriatric—pertaining to old age or the aging process
- gyrus (*plural* = gyri)—a convolution or raised area between grooves
- hypothalamus—the part of the brain that links the endocrine system to the nervous system
- impulse—an electrical signal that travels along an axon
- kyphosis—abnormal convex curvature of the spine
- myelin—a fatty, white substance that surrounds some axons and is produced by special cells in the central nervous system
- pia mater—"delicate, soft mother"; the thin, innermost membrane covering the brain
- pituitary—the master endocrine gland that affects nearly all hormonal activity in the body
  - It receives hormone-releasing and -inhibiting factors from the hypothalamus.
  - Pituitary literally means "relating to mucus" because it was thought that the pituitary channeled mucus to the nose.
- potential space—the space or cavity that can exist between two adjacent body parts that are not tightly adjoined; does not appear during normal functioning
- sulcus (*plural* = sulci)—a groove
- synapse—the junction across which a nerve impulse passes from an axon to another neuron, a muscle cell, or a gland cell
- syrinx—a pathological tube-shaped lesion in the brain or spinal cord
- thalamus—the part of the brain that relays sensory impulses to the cerebral cortex

EXERCISE 11-1 *Recall It!*

Repetitive use of terms that defy word analysis will help you commit them to memory.
In preparation for a better understanding of the nervous system, match the best answers
from words in the right column to their descriptions in the left column.

1. _Cerebrum_ largest portion of the brain

2. _~~Cortex~~ Dura matter_ outer covering of the brain

3. _Mylein_ fatty white substance that surrounds some axons

4. _sulcus_ a groove in the brain

5. _cerrebellum_ second largest part of the brain

6. _neuron_ a nerve cell

7. _cortex_ outer layer of nervous tissue in the brain

8. _efferent_ "to carry away" from a place

9. _pituitary_ the master endocrine gland

10. _ganglion_ cluster of nerve cells in the peripheral nervous system

cerebellum

cerebrum

cortex

dura mater

efferent

ganglion

myelin

neuron

pituitary

sulcus

Check your answers at the end of the chapter, Answers to Exercises.

The Central Nervous System (CNS)

The central nervous system is made up of the **brain** and the **spinal cord.** The CNS lies in the dorsal body cavity. Like all other parts of the body, these structures are made up of cells. The brain contains billions of cells that receive, analyze, and store information and control conscious and unconscious thoughts. For all the work that a brain does, it is not a giant organ encased in a giant head. A human brain weighs 1300 to 1400 grams. Compare that with the brain of a horse at 532 grams, a cow at 425 to 458 grams, a Beagle dog at 72 grams, and a goldfish at 0.097 gram.

Two basic types of cells are present in the central nervous system: neurons and glial cells. A neuron is made up of three parts (Figure 11-1):
• perikaryon
   ▪ This is the cell body.
   ▪ It contains the nucleus and all organelles in the cytoplasm necessary for cellular metabolism.
• dendrites
   ▪ These short, fine branching fibers extend from the cell body.
   ▪ They collect electrical signals from other neurons and set up an electrical impulse that will pass through the neuron to the next neuron.
• axon
   ▪ This single long fiber extends from the cell body. It can be up to several feet long.

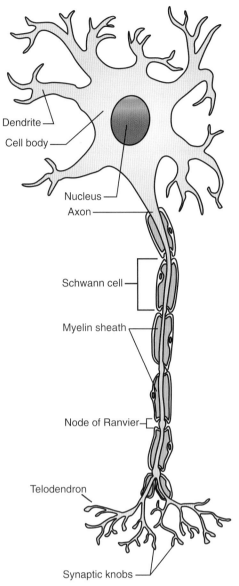

FIGURE 11-1 Structure of a neuron. (From Colville TP: *Clinical Anatomy and Physiology for Veterinary Technicians,* ed 2, St Louis, 2009, Mosby.)

- The electrical impulse flowing through the neuron leaves the neuron via the axon to travel to another neuron or to an **effector cell** (a cell that does something when stimulated, e.g., a muscle contraction).

A neuron transmits electrical signals **(impulses),** much as electricity travels along a wire. However, for the impulse to pass from one neuron to another neuron, some sort of connection must be present between them. This is the **synapse.** The impulse from one neuron passes down the axon until it reaches the end of the axon. At the end of the axon are packets of chemical **neurotransmitters,** which are released into the synapse when the impulse reaches them. These neurotransmitters carry the impulse across the synapse. The impulse is then picked up by the dendrites of other neurons.

Neurons are further classified according to their function. **Sensory neurons** carry information from the senses (i.e., taste, smell, hearing, vision, touch) toward the central nervous system. **Motor neurons** carry impulses away from the central nervous

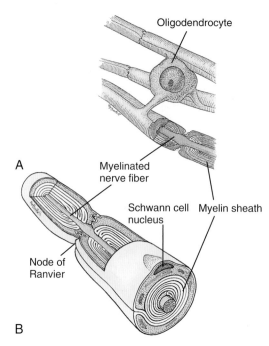

FIGURE 11-2 Myelinated nerve fibers (axons) of **(A)** the central nervous system, and **(B)** the peripheral nervous system. (Adapted from Patton K: *Anatomy and Physiology,* ed 7, St Louis, 2010, Mosby.)

system and toward the muscles and glands; they relay information regarding an action to be done (e.g., to activate a muscle contraction).

The other type of cell within the central nervous system is the **glial** cell. Its function is to supply nutrition and provide support for the neurons. Three types of glial cells have been identified:

- oligodendrocytes (oligodendroglia)
  - They secrete a fatty substance called **myelin** (Figure 11-2), which surrounds axons in a sheath, like an insulator. The myelin sheath allows the electrical signal to travel more quickly down the axon.
  - Some axons have a very thin layer of myelin; these neurons are referred to as **nonmyelinated.**
  - In the peripheral nervous system, the myelin is an extension of the cell membrane of a **Schwann cell,** a type of supporting cell that is not part of the central nervous system. Between the myelin sheath of each Schwann cell is a bare spot of axon called a **node of Ranvier** (see Figure 11-2). As an electrical signal passes down the axon, it has to jump across the section of myelin sheath from one node of Ranvier to another.
- astrocytes
  - These cells are not fully understood.
  - They are believed to play a role in the selective exchange of chemicals between the circulatory system and the central nervous system.
  - Astrocytes help to form a **blood–brain barrier,** which provides the basis for this selective exchange. Not every medication that enters the circulatory system will automatically enter the central nervous system.
- microglial cells
  - These cells are the macrophages of the central nervous system.
  - They destroy pathogens and get rid of dead neurons.

CASE STUDY 11-2   #2003-307 YODA

Signalment and History: An 11-year-old **M** Pekingese named Yoda was brought to the Frisbee SA Clinic because he was exhibiting a head tilt. Five months ago, Yoda had been examined by another veterinarian because of a right-sided head tilt. At that time, a tentative **dx** of a **geriatric** inner ear disease was made. The head tilt had resolved on its own, according to the owner. Two months ago, Yoda was brought to the Frisbee SA Clinic because of coughing and **emesis.** At that time, Dr. Frisbee noted in Yoda's chart a right-sided head tilt, **ataxia,** and **scoliosis** with concave deviation of the **vertebral column.** The owner elected to forego further neurological diagnostic testing at that time.

Physical Examination: Jess performed the initial examination and found that Yoda was BAR but would easily fall asleep if he was left alone. Other **neurological** abnormalities noted included a right-sided head tilt, marked ataxia, and scoliosis of the **cervicothoracic** portion of the vertebral column with concave deviation to the right. The extent of the scoliosis had remained unchanged over the past 2 months. Signs of involvement suggested that damage was localized to the **brainstem.**

Diagnosis: Results of a **CBC** and serum biochemistry profile were within expected reference ranges. A magnetic resonance imaging (MRI) scan of the brain was recommended and was performed at a private facility. Assessment of these images revealed a 2 × 2-cm **extra-axial,** wide-based mass on the floor of the brainstem, primarily on the right side. It extended from the **caudal** portion of the midbrain to the caudal aspect of the **medulla.** It was easily identified and was surrounded by moderate **edema.** A **cerebellar herniation** was also detected. An enlargement of the **central canal** was observed in the first part of the cervical spinal cord and in a portion of the second part. Unfortunately, other **cervical** segments of the spinal cord were not included in this MRI scan.

The brainstem lesion was highly suggestive of a **neoplastic** process. Because of the extra-axial location of the mass, Dr. Frisbee made a tentative **dx** of **meningioma.** A **ddx** of other tumors such as **astrocytoma** or **oligodendroglioma** was also considered. Other less likely ddx included **abscess** and **granuloma** formation.

Treatment: Yoda was started on **IV** (0.25 **mg/kg**) anti-inflammatory medication followed by oral anti-inflammatory medications (0.5 mg/kg) **PO q24h.** Dr. Frisbee decided that surgical treatment was impractical because of the tumor's location. Radiation therapy was started 2 weeks after Yoda's initial diagnosis. He received 10 treatments over a 4-week period. No adverse effects of radiation treatment were seen, other than mild **dermatitis** at the irradiated site and within the right ear canal.

Dr. Frisbee performed a complete neurological evaluation 1 and 4 weeks post radiation therapy. One week after treatment, mild ataxia and the head tilt were still present. By the fourth week, the head tilt was gone but mild ataxia persisted. Yoda was **neurologically** normal 2 months after receiving radiation therapy. He had had no other bouts of coughing or emesis.

EXERCISE 11-2 *Case It!*

Read Case Study 11-2. Did you understand all of the words so that you can define them?

1. neurological = _____

2. geriatric = _____

3. PO q24h = _____

4. edema = _____

5. caudal = _____

6. astrocytoma = _____

7. scoliosis = _____

8. abscess = _____

9. extra-axial = _____

10. cervicothoracic = _____

11. CBC = _____

12. neoplastic = _____

13. herniation = _____

14. cerebellar = _____

15. mg/kg = _____

16. meningioma = _____

Check your answers at the end of the chapter, Answers to Exercises.

TABLE 11-2	Abbreviations	
Abbreviation	**Meaning**	**Example**
CNS	central nervous system	Starfire was exhibiting signs of neck and back pain, so the veterinarian was concerned that they may be signs of a CNS problem.
CSF	cerebrospinal fluid	A CSF sample was obtained from Starfire's spinal cord to help rule out meningitis.

CNS

CSF

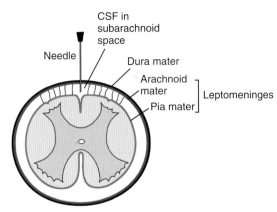

FIGURE 11-3 Diagram shows the relationship between the meninges and the CSF surrounding the spinal cord. (From Taylor SM: *Small Animal Clinical Techniques,* St Louis, 2010, Saunders.)

Anatomy of the CNS

Both the brain and the spinal cord are encased in the dorsal body cavity within bony structures that protect them: the brain in the skull, and the spinal cord in the canal that runs through the vertebrae (the spine or the vertebral column).

Between the nervous tissue and the bony tissue are three layers of connective tissue membranes (Figure 11-3), which are collectively called the **meninges:**

- dura or dura mater
  - This tough fibrous membrane is loosely connected to its bony surroundings.
  - This outermost layer of the meninges helps restrict movement of the brain and spinal cord.
  - The **epidural space** is the potential space between the dura and the bone.
- arachnoid
  - This is the middle layer.
  - As its name implies, it looks like a spider web. The web-like appearance is due to the delicate fibers of the arachnoid, which extend down through the subarachnoid space and attach to the pia mater.
  - The **subarachnoid space** lies between the arachnoid and the pia. This space contains **cerebrospinal fluid (CSF)** and all the blood vessels that enter the brain.
- pia mater or pia
  - This innermost layer is tightly adhered to the nervous tissue.
  - It is involved in the production of cerebrospinal fluid.
  - The pia mater and the arachnoid are sometimes referred to as one structure, called the **leptomeninges.**

The **cerebrospinal fluid (CSF)** is produced in the **ventricles** of the brain. The ventricles and canals that run through the central nervous system distribute cerebrospinal fluid throughout the central nervous system, to support and buffer the brain against blows to the head. Cerebrospinal fluid also carries away waste materials and dumps them into the blood. If too much fluid builds up inside the brain, a condition called **hydrocephalus** can develop.

The brain and the spinal cord are each divided into sections (Figure 11-4). The spinal cord is divided and identified by the vertebrae through which it is passing. The brain is a little more complicated. The brain has four major divisions: cerebrum, cerebellum, diencephalon, and brainstem.

The **cerebrum,** the largest part, is in charge of the "higher" functions of language, conscious thought, hearing, touch, memory, personality, and vision. The cerebrum is divided into four lobes: frontal, parietal, temporal, and occipital. Each lobe receives and processes different types of information.

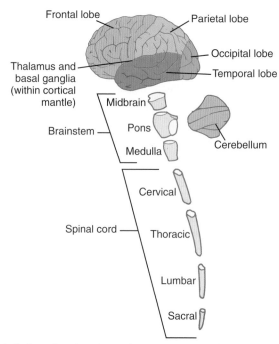

FIGURE 11-4 Exploded view showing the major components of the central nervous system. Also shown are four of the major divisions of the cerebral cortex: the frontal, parietal, occipital, and temporal lobes. (From Koeppen BM and Stanton BA: *Berne & Levy Physiology,* ed 6, Philadelphia, 2010, Mosby.)

If you could lift off the top of your animal's head, you would see the cerebrum. It looks somewhat like half of a shelled walnut because the surface is all wrinkled and folded. The many folds **(gyri)** and shallow grooves **(sulci)** increase the surface area of the cerebrum, thus allowing for more neurons. At one point, it was thought that you could tell the intelligence of an animal by the number of gyri and sulci found in the cerebrum.

Like a walnut, the cerebrum consists of two halves, which are mirror images of each other. These halves are the **right and left hemispheres,** and they are divided by the **longitudinal groove.** The right and left hemispheres communicate with each other through the **corpus callosum,** a group of nerve fibers located between the hemispheres.

When the cerebrum is transected, you will see two colors of tissue (Figure 11-5). The outer, darker tissue is composed of unmyelinated nerve fibers and neuron cell bodies. This is called the **gray matter** and is what forms the **cerebral cortex.** Information from the senses (i.e., taste, smell, hearing, vision, touch) comes from the spinal cord to the cerebral cortex for analysis and distribution to other parts of the brain. The inner, lighter colored material is called the **white matter** and is composed of axons with their myelin sheaths.

The **cerebellum** sits just caudal to the cerebrum. It is the second largest section of the brain and is in charge of coordinating movement, balance, posture, and complex reflexes. Like the cerebrum, it is divided into right and left hemispheres and is made up of gray and white matter. The cerebral cortex may tell the animal to move, but it is the cerebellum that allows the animal to move smoothly and in a coordinated manner. **Hypermetria** is a condition that results from damage to the cerebellum seen when movements become exaggerated and jerky. **Cerebellar hypoplasia** in newborn animals can result in the same condition.

Cerebrum and cerebellum are easily confused. One way to keep them straight is to remember that the one with the shorter name is the bigger section, and vice versa.

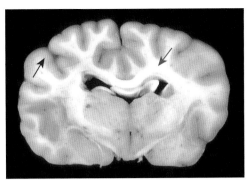

FIGURE 11-5 **Organization of the brain, gray matter, and white matter.** A transverse section of the cerebrum of dog. Gray matter *(blue arrow, darker areas)* of the cerebral cortex lies beneath the leptomeninges on the external surface of the brain. Major white matter areas *(red arrow, light areas)* lie internally. (Courtesy of Dr. J.F. Zachary, College of Veterinary Medicine, University of Illinois. In McGavin MD: *Pathologic Basis of Veterinary Disease,* ed 4, St Louis, 2007, Mosby.)

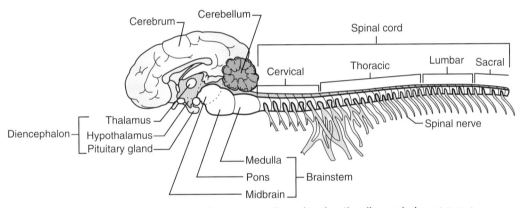

FIGURE 11-6   **Anatomy of the central nervous system showing the diencephalon.** (Adapted from Colville TP: *Clinical Anatomy and Physiology for Veterinary Technicians,* ed 2, St Louis, 2009, Mosby.)

The **diencephalon** (Figure 11-6) is made up of many structures that provide a pathway between the primitive brainstem and the cerebrum. Three important structures in the diencephalon are:

- thalamus
  - This mass of gray matter directs sensory input to the sensory area of the cerebral cortex.
  - All signals from the cerebellum pass through the thalamus on their way to the motor area of the cerebral cortex.
- hypothalamus
  - This links the nervous system and the endocrine system (hormones).
  - It helps to control functions like body temperature, thirst, hunger, water balance, and sexual function.
- pituitary gland
  - This is the master endocrine gland.
  - The hypothalamus is physically connected to the pituitary gland by a short stalk containing nerve fibers and blood vessels, and it tells the pituitary gland which hormones to release.
  - Two distinct areas of the pituitary gland have been noted: one is controlled by hormone-releasing and -inhibiting factors from the hypothalamus, and the other is controlled by direct nerve stimulation from the hypothalamus.

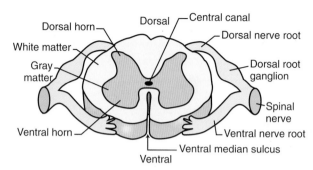

FIGURE 11-7 **Cross section of the spinal cord.** (From Colville TP: *Clinical Anatomy and Physiology for Veterinary Technicians*, ed 2, St Louis, 2009, Mosby.)

The **brainstem** provides the connection between the brain and the spinal cord. All nerve fibers leaving the brain must travel through the brainstem to get to the spinal cord. Grossly, it looks like a stem coming off the rest of the brain; this is why it was named the brain*stem*. The three parts of the brainstem are:
• medulla oblongata
• pons
• midbrain

The brainstem is the most primitive part of the brain. It controls the most basic body functions—the functions necessary for life that take place at the subconscious level (autonomic control). Some of the activities that are completely or partially controlled by the brainstem include functioning of the heart, respiration, blood pressure, hunger, thirst, and sleep patterns.

The spinal cord, along with the brain, makes up the central nervous system. The function of the spinal cord is to conduct sensory information and motor instructions between the rest of the body and the brain.

The **spinal cord** is a thick, white bundle of nerve fibers that is a continuation of the brainstem. It runs down the spine through the spinal canal. If you look at a cross section of the spinal cord grossly (Figure 11-7), you will notice that it has two colors, just as the cerebrum and the cerebellum do. However, these colors are reversed in the spinal cord. This means that the white matter (made up of myelinated nerve fibers [axons]) makes up the outer layer of the spinal cord. The inner layer, the gray matter, is shaped like a butterfly and consists mostly of unmyelinated nerve fibers and neuron cell bodies. Running down the center of the gray matter is the **central canal,** through which cerebrospinal fluid circulates and nourishes nerve cells.

CASE STUDY 11-3 | **#2011-1547 MULE DEER 1; #2011-1548 MULE DEER 2**

Signalment and History: Dr. Murdoch and Pat were called to the local zoo to examine two juvenile **M** mule deer exhibiting **signs** of acute **bilateral pelvic limb paresis, ataxia,** and urinary incontinence. The mule deer were part of a small herd housed in a prairie exhibit with a small herd of white-tailed deer. One week before this date, a **yearling** mule deer from the same herd had been found dead, but no necropsy was performed. Because these two mule deer had developed such severe clinical signs so close to the time the yearling mule deer had died, Dr. Murdoch believed it was essential to determine a **dx ASAP** to minimize the risk that other animals in the exhibit might become ill. Dr. Murdoch and the zoo curator decided that the best course of action would be to **euthanize** the two mule deer. Dr. Murdoch **sedated** each of them with 1.5 mL of a potent sedative delivered **IM** with a plastic dart from a CO_2 dart pistol. When they were **recumbent,** the animals were euthanized with an **IV** euthanasia solution.

Outcome: Dr. Murdoch and Pat loaded the two deer into a trailer and hauled them to the state diagnostic laboratory for **necropsy.** The report from the diagnostic lab indicated that no gross abnormalities were seen in either animal. In both animals, initial **histological** examination of the **CNS** revealed generalized eosinophilic **meningoencephalitis** with moderate multifocal aggregates of **eosinophils** and **mononuclear** cells in the **perivascular** regions of the **meninges** and **gray matter** of the **cerebrum, cerebellum,** and **brainstem.** The severity of the lesions varied from one region of the spinal cord to another, with the **cranial cervical** and **caudal lumbar** regions of the cord being most severely affected. This was suggestive of a parasitic infection. Further histological examination of sections of the brains from both deer revealed the presence of parasitic worm sections and **aberrant** parasite migration. The pathologist at the diagnostic lab stated that she thought the parasite was the brain-worm that normally infects white-tailed deer (which show no signs of infection). In this instance, the mule deer were accidental, dead-end hosts for the parasite, which had undergone CNS migration.

Dr. Murdoch advised the zoo curator that the mule deer and the white-tailed deer should be exhibited separately. A **fecal** examination of the white-tailed deer tested positive for parasite eggs, and they were treated accordingly. No other mule deer have become ill to this date.

EXERCISE 11-3 *Case It!*

Complete the following statements regarding information you have read about in Case Study 11-2.

1. Acute onset means that the signs appeared _____.

2. Bilateral means that the signs appeared _____.

3. Necropsy was performed after _____.

4. The cranial cervical region of the spinal cord is where? _____

5. The caudal lumbar region of the spinal cord is where? _____

6. What is an eosinophil? _____

7. What is a yearling deer? _____

8. To administer drugs IM by a metal dart is to _____.

9. What are meninges? _____

10. The gray matter of the cerebrum is the _____.

11. What do paresis and ataxia signify? _____

12. Aberrant migration refers to _____.

Check your answers at the end of the chapter, Answers to Exercises.

The Peripheral Nervous System (PNS)

The peripheral nervous system is that part of the nervous system that lies outside the brain and spinal cord. It contains sensory receptors that are activated by an internal or external stimulus (e.g., from senses of taste, smell, hearing, vision, and touch), sensory neurons that carry the impulse to the central nervous system, and motor neurons that relay an action message back out to the body.

A **spinal nerve** comes off each side of the spinal cord at the junction between vertebrae (see Figure 11-6). This nerve connects the peripheral nerves to the spinal cord. The **dorsal nerve roots** of the spinal nerve feed sensory **(afferent)** impulses to the **dorsal horns** of the gray matter, which then send it to the brain. The **ventral horns** of the gray matter relay motor **(efferent)** impulses generated within the brain to the **ventral nerve roots,** which in turn relay the impulse to the muscles and glands.

The peripheral nervous system is subdivided into the somatic (voluntary) nervous system and the autonomic (involuntary) nervous system.

The **somatic nervous system** consists of (1) peripheral nerve fibers (nerves coming directly off the spinal cord [spinal nerves] or the brain **[cranial nerves]**) that send sensory information to the central nervous system, and (2) motor nerve fibers that relay messages to **effector cells.** *Effector* cells are the cells in the body on which the motor nerve fibers will have an *effect* (e.g., skeletal muscle). The cell bodies for somatic nerves are located in the brain or the spinal cord, and the (sometimes very long) axon travels directly to the effector cell. An animal's conscious awareness of its external environment and the motor reaction to deal with it are coordinated through the somatic nervous system. In a simple or **monosynaptic reflex** reaction, the sensory impulse does not have to travel all the way to the brain. The spinal cord connects the sensory input directly to a motor neuron that sends out a motor response. This type of reflex is similar to that seen when a cat puts its paw on something very hot and immediately pulls it away. The "knee jerk" reflex is also an example of a reflex action that is mediated by the spinal cord.

The function of the **autonomic nervous system** is to maintain homeostasis. The autonomic nervous system (literally "self-law") controls the smooth muscles of the viscera via actions that are automatic or involuntary. It consists of (1) receptors within the viscera, (2) afferent nerves that carry information to the central nervous system, and (3) efferent nerves that relay messages to the effector cells, such as smooth muscle, cardiac muscle, and glands.

The autonomic nervous system is further divided into the sympathetic and the parasympathetic systems. The **sympathetic system** (Does it feel sympathy for the animal?) prepares it to "fight or take flight" when presented with a stressful situation. By controlling the smooth muscle of the viscera, it can dilate eye pupils and increase blood pressure, pulse, breathing rate, and blood flow to muscles. It does this by decreasing digestion, elimination, and other processes that are not necessary for fight/flight.

The **parasympathetic system** is the "rest and digest" part of the autonomic nervous system. It calms the animal by slowing the heartbeat and breathing, by lowering blood pressure, and by increasing digestion and elimination.

EXERCISE 11-4   *Have Fun!*

So far you have been working very hard learning clinical veterinary language. Now it is time to have a little fun with your new knowledge. The list below contains common sayings that have some body part in them. Just for fun, see how many of these sayings you can translate into clinical veterinary language. There are no right or wrong answers; be creative. You can always start with "a condition of…" One saying is done for you, with one possible answer.

    Example: *avian intrametacarpalia* could be *a condition of a bird in the hand*

1. tear your hair out _____

2. a pain in the neck _____

3. two-faced _____

4. cold hands, warm heart _____

5. tongue-tied _____

6. stomach in a knot _____

7. heart-to-heart _____

8. sweet tooth _____

9. get the monkey off your back _____

10. cat got your tongue _____

11. elbow grease _____

12. green thumb _____

13. big mouth _____

14. horse of a different color _____

15. no skin off your nose _____

16. by the skin of your teeth _____

17. stiff upper lip _____

18. scarce as hen's teeth _____

Check your answers at the end of the chapter, Answers to Exercises.

CASE STUDY 11-1   #2002-1296 BELLA

Signalment and History: A 9-year-old **F(S)** Golden Retriever named Bella was brought to the Frisbee SA Clinic because of a **chronic** history of progressive right **pelvic limb** lameness. The owner reported that occasionally, over the past 3 years, Bella would not bear weight on this leg. Within the past 4 months, Bella had episodes of **fecal** and urinary incontinence while asleep. About 4 weeks ago, Bella displayed **paresis** of the left pelvic limb, and the right pelvic limb had become progressively weaker. Bella was taken to another veterinarian, who prescribed an **anti-inflammatory** drug regime. Bella's owner had also been giving her glucosamine supplements **PO.**

Physical Examination: Jess performed a routine physical exam on Bella, and all parameters were within expected reference ranges. She also collected blood and urine samples from Bella. **Palpation** of both pelvic limbs revealed mild, diffuse **atrophy** of the musculature. Dr. Frisbee performed a complete **neurological** examination and discovered that Bella was **paraparetic** and had exaggerated **patellar** reflexes. She also detected mild **bilateral** atrophy of the **hamstring** muscles. Bella's **cranial nerve reflexes** were normal. Dr. Frisbee made a tentative diagnosis of right CCL (cranial cruciate ligament) rupture and a spinal cord abnormality involving the region from **T3 to L3.** The **ddx** for the spinal cord abnormality included **neoplasia, intervertebral** disk disease, **meningitis, myelitis,** and **diskospondylitis.** The **hemogram,** serum biochemical test findings, and urinalysis results were all within expected reference ranges.

Diagnosis: X-rays of both **stifle joints,** the **vertebral column** from **T2** to the **sacrum,** and the **thoracic cavity** were taken. The left stifle joint appeared unaffected. A **chronic** degenerative excavation of **subchondral** bone of the right stifle joint was noted, with calcification of the soft tissues in the joint. Dr. Frisbee indicated that these changes were consistent with a CCL rupture and chronic degenerative joint disease. The thoracic cavity appeared normal.

Magnetic resonance imaging (MRI) of the thoracic and lumbar portions of the vertebral column was performed at an off-site imaging facility. For this evaluation, Bella was anesthetized and was placed in **sternal** recumbency in a 1.0-Tesla magnetic resonance scanner. Results showed **lesions** of the spinal cord overlying the T6-T7 intervertebral space. **CSF** from the **lumbar** area contained a high protein concentration (121.9 **mg/dL**). A ddx for the spinal cord abnormality that was considered based on the MRI included neoplasia, **hemorrhage,** vascular **anomaly,** parasite migration, and myelitis.

Treatment: Dr. Frisbee decided that surgery was necessary for further clarification of the lesion and for collection of tissues for histological evaluation. Bella was prepared for surgery. Parts of the T5 to T7 vertebrae were removed. When the spinal canal was entered, the dural tube appeared larger than normal, and increased **vascularization** of the **dura** overlying the T7 spinal cord segment was noted. Dr. Frisbee performed a **durotomy.** The exposed spinal cord in this area was focally discolored and enlarged. She next performed a **lateral,** longitudinal **myelotomy** over this spinal cord segment. Within the spinal cord, she found a firm, gray, 1 × 1-**cm** mass that contained numerous blood vessels. She removed the mass with blunt dissection using **microsurgical** instruments and an operating **microscope.**

Outcome: Bella recovered from anesthesia without complications and was walking with sling support the day after surgery. Urination and defecation were normal, and Bella was discharged 3 days after surgery. At the time of discharge, Bella needed assistance to stand from a recumbent position but was able to walk with minimal support. At her 1-month recheck examination, Bella was standing and walking normally.

EXERCISE 11-5 *Case It!*

In Case Study 11-1, you read that **cranial nerve reflexes** were normal. Cranial nerves are represented by Roman numerals (e.g., III is the name of the third cranial nerve). Spinal nerves are named by where they arise from in the spinal cord, using the same letter abbreviations as are used for the names of the vertebrae where the nerves exit the cord (e.g., C3 represents the third cervical vertebra, as well as the third cervical spinal nerve). Nerves are also named for the area or function they serve. You will recognize familiar word roots in the following list of names of nerves. What does each name tell you about where to look for this nerve?

1. cranial nerve _____

2. digitalis palmaris medialis _____

3. femoral _____

4. glossopharyngeal nerve _____

5. intercostals _____

6. interosseous antebrachial _____

7. L4 _____

8. lateral cutaneous femoral _____

9. lumbar splanchnic _____

10. mandibular alveolar _____

11. median _____

12. sublingual _____

13. suprascapularis _____

14. thoracodorsal _____

15. vertebral _____

16. VII _____

Check your answers at the end of the chapter, Answers to Exercises.

ANSWERS TO EXERCISES

Exercise 11-1

1. cerebrum
2. dura mater
3. myelin
4. sulcus
5. cerebellum
6. neuron
7. cortex
8. efferent
9. pituitary
10. ganglion

Exercise 11-2

1. neurological = pertaining to the study of nerves, or having knowledge of them
2. geriatric = pertaining to old age or the aging process
3. PO q24h = by mouth once a day
4. edema = swelling caused by fluid in the body tissues
5. caudal = toward the tail end of the body
6. astrocytoma = tumor or abnormal new growth composed of star-shaped cells (astrocytes)
7. scoliosis = spine is curved from side to side
8. abscess = a collection of pus in any part of the body, usually causing swelling and inflammation around it
9. extra-axial = "off the axis"; term applied to intracranial lesions that do not arise from the brain itself
10. cervicothoracic = referring to the neck and the chest (thorax)
11. CBC = complete blood count
12. neoplastic = new growth, development, or formation
13. herniation = protrusion of an organ or a part of an organ through the wall of the cavity that normally contains it
14. cerebellar = pertaining to the second largest portion of the brain
15. mg/kg = milligrams per kilogram
16. meningioma = a tumor or new abnormal growth of the meninges (the three membranes that cover the brain and spinal cord)

Exercise 11-3

1. rapidly, in a short time
2. on both sides of the body, both hind legs
3. after euthanization or death
4. in the neck toward the head end
5. in the loin toward the tail end
6. a blood cell whose granules in its cytoplasm stain red
7. intact male who has not been castrated/neutered and who is nearly or is just turning 1 year old
8. inject them into a muscle
9. the membranes that enclose the brain and spinal cord
10. outer darker tissue composed of unmyelinated neuron fibers and cell bodies
11. paresis is a slight or incomplete paralysis; ataxia is lack of coordination
12. abnormal movement to another place; deviation from the usual or ordinary location

Exercise 11-4

Remember? There are no right or wrong answers. Did you have fun?

Exercise 11-5

1. head or skull
2. dorsum of the pastern and hoof of the foreleg
3. femur bone
4. tongue and throat
5. between the ribs
6. upper foreleg
7. fourth lumbar vertebra
8. side of the femur
9. loin
10. lower jaw
11. toward the center of the body
12. under the tongue; ventral surface of tongue and floor of mouth
13. scapula
14. on the back in the thorax area
15. vertebrae or spinal column
16. head (7th cranial nerve)

Chapter 12
The Senses

A pine needle dropped in the forest. The deer heard it. The eagle saw it. The bear smelled it.

Unknown

WORD PARTS

acous/o	ah-**koo**-sō	-esthesia	ehs-**thē**-zē-ah	noci-	**nō**-sē	palpebr/o	**pahl**-peh-brō
aqua-	**ah**-kwah	eu-	ū	ocul/o	**ohk**-ū-lō	propri/o	**prō**-prē-ō
aque/o	**ah**-kwē-ō	gust/o	**guh**-stō	odor/o	**ō**-dər-ō	retin/o	**reht**-ih-nō
audi/o	**ahw**-dē-ō	-ile	īl	olfact/o	ohl-**fahck**-tō	rhin/o	**rī**-nō
blephar/o	**blehf**-ər-ō	irid/o	ihr-ih-**dō**	ophthalm/o	**ohf**-thahl-mō	tact-	tahckt
cor/o	**kohr**-ō	-ity	**ih**-tē	opt/o	**ohp**-tō	tympan/o	**tihm**-puh-nō
corne/o	**kohr**-nē-ō	kerat/o	**kehr**-ah-tō	osm/o	**ohz**-mō		
dacry/o	**dahck**-rē-ō	lacrim/o	**lahck**-rih-mō	oss/o	**ohs**-sō		
esthesi/o	ehs-**thē**-zē-ō	myring/o	**mihr**-ihng-ō	ot/o	**ō**-tō		

OUTLINE

THE SENSES

GENERAL SENSES

THE SPECIAL SENSES
    Taste
    Smell
    Hearing
    Equilibrium
    Vision

LEARNING OBJECTIVES

When you have completed this chapter, you will be able to:

1 Understand the components and functions of the senses.

2 Identify and recognize the meanings of word parts related to the senses, using them to build or analyze words.

3 Apply your new knowledge and understanding of clinical veterinary language in the context of medical reports.

CASE STUDY 12-1 #2010-2747 ONAM

Signalment and History: An 18-year-old Arabian **gelding** named Onam was brought to the Frisbee Large Animal Clinic because of a **chronic unilateral mucoid nasal** discharge. Onam was still eating and drinking. His vaccinations were all current. Onam was admitted to the hospital for diagnostic evaluation.

Physical Examination: Pat performed an initial physical examination and found that Onam was BAR with a TPR within expected reference ranges, but respiratory noises were audible when he listened to Onam inhale and exhale. There was no sign of **dyspnea.** The right **submandibular** lymph nodes were enlarged and **palpable.** An obvious deformity on Onam's face ran from the caudal aspect of the right **naris** up to the right medial canthus. The rest of the examination was unremarkable. Onam weighed 981.2 lb. Pat drew blood samples for a CBC and serum biochemical testing and collected feces and urine for analysis. Dr. Murdoch examined the face, nose, and mouth. He found a large **intranasal** mass at the **rostral** end of the right naris. The mass appeared to be covered with normal nasal mucous membrane. When he opened Onam's mouth and examined the **oral cavity,** he found that the caudal part of the hard palate was pushed down **ventrally.** Onam was sedated with an **equine** sedative (0.5 **mg/kg** [0.23 mg/lb] of body weight **IV**). An **endoscope** was passed through the left naris with no trouble, but it could not be passed through the right naris without possibly causing trauma. He also noted a **nasal septum** deviation to the left. The **pharynx, glottis,** and **proximal tracheal** regions appeared normal.

(See the rest of the story later in the chapter.)

THE SENSES

In Chapter 11, you learned about sensory nerves and sensory impulses. In this chapter, you will explore the senses that stimulate the sensory nerves and make your prototype animal aware of its surroundings. The degree to which animals will perceive their environment and the senses with which they do so will vary a lot among species. Some species have a keen sense of smell but cannot see very well. Other species can see in low light, but hearing is not their strongest sense.

How do animals sense? Sensory receptors are present all over an animal's body, inside and out. These receptors are actually specialized dendrites on sensory neurons. When stimulated, these specialized dendrites pick up the signal and the sensory neurons transmit the impulse to the brain. Most animals will respond to four general types of stimuli. With these stimuli, the animal can sense its entire world:
- mechanical stimuli (touch, hearing, balance)
- chemical stimuli (taste, smell)
- thermal stimuli (hot, cold)
- electromagnetic stimuli (sight)

Animals rely on 10 different senses, to varying degrees, to survive. The senses are divided into two groups: general senses (Table 12-1) and special senses (Table 12-2).

BOX 12-1 Terms That Defy Word Analysis

- allodynia—a painful response to a normally nonpainful stimulus
- heatstroke—a considerable elevation in body temperature (hyperthermia)
- hyperesthesia—an increased response to a painful stimulus
- perception—conscious interpretation of sensory information
- sedative—a drug that depresses (makes it quieter) an animal and slows down body functions; no painkilling action
- sensation—awareness of stimuli from the environment
- tranquilizer—a drug that makes the animal less anxious; no painkilling action

TABLE 12-1   Word Parts Associated with the General Senses

Word Part	Meaning	Example and Definition	Word Parts	
noci-	injury, pain, harm	**nociperception** the recognition by the nervous system of an injury or painful stimulus	noci- = injury, pain, harm perception = interpretation of sensory information	noci-
propri/o	self, one's own	**proprioception** scientific term for the physical feeling of your moving body *If you were to appropriate your neighbor's car, you would make use of it exclusively for yourself, often without permission.*	propri/o = self, one's own (per)ception = interpretation of sensory information	propri/o
-esthesia esthesi/o	feeling, experience, sensation	**anesthesia** without feeling (sometimes induced to permit the performance of surgery and other painful procedures)	an- = without, no, not -esthesia = feeling, experience, sensation	-esthesia
		esthesiogenesis the production of a feeling or sensation, especially having to do with the nervous system	esthesi/o = feeling, experience, sensation gen/o = formation or beginning -esis = process of an action	esthesi/o
-ile -ity	capable of, pertaining to	**infantile** childish, pertaining to infants	infant = the very young offspring of an animal -ile = capable of, pertaining to	-ile
		abnormality state or condition of not being typical or usual	ab- = away from norm/o = normal -al = pertaining to -ity = capable of, pertaining to	-ity
tact-	touch	**tactile agnosis** the inability to recognize objects by handling them	tact- = touch -ile = capable of, pertaining to a- = without, no, not -gnosis = knowledge	tact-

General senses have receptors located all over the body, but all receptors for the special senses are located in the head in specialized sensory organs.

GENERAL SENSES

Although they are important to the well-being of an animal, the general senses are rarely involved in clinical disease or treatment, except for the sensation of pain. The general senses are as follows:

- visceral sensation
  - These are the sensations from the animal's interior or viscera. They include the sensations produced in the hollow visceral organs (e.g., gastrointestinal [GI] tract, urinary tract, reproductive tract). Most of the sensory receptors in hollow organs are stretch receptors that respond to the walls of the organs stretching as the organs fill.
  - Sensations from the pleural and peritoneal membranes are included in this group.

- Visceral sensations also include those of hunger and thirst, which tell an animal that it is time to eat or drink.
- touch and pressure sensation
  - Touch is the **tactile** sense.
  - These sensory receptors are located in the dermis. They tell the animal's body when it is in contact with another surface or object. Pressure is a measure of how much force is being exerted by something touching the animal.
  - An injectable **local anesthetic** blocks the nerves around the injection site so the animal cannot feel the touch of stitches being sewn, a small tumor being removed, or any other localized superficial procedure. A local anesthetic does not affect the brain.
- temperature sensation
  - This sense involves monitoring the animal's body temperature.
  - The central temperature receptors are located within the hypothalamus. Superficial temperature receptors are present in the skin.
  - An animal can control its internal body temperature to varying degrees by responding to the sensory input from central and superficial receptors.
- pain sensation
  - **Nociception** is the ability to take a painful stimulus and translate it into a nerve impulse that will travel to the brain for interpretation and reaction.
  - Some areas of the body are more sensitive to pain because they contain a greater number of nerve endings (dendrites).
  - **Windup phenomenon** causes untreated pain to get worse because the nerve fibers become more effective in transmitting pain impulses to the brain. Over time, the brain becomes more sensitive to the pain, and the pain seems to get worse.
- body position and movement sensation
  - Another name for this sensation is **proprioception**, sometimes called *proprioreception*.
  - This sensation is the ability of an animal to know where its body is and what the muscles, tendons, ligaments, and joints are doing.
  - The brain can then send out appropriate signals to keep the animal standing, walking, or doing whatever is required.

TABLE 12-2	Word Parts Associated with Special Senses		
Word Part	**Meaning**	**Example and Definition**	**Word Parts**
gust/o	taste	**gustation** taste; also known as *gust*	gust/o = taste -ation = state, condition, action, process, or result
		If you do something with a lot of gusto, *you are enthused about it—you have a "taste" for it!*	
eu-	good, well, normal	**eupepsia** normal digestion	eu- = good, well, normal peps/o = digestion -ia = pertaining to
rhin/o	nose	**rhinitis** inflammation of the upper respiratory tract, especially the nose	rhin/o = nose -itis = inflammation

gust/o

eu-

rhin/o

TABLE 12-2	Word Parts Associated with Special Senses—cont'd		

Word Part	Meaning	Example and Definition	Word Parts
olfact/o odor/o osm/o	smell	**olfactory nerve** a nerve that sends the impulses for the sense of smell from the nose to the brain	olfact/o = smell -ory = pertaining to nerve = nerve
		malodorous a terribly bad smell or odor	mal- = diseased, bad, abnormal, defective odor/o = smell -ous = pertaining to
		aosmia inability to smell; also known as *olfactory anesthesia*	a- = without, no, not osm/o = smell -ia = pertaining to
		⚠ *Do not confuse this* osm/o *with the* osm/o *that means thrust, push, or impel.* **osmosis** tendency of a fluid (usually water) to pass through a membrane to equalize the concentrations of materials on either side of the membrane	osm/o = thrust, push, impel -osis = disease or abnormal condition
ot/o	ear	**otorhinolaryngology** branch of medicine concerned with the ears, nose, and throat; ENT	ot/o = ear rhin/o = nose laryng/o = larynx -logy = to study, or to have knowledge of
		💡 *It is this type of medical specialty that can frustrate a nonmedical person when trying to pronounce the word properly—and when trying to figure out what it means. No wonder these doctors list their specialty as ENT in the yellow pages of the phone book.*	
tympan/o myring/o	eardrum	**tympanocentesis** surgical puncture of the eardrum to remove fluid from the middle ear 💡 *You are familiar with the big kettle drums in the orchestra—the* tympan*i. They definitely have big eardrums.*	tympan/o = eardrum -centesis = surgical puncture
		myringectomy surgical removal of the eardrum	myring/o = eardrum -ectomy = surgical removal
acous/o	hearing, listening	**acoustics** the science of sound and the phenomenon of hearing	acous/o = hearing, listening -tic = pertaining to -s = *plural*
audi/o	sound	**audiology** the study of hearing disorders and the treatment of patients with hearing impairments	audi/o = sound -logy = to study, or to have knowledge of

Continued

ocul/o

ophthalm/o

opt/o

blephar/o

palpebr/o

lacrim/o

dacry/o

kerat/o

corne/o

irid/o

TABLE 12-2	Word Parts Associated with Special Senses—cont'd		
Word Part	**Meaning**	**Example and Definition**	**Word Parts**
ocul/o ophthalm/o opt/o	eye	**oculocutaneous** pertaining to the eyes and the skin; referring to type of albinism that involves the eyes	ocul/o = eye cutane/o = skin -ous = pertaining to
		ophthalmologist physician who specializes in the diagnosis and treatment (with drugs and surgery) of diseases of the eye	ophthalm/o = eye log/o = to study, or to have knowledge of -ist = a person or thing that does something specified
		⚠ *When you spell ophthalmologist, do not forget the first h.*	
		optometrist person specially licensed to test for vision defects and to prescribe and fit glasses—without prescribing drugs or performing surgery	opt/o = eye metr/o = measure -ist = a person or thing that does something specified
blephar/o palpebr/o	eyelid	**blepharospasm** an abnormal contraction of the eyelid; a twitch	blephar/o = eyelid spasm = intermittent involuntary abnormal contraction
		palpebration abnormal repeated and frequent winking or blinking, as from a tic	palpebr/o = eyelid -ation = state, condition, action, process, or result
lacrim/o dacry/o	tears	**nasolacrimal duct** the duct that runs from the lower eyelid area to the nose; the reason why your nose runs when you cry	nas/o = nose lacrim/o = tears -al = pertaining to
		dacryopyorrhea flow of tears mixed with pus	dacry/o = tears py/o = pus -rrhea = flow
		💧 *It will help you to remember that lacrim/o and dacry/o mean "tears" if you can see "cry" in the middle of them.*	
kerat/o corne/o	cornea	**keratitis** inflammation of the cornea ⚠ *Did you remember that kerat/o also refers to the hard, horn-like tissue found in the outer layer of the skin?*	kerat/o = cornea -itis = inflammation
		corneitis inflammation of the cornea; keratitis	corne/o = cornea -itis = inflammation
irid/o	iris (*plural* = irides)	**iridocele** protrusion of a portion of the iris through a defect in the cornea	irid/o = iris -cele = protrusion, hernia

| TABLE 12-2 | Word Parts Associated with Special Senses—cont'd | | |
Word Part	Meaning	Example and Definition	Word Parts
cor/o	pupil of the eye	**corectasis** abnormal dilation of the pupil of the eye ⚠️ *You have met cor/o before. Remember the corium? It is the dermis, the layer of skin just below the epidermis. Also some words about the heart will contain the combining form of cor/o.* 💡 *If you look up dilatation and dilation, they have the same meaning. The original English word is dilatation, but it has been shortened by Americans to dilation—and the rest of the world has agreed that this is acceptable.*	cor/o = pupil of the eye -ectasis = expansion, dilation, or distention
retin/o	retina	**neuroretinitis** an inflammation affecting both the optic nerve and the retina	neur/o = nerve retin/o = retina -itis = inflammation
oss/o	bone	**ossicle** a small bone 🔍 *This would be a good time to recall the other word parts that you have already learned that mean "bone": os and oste/o.*	oss/o = bone -ic = pertaining to -(u)le = indicating something small
aque/o aqua-	water, watery solution	**aqueous** pertaining to water	aque/o = water, watery solution -ous = pertaining to
		aquatic of, in, or pertaining to water	aqua- = water, watery solution -(t)ic = pertaining to

cor/o

retin/o

oss/o

aque/o

aqua-

BOX 12-2 **Terms That Defy Word Analysis**

- amplify—increase in size, effect, volume, extent, or amount
- amplitude—the loudness of a sound
- canthus—the corner of each eye formed by the junction of the upper and lower eyelids
  - There is a lateral and a medial canthus for each eye.
- cochlea = snail shell—spiral organ in the inner ear that turns sound waves into sensory impulses
- conjunctiva—the mucous membrane that lines the exposed portion of the eyeball and the inner surface of the eyelids
  - *Conjunctivitis* is the medical term for "pink eye."
- eustachian tube—also known as the *auditory canal;* a canal that runs from the middle ear to the pharynx
- frequency—the pitch of a sound
- humor—an antiquated word meaning any one of the four cardinal fluids in the body: blood, phlegm, yellow bile, and black bile
  - Humors were thought to determine a person's emotional and physical state. A person would be healthy as long as his humors were in balance.
- matrix—a surrounding-substance in which something else is contained

For more than 2500 years until modern medicine intervened, bloodletting (phlebotomy) was the standard of the "humoral" medical practice for curing all ailments of the body. The belief was that when a person was sick, his humors were out of balance. Bloodletting would put him back in balance. Many times it did more harm than good.

Continued

> **BOX 12-2**   **Terms That Defy Word Analysis—cont'd**
>
> - miosis (myosis)—prolonged constriction of the pupil of the eye
> - modulate—change, regulate, adjust
> - mydriasis—prolonged dilation of the pupil of the eye
> - neural transmission—passage of a nerve impulse across a synapse
> - nocturnal—active at night
> - papilla (*plural* = papillae)—a small, round, or cone-shaped projection or peg on the top of the tongue that may contain taste buds
> - pheromone—a liquid substance released in very small quantities by an animal that causes a specific response if it is detected by another animal of the same species
> - pinna—ear flap
> - sensory receptor—a nerve ending that responds to a stimulus, found in the internal or external environment of an animal; sends an impulse to the brain
> - sensory transduction—conversion of a signal from one form (e.g., light) to another (e.g., electrical impulse)
> - vitreous—resembling glass

THE SPECIAL SENSES

The special senses are taste, smell, hearing, equilibrium, and vision. In contrast to the general senses, all receptors for special senses are localized in specialized sensory organs in the head and include the tongue, nose, ear, and eye. These specialized organs are often involved in clinical illnesses because of their location, structure, and function.

Taste is the **gustatory sense.** Taste involves detection in the mouth of the concentration of chemical molecules found in food. The receptors are the **taste buds,** which contain hundreds of microscopic sensory taste receptor cells. When appropriate chemical molecules come in contact with the receptors, nerve impulses are generated that travel to the brain to be interpreted as particular tastes.

Most of the taste buds are located on the **tongue** on macroscopic **papillae** (Figure 12-1), but a few are found in the walls of the oral cavity. Every mammal, bird, reptile, amphibian, and fish has a tongue, and every tongue has taste buds. Herbivores have the greatest number of taste buds, which enable them to distinguish between good and toxic foods.

Five types of taste are recognized by humans:
- sweet = high-energy foods
- sour = acidic foods
- salty = electrolyte-modulating foods
- bitter = toxic or "bad" foods
- umami = protein-rich foods
  - This recently identified type of taste, also known as *savory*, is based on the natural presence of monosodium glutamate in foods such as meat and aged cheese.

We cannot know how animals perceive taste. Perhaps it is categorized by them as pleasant, unpleasant, or indifferent. Research has shown that cats cannot taste sweet flavors, and pigs are partial to bitter flavors. Animals prefer to eat foods that taste like the food they would consume in their natural environment.

Smell is the **olfactory sense.** Smell, together with taste, is thought to be the most primitive of the senses. Smell plays an important role in taste because it is partially through smell that the flavor of a food is sensed. **Olfaction** is controlled by areas of specialized sensory receptors located high in the nasal passages (Figure 12-2). The olfactory cells have hair-like projections (cilia) on their surfaces that project into the surface mucus, which is produced by special cells in the lining of the nasal cavity.

A 6-inch catfish has as many as 250,000 taste buds, but they aren't located just on its tongue. They cover its entire body, including tail, fins, back, and belly. Does this make it a swimming tongue?

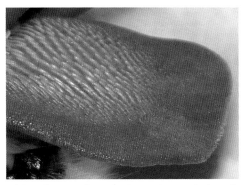

FIGURE 12-1 Caudally pointing firm papillae on the cat's rough dorsal tongue surface. (From Little S: *The Cat: Clinical Medicine and Management,* St Louis, 2012, WB Saunders.)

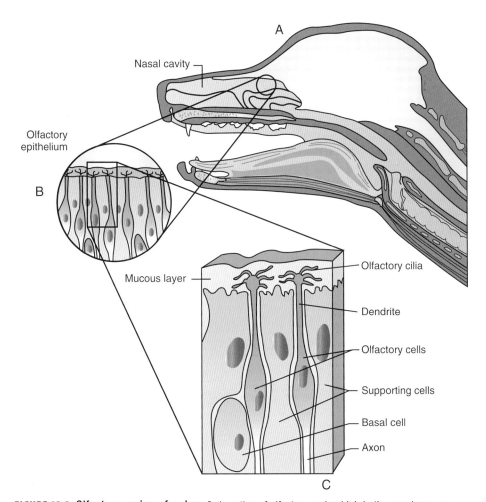

FIGURE 12-2 Olfactory region of a dog. A, Location of olfactory region high in the nasal passage. **B,** Olfactory epithelium. **C,** Detail of olfactory epithelium showing olfactory cilia projecting up into the overlying mucous layer. (From Colville TP: *Clinical Anatomy and Physiology for Veterinary Technicians,* ed 2, St Louis, 2009, Mosby.)

The cilia are actually modified dendrites that detect airborne odor molecules (**odorants**) that have dissolved in the mucus. Nerve impulses are generated and transmitted to the brain to be interpreted as particular smells.

Two distinct olfactory systems are present in most animals, other than humans and some primates. The primary olfactory system was described earlier. An accessory olfactory system detects fluid-phased stimuli and is based in a specialized organ located between the nose and the mouth called the *VNO*, or *vomeronasal organ*. A snake uses this system to smell prey, sticking its tongue out and then touching it to the VNO. Other mammals use a facial expression to direct stimuli to the VNO. Have you ever seen a horse tilt up its head and curl its upper lip in a "horse laugh"? Or have you watched a cat smell something and then wrinkle its nose and hold its mouth open like it smells bad? Although these expressions are amusing, they actually have a practical purpose. The posture is called **flehmen** (testing), and it appears to help animals trap **pheromone** scents in the VNOs so they can be analyzed more closely. Pheromones act as a chemical means of social communication between animals of the same species. Different pheromones elicit different responses, such as alarm, sexual arousal, lay your eggs someplace else, mother/baby bonding, respect my territory, and back off. Remember the foul-smelling secretions from the anal glands of some small mammals (dogs and cats included)? That smell is believed to contain pheromones that either attract or repel other members of the same species. The presence of human pheromones and what, if any, effect they may have is the subject of current debate and research.

With their sense of smell, animals are able to locate prey, navigate, recognize and communicate with others of their species, and mark their territory. Most animals, other than humans and some primates, have a sense of smell that has been highly developed as a means of survival. The bear is thought to have the best sense of smell of any land animal. The area in the bear's brain that is devoted to smell is 5 times larger than it is in the human brain. In water, the distinction for the best sense of smell goes to the shark, which can smell one drop of blood in the water from more than a mile away. Rats have been successfully trained to sniff out land mines. Bloodhounds can follow a scent several days after a person has walked through high-traffic pedestrian areas. Some dogs can smell explosives, drugs, and even cancer.

> Ants use pheromones to make a trail from a food source to the nest. Certain ants make the initial trail that attracts other ants to follow. The trail must be constantly renewed as long as the food source is present.

CASE STUDY 12-1 #2010-2747 ONAM

Signalment and History: An 18-year-old Arabian **gelding** named Onam was brought to the Frisbee Large Animal Clinic because of a **chronic unilateral mucoid nasal** discharge. Onam was still eating and drinking. His vaccinations were all current. Onam was admitted to the hospital for diagnostic evaluation.

Physical Examination: Pat performed an initial physical examination and found that Onam was BAR with a TPR within expected reference ranges, but respiratory noises were audible when he listened to Onam inhale and exhale. There was no sign of **dyspnea.** The right **submandibular** lymph nodes were enlarged and **palpable.** An obvious deformity on Onam's face ran from the caudal aspect of the right **naris** up to the right medial canthus. The rest of the examination was unremarkable. Onam weighed 981.2 lb. Pat drew blood samples for a CBC and serum biochemical testing and collected feces and urine for analysis. Dr. Murdoch examined the face, nose, and mouth. He found a large **intranasal** mass at the **rostral** end of the right naris. The mass appeared to be covered with normal nasal mucous membrane. When he opened Onam's mouth and examined the **oral cavity,** he found that the caudal part of the hard palate was pushed down **ventrally.** Onam was sedated with an **equine** sedative (0.5 **mg/kg** [0.23 mg/lb] of body weight **IV**). An **endoscope** was passed through the left naris with no trouble, but it could not be passed through the right naris without possibly causing trauma. He also noted a **nasal septum** deviation to the left. The **pharynx, glottis,** and **proximal tracheal** regions appeared normal.

X-rays of the nasal and sinus regions of the head showed a soft tissue mass in the right nasal cavity that extended from the rostral area of the nasal cavity to the **ventrocaudal** area of the maxillary and frontal **sinuses.** No bone **lysis** was evident.

Onam was **anemic, leukopenic, neutropenic,** and slightly **hyperfibrinogenemic** according to the **hemogram.** Dr. Murdoch performed a fine-needle aspiration of the nasal mass, and **cytological** examination revealed an accumulation of **RBCs,** a few mature **PMNs,** and some bacteria. No evidence of **neoplasia** was noted.

Three days after admission to the Frisbee LA Hospital, Onam rubbed his nose on the wall of his stall and dislodged a segment of the mass, causing self-limiting **epistaxis.** Dr. Murdoch repeated the endoscopy and found that there was still a large mass in the right nasal cavity, from which he took a bx. The facial deformity receded over the next 2 days.

Histological evaluation of the bx of the mass revealed a **hematoma** that contained immature granulation tissue, **hemorrhage,** and large areas of **necrosis.** After discussion with the owner, Dr. Murdoch planned a surgical **resection** of the mass, with future **intralesional** injections of formalin. Surgery was delayed for 3 days to wait for the leukopenia to resolve.

On the day of surgery, anesthesia was induced and maintained. Onam was positioned in **left lateral recumbency.** The region over the right maxillary and frontal sinuses was **aseptically** prepared, as was the cranial aspect of the ventral cervical region over the trachea. A temporary **tracheotomy** was performed here. A self-retaining **tracheostomy** tube was placed to establish an open airway. A standard flap **sinusotomy** of the right frontomaxillary sinus was performed, and the hematoma was **resected.** The sinus and nasal cavities were packed with sterile gauze, and the sinus-otomy flap was routinely closed. Anesthetic recovery was without complications. The gauze packing and the tracheotomy tube were removed 48 hours after surgery without incident. **Antibiotics** were administered IV for 7 days post surgery. After removal of the gauze packing, all of Onam's vital signs were within expected reference ranges. He still had a slight blood-tinged **mucoid nasal discharge.** Onam was discharged from the hospital 8 days after surgery, and antibiotics were administered IM by the owner for an additional 10 days. When Onam returned for suture removal, the nasal discharge was gone. Endoscopy indicated a restricted but functional right nasal airway.

EXERCISE 12-1 *Case It!*

Case Study 12-1 will give you the opportunity to apply your new knowledge and understanding of clinical veterinary language in the context of a medical report. Write the word, words, or abbreviations found in the Case Study in the blanks that correspond to their definitions. *Hint:* All answers are bolded words found in the Case Study.

1. _____ pertaining to the study of cells

2. _____ difficult or labored breathing

3. _____ pertaining to the lack or deficiency of white blood cells

4. _____ lying down, reclining

5. _____ pertaining to the study of tissues

6. _____ pertaining to the nose

7. _____ surgical incision into the windpipe

8. _____ instrument used to view the inner part of a body

9. _____ intravenous administration of a drug

10. _____ the vocal cords and the space between them

11. _____ situated near to the point of attachment to the body

12. _____ blood cell that carries oxygen to the body cells

13. _____ literally, a "swelling or tumor of blood"

14. _____ death of a portion of body tissue

15. _____ a nosebleed

16. _____ surgical creation of a new permanent opening in the windpipe

17. _____ resembling mucus

18. _____ situated within the nose

19. _____ cavities or passageways in hollow bones

20. _____ bleeding; a profuse discharge of blood

21. _____ capable of being handled, touched, or felt

22. _____ located on only one side

23. _____ destruction or breakage

24. _____ surgical removal of all or part of an organ or tissue

25. _____ direction toward the tip of the nose when referring to the head

Check your answers at the end of the chapter, Answers to Exercises.

Hearing is the **auditory sense.** It is the ability to identify sound by detecting vibrations of air molecules or sound waves through the ear. The function of the ear is to gather sound waves that are speeding through the air, funnel them into the middle and inner ear, and convert them to electrical impulses that will travel to the brain to be interpreted as sound. Each structure in the ear plays a critical role (Figure 12-3).

The **pinna** (_plural_ = pinnae) is the ear flap. It acts as a funnel to catch sound waves and direct them into the **ear canal** or **external auditory canal.** Have you ever noticed how a dog, horse, or cat "listens"? Many animals have large, movable pinnae so they

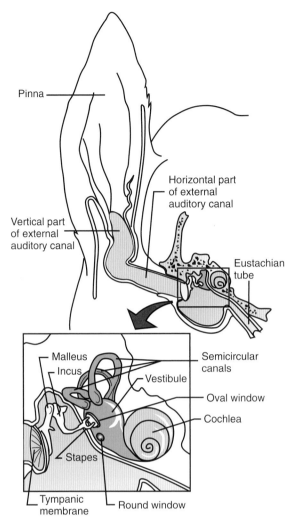

FIGURE 12-3 Structures of the middle ear and inner ear. (From Colville TP: *Clinical Anatomy and Physiology for Veterinary Technicians,* ed 2, St Louis, 2009, Mosby.)

can hear sounds from all directions. Humans have fixed pinnae and hear best the sounds coming from the front.

At the medial end of the ear canal, the **tympanic membrane** or **eardrum** is tightly drawn across the canal. When sound waves hit the eardrum, it starts to vibrate.

On the medial side of the eardrum, the **middle ear** begins. In the middle ear is the **eustachian tube,** a tube that connects the middle ear to the pharynx. It regulates air pressure in the middle ear so that the pressure is equal on both sides of the eardrum. Also in the middle ear are three tiny bones called the **ossicles.** They are named the **malleus** (hammer), **incus** (anvil), and **stapes** (stirrup). The malleus is connected to the eardrum. The malleus forms a joint with the incus, which in turn forms a joint with the stapes. The stapes is connected to another membrane called the **oval window.** When the eardrum starts to vibrate, so does the malleus. When the malleus vibrates, it sets up a series of vibrations that act as a system of levers when vibrations pass through the incus and stapes. This causes the vibration to be **amplified.**

The other side of the oval window marks the beginning of the **inner ear.** One of the structures here is the **cochlea.** The cochlea is a spiral tube filled with fluid and lined with hair cells (specialized dendrites) that project into the fluid. Cilia in different areas of the cochlea detect vibrations of different frequency. When the membrane of the oval window vibrates, this causes the fluid in the cochlea to vibrate. These vibrations are detected by the tiny hair cells and are converted to electrical impulses. So the cochlea is the animal's microphone. It takes the amplified sound waves that entered the ear canal and traveled through the middle ear and converts them to electrical impulses that are transmitted to the brain and are interpreted as sounds.

The more cilia are stimulated, the greater is the number of electrical impulses transmitted to the brain, and the louder is the sound perceived. Each species has a range of normal hearing for loudness (amplitude) and pitch (frequency). Frequencies normally heard by humans are called **audio** or **sonic** frequencies. Have you ever heard a sonic boom from a speeding aircraft? Frequencies higher than sonic are called **ultrasonic** frequencies, or **ultrasound.** Bats use ultrasound for **echolocation** during flight. Dogs can hear ultrasonic frequencies produced by "silent" dog whistles. Frequencies lower than sonic are called **infrasonic** frequencies, or **infrasound.** Whales, giraffes, dolphins, and elephants use infrasound to communicate.

EXERCISE 12-2 *Hear It!*

An old joke asks, If a tree falls in a forest and nobody is around to hear it, does it make a sound? What do you think? Well, a tree fell in the forest and Bambi was there to hear it. The tree produced sound waves that were picked up by Bambi's ears. But before he could hear the tree fall, the waves had to pass through many structures to be converted to an electrical impulse that would go to the brain to be interpreted as a sound. Below is a list of the common names for the structures through which the sound traveled. In the spaces provided, put the anatomical name of each structure. Then place them in the order through which the sound wave would travel. The first structure is done for you.

common name	anatomical name
anvil	
ear canal	
eardrum	
ear flap	*pinna*
hammer	
oval window	*oval window*
snail shell	
stirrup	

structure order

1. *pinna*
2. _____
3. _____
4. _____
5. _____
6. _____
7. _____
8. _____

Check your answers at the end of the chapter, Answers to Exercises.

Equilibrium is what helps an animal keep its balance by tracking the movement and position of its head. An animal keeps its balance by interpreting input from the ears, the eyes, and muscles throughout the body.

The structures of equilibrium in the ear are found in the inner ear (see Figure 12-3). They are the vestibule and the **semicircular canals.** The **vestibule** is made up of two structures: the **utricle** and the **saccule.** The utricle and the saccule are fluid-filled sacs that function alike. Each has a raised patch of sensory epithelium called the **macula,** which is covered by supporting cells and hair cells that project tiny hairs into its gelatinous matrix. Also found in the gelatinous matrix are tiny calcium carbonate crystals, called **otoliths.** The otoliths are in contact with the hairs of the hair cells, which in turn create a sensory impulse that is transmitted to the brain. Gravity causes the otoliths to put constant pressure on the hairs, as long as the head stays still. Movement of the head causes the otoliths to move, bending the hairs. This then creates a different impulse that is transmitted to the brain. The brain learns that the head has moved and responds accordingly.

EXERCISE 12-3 *Stoned!*

You may hear of a stone referred to as a **calculus.** This is spelled the same as the mathematical calculus. Both came to be called the same because the early Romans used stones in counting. An otolith is a stone in the inner ear and is important for sensing gravity. Stones can be formed in many places in the body as the result of a pathological condition. Define the following words about "stones."

1. arteriolith = _____

2. arthrolithiasis = _____

3. broncholith = _____

4. cardiolith = _____

5. choledocholithiasis = _____

6. cholelith = _____

7. cholelithotomy = _____

8. coprolith = _____

9. enterolith = _____

10. gastrolith = _____

11. hepatolith = _____

12. hypodermolithiasis = _____

13. hysterolith = _____

14. lithiasis = _____

15. lithoclasty = _____

16. lithogenesis = _____

17. lithologist = _____

18. litholysis = _____

19. lithometer = _____

20. lithoscope = _____

21. lithotome = _____

22. lithotomist = _____

23. lithotomy = _____

24. lithous = _____

25. microlithiasis = _____

26. pancreatolithectomy = _____

27. phlebolith = _____

28. pneumolithiasis = _____

29. ptyalolith = _____

30. rhinolith = _____

31. rhinopharyngolith = _____

32. sebolith = _____

33. sialolithotomy = _____

34. tricholith = _____

Check your answers at the end of the chapter, Answers to Exercises.

The **semicircular canals** are three curved, bony, fluid-filled canals, each of which contains a fluid-filled tube (Figure 12-4). Each canal, and therefore each tube, is set at right angles to the other two canals. Look at the ceiling in the corner of a room. This will give you an idea of how the three canals are oriented to each other. Within each tube is a raised area called the **ampulla,** which contains a sensory patch of epithelium called the **crista,** which functions very similarly to the macula of the utricle. However, there are no otoliths in the semicircular tubes. The hair cells are covered with a gelatinous structure called the **cupula** that "floats" in the fluid that fills the tubes. The semicircular canals detect acceleration. As the animal's head moves, the cupulae floating in the fluid stimulate the hairs of the crista. The stimulus is translated into a sensory impulse that is transmitted to the brain. The brain reacts by sending motor impulses to muscles that react to keep the animal balanced.

Vision or **sight** is the **ophthalmic sense,** which originates in the eye. The main structures of the eye are the eyelids, cornea, anterior chamber, iris, lens, posterior

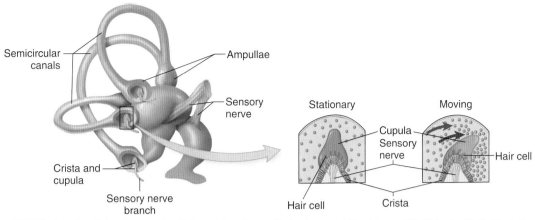

FIGURE 12-4 Semicircular canals. (Adapted from Patton K: *Anatomy and Physiology,* ed 7, St Louis, 2010, Mosby.)

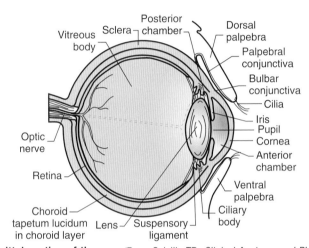

FIGURE 12-5 Sagittal section of the eye. (From Colville TP: *Clinical Anatomy and Physiology for Veterinary Technicians,* ed 2, St Louis, 2009, Mosby.)

chamber, retina, optic nerve, and sclera (Figure 12-5). These structures work together to gather and focus light rays on the sensory cells at the back of the eye to create a sensory impulse that is transmitted to the brain and interpreted as an image.

Eyelids close over the eyeball to protect the eye from physical damage or from excess light. Mammals have an upper and a lower **eyelid.** Birds and some reptiles have a third eyelid called the **nictitating membrane.** Dogs and cats have nictitating membranes that are not normally visible. Tears (**lacrimal fluid** from the **lacrimal gland)** are spread over the eye every time an animal blinks. This clears away dust and moistens the cornea.

The **sclera** is a tough, leathery connective tissue made up of collagen fibers. It protects the eyeball and helps it keep its shape. The sclera forms the "whites" of the eyes that you can see. However, the sclera actually covers the entire eyeball. At the front of the eye, the sclera is continuous with the transparent cornea. Through **extraocular muscles** attached by tendons to the sclera, the eyeball is moved up, down, left, right, and diagonally.

The **conjunctiva** is a transparent membrane that covers the rostral portion of the sclera. It also lines the inner surfaces of the eyelids. Many blood vessels are found in the conjunctiva. When the eye is injured, these blood vessels dilate and make the white part of the eye look red.

The **cornea** is a clear, protective covering on the front of the eyeball. It is made up of collagen fibers, like the sclera, but its higher water content makes it transparent. If the water content is too high or too low, it loses its transparency. The cornea admits light to the interior of the eye, helps focus the light rays on the retina, and filters out ultraviolet light. It gets its oxygen directly from the air. However, it does contain many nerve endings, so it is very sensitive to pain stimuli, such as those that happen when the cornea is scratched.

The **iris** is the thin sheet of muscle tissue that forms the colored part of the eye. The iris is the structure that controls the amount of light that enters the eye. In the middle of the iris is the **pupil,** a hole through which the light passes. The iris can open or close the hole by means of dilator and constrictor muscles. In a normal animal, the pupils should be the same size and should react to light stimulus in the same manner. **Anisocoria** is an abnormal condition wherein the pupils are two different sizes. The **pupillary light reflex** (PLR) controls the size of the pupil in response to the intensity of the light being sent to the retina.

During the course of a 24-hour cycle, the amount of light in the environment will change. The iris adjusts accordingly. Animals with excellent night vision (nocturnal animals) can open their pupils to a greater degree than animals that are active during the day. If the pupil of an animal is dilated by drugs or disease, the condition is called **mydriasis.** In a clinical situation, this is usually done to inspect the interior of the eye. If the pupil is constricted by drugs or disease, the condition is called **miosis (myosis).** Drugs that inhibit the sympathetic nervous system will cause miosis.

Right behind the pupil is the **lens,** a clear structure attached to the **ciliary body** by suspensory ligaments around its periphery. As the ciliary body muscles contract and relax, the suspensory ligaments are able to change the shape of the lens. This is called **accommodation,** or changing the focus (i.e., adjusting the shape of the lens to allow near and far vision). Most animals have poor lens accommodation and have developed other methods to allow for near and far vision.

A **cataract** is an abnormal condition wherein the lens becomes cloudy, thus producing a blurred image. Cataracts can be caused by genetic disposition, trauma, disease, and old age. The thicker and more opaque the cataract becomes, the more likely the animal will become blind.

The **anterior compartment** lies in front of the lens and is filled with **aqueous humor.** The **anterior chamber** lies between the cornea and the iris. The **posterior chamber** is located between the iris and the lens. The **posterior compartment** is located behind the lens. It contains a clear, gelatinous substance called **vitreous humor** (vitreous body) that fills the space between the back of the lens and the retina.

The **retina** is the light-receptive layer of the eye. It is covered with **photoreceptive** cells, which are actually sensory dendrites that will create electrical impulses from the light that strikes them. As light strikes the photoreceptive cells, each cell sends an impulse to the brain. The brain interprets all of these dots of light and blends them together into one image. The more photoreceptors per square millimeter, the greater is the ability of an animal to distinguish objects at a distance. An eagle, for example, has about one million receptors per square millimeter. Hunting for supper is much easier for an eagle than for a human, who has only about 200,000 receptors per square millimeter. Besides, humans cannot fly on their own to find supper.

The photoreceptive cells are called **cones** and **rods.** Cones are detail- and color-sensitive and allow animals to distinguish between colors to some extent. However, cones do not function well in dim light. Rods are located mostly toward the periphery of the retina. They are more sensitive to small amounts of light and are therefore better for night vision, although the image will be black and white. Some nocturnal animals (e.g., opossums) have only rods in their retinas. The rods make their eyes very sensitive to light, but the image produced is black and white and is not very sharp.

Because of the greater number of rods in the retina, nocturnal animals have enhanced night vision. Night vision is augmented by two other mechanisms. Opening the iris (dilating the pupil) lets in more light. A third system is provided by a layer of cells, called the **tapetum** or **tapetum lucidum,** located just behind the retina. These cells reflect light back through the layer of rods and cones in the retina, giving the rods and cones a second chance to be stimulated by the light. The reflected light keeps on going right out of the pupil, so when a light shines on these eyes at night, they seem to be shining back at you. Think of cat eyes or raccoon eyes shining in the night when a flashlight shines on them, or your headlights shining on a fox's eyes.

Axons from the neurons of the rods and cones come together to form the **optic nerve.** At the point of convergence, no photoreceptive cells are present, so a blind spot **(optic disk)** is created on the retina. The blood vessels of the retina spread out from the area of the optic disk.

The **fundus** of the eye is its inner surface, opposite the lens. The retina and the optic disk are part of the fundus. The eye's fundus is the only part of the body where blood vessels can be observed directly (with an ophthalmoscope).

EXERCISE 12-4 *Where Am I?*

You have learned that the many receptors for the special senses are localized in specialized sensory organs. Name the sensory organ in which the following structures are located.

1. _____ ampulla

2. _____ cochlea

3. _____ iris

4. _____ lacrimal gland

5. _____ malleus

6. _____ otolith

7. _____ papillae

8. _____ pinnae

9. _____ retina

10. _____ saccule

11. _____ semicircular canals

12. _____ stapes

13. _____ tympanic membrane

14. _____ utricle

15. _____ vomeronasal organ

Check your answers at the end of the chapter, Answers to Exercises.

CASE STUDY 12-2 #2003-1208 SHERPA

Signalment and History: A 1-year-old, 32-lb F(S) Border Collie named Sherpa was brought to the Frisbee SA Clinic because of an acute onset of blindness accompanied by a reduced level of consciousness (obtundation). Her previous history was unremarkable, and her vaccinations were current.

Physical Examination: Jess found that except for neurological signs, Sherpa appeared to be in good condition. Her **TPR** was within expected reference ranges. Jess drew blood samples for a **CBC** and serum biochemical testing. Dr. Frisbee performed a neurological examination and found mild **obtundation** and **mydriasis** in **ambient** light and an incomplete **pupillary light reflex** (PLR) in both eyes. **Anisocoria** was not evident. Sherpa behaved as if she was blind. In both eyes, **palpebral** reflexes were complete, and eyeball position and movements were normal. Dr. Frisbee also found that Sherpa's gait, postural reactions, segmental reflexes, and vertebral column were within acceptable ranges.

A complete **ophthalmic** examination involving **binocular** indirect **ophthalmoscopy** was conducted by Dr. Beauregard, a veterinary **ophthalmologist.** He reported that there was no obvious **ocular** discharge or facial asymmetry. Other than a subtle **subcapsular cataract** in the left eye, he detected no abnormalities in the **anterior chamber** or **vitreous humor** of either eye. Examination of the **fundus** revealed abnormal multifocal, blurry, white-gray opacities within the **retina,** which he identified as **retinal edema.** The **optic nerve, tapetum,** and retinal **vasculature** appeared normal in both eyes. Sherpa had been examined for an unrelated problem 5 months before this examination, and her PLRs were recorded as normal. There was no record of a fundus examination at that time.

Diagnosis: On the basis of the neurological and ophthalmic examinations, Dr. Frisbee arrived at a diagnosis of **intracranial** disease. The primary **ddx** were infectious disease, inflammatory response, toxicity, and metabolic disease. The **hemogram** was unremarkable. Dr. Frisbee performed an abdominal **ultrasound,** which revealed a moderate **splenomegaly.**

After **pupil dilation** with a topically applied **mydriatic,** Dr. Beauregard performed an **electroretinography** (ERG) to determine whether the retinas were functioning properly. Sherpa's retinal response was < in both eyes.

Upon further questioning, Jess discovered that Sherpa's owner also owned horses that had been dewormed with an antiparasitic paste 1 day before Sherpa developed clinical signs. The paste contained a drug, ivermectin, with known toxic effects in dogs. The owner also indicated that Sherpa was quite a scavenger. With this further information, Dr. Frisbee concluded that Sherpa probably had been poisoned by the antiparasitic paste upon eating horse feces or spilled paste. The day after Sherpa's initial examination (2 days after her suspected exposure), Jess drew another blood sample for ivermectin analysis. The serum ivermectin level in Sherpa's blood confirmed exposure to ivermectin.

Treatment: Dr. Frisbee did not prescribe any specific treatment because Sherpa appeared to be clinically improving. Her ivermectin level was rechecked again the next day, at which time it had greatly decreased. Two days after her initial evaluation (4 days after her supposed exposure), Sherpa was **BAR** and her **PLRs** were improving. Sherpa was discharged from the hospital and was brought back to the clinic for reexamination 1 week later. The owner reported improvement in Sherpa's vision and described that it was near normal.

EXERCISE 12-5 *Case It!*

Case Study 12-2 will definitely give you another opportunity to apply your new knowledge and understanding of clinical veterinary language in the context of a medical report. Write the word, words, or abbreviations found in the Case Study in the blanks that correspond to their definitions.

1. _____ the size of the pupils is not equal

2. _____ pertaining to both eyes

3. _____ cloudy lens, producing a blurred image

4. _____ abnormal accumulation of fluid in the cavities and intracellular places in the body

5. _____ inner part of the back of the eye where blood vessels may be observed

6. _____ less than

7. _____ the pupil is dilated by drugs or disease

8. _____ reduced level of consciousness

9. _____ procedure to examine the eye

10. _____ all the axons from the neurons of the rods and cones

11. _____ pertaining to the eyelids

12. _____ reduction of the size of the pupil in response to light

13. _____ light-receptive layer of the eye

14. _____ an enlarged spleen

15. _____ layer of cells behind the retina that reflects light

16. _____ gelatinous substance that fills the space between the back of the eye and the retina

Check your answers at the end of the chapter, Answers to Exercises.

TABLE 12-3	Abbreviations	
Abbreviation	**Meaning**	**Example**
PLR	pupillary light reflex	Dr. Frisbee checked Lady's PLR with a penlight after Lady was HBC in the head. Everything was OK.

PLR

ANSWERS TO EXERCISES

Exercise 12-1

1. cytological
2. dyspnea
3. leukopenic
4. recumbency
5. histological
6. nasal
7. tracheotomy
8. endoscope
9. IV
10. glottis
11. proximal
12. RBC
13. hematoma
14. necrosis
15. epistaxis
16. tracheostomy
17. mucoid
18. intranasal
19. sinuses
20. hemorrhage
21. palpable
22. unilateral
23. lysis
24. resection
25. rostral

Exercise 12-2

common name	anatomical name
anvil	incus
ear canal	auditory canal
eardrum	tympanic membrane
ear flap	pinna
hammer	malleus
oval window	oval window
snail shell	cochlea
stirrup	stapes

structure order

1. pinna
2. auditory canal
3. tympanic membrane
4. malleus
5. incus
6. stapes
7. oval window
8. cochlea

Exercise 12-3

1. arteriolith = stone in an artery
2. arthrolithiasis = pathological condition that results from a stone in a joint
3. broncholith = stone in a bronchus
4. cardiolith = stone in the heart
5. choledocholithiasis = pathological condition that results from a stone in the bile duct
6. cholelith = a stone of bile; a gall stone
7. cholelithotomy = incision into a gall stone
8. coprolith = stone formed around fecal matter
9. enterolith = stone in the intestines
10. gastrolith = stone in the stomach
11. hepatolith = stone in the liver
12. hypodermolithiasis = pathological condition that results from a subcutaneous stone
13. hysterolith = stone in the uterus
14. lithiasis = pathological condition that results from a stone
15. lithoclasty = crushing of a stone into fragments that may pass through natural channels
16. lithogenesis = process of the formation or beginning of a stone
17. lithologist = a person who studies or has knowledge of stones
18. litholysis = destruction, dissolving, or breakage of a stone
19. lithometer = instrument used to measure a stone
20. lithoscope = instrument used for visual examination of a stone in a body organ
21. lithotome = surgical instrument specifically designed to perform incisions into a duct or body organs for the purpose of removing stones
22. lithotomist = a person who removes stones (i.e., a person who cuts or uses a tome)
23. lithotomy = surgical incision into a stone
24. lithous = pertaining to a stone
25. microlithiasis = pathological condition that results from a very small stone
26. pancreatolithectomy = surgical removal of a stone in the pancreas
27. phlebolith = stone in a vein
28. pneumolithiasis = pathological condition that results from a stone in the lung
29. ptyalolith = stone in a salivary gland
30. rhinolith = stone in the nose
31. rhinopharyngolith = stone in the nose and throat
32. sebolith = stone in a sebum gland
33. sialolithotomy = surgical incision into the salivary gland to remove a stone
34. tricholith = a calcified hairball

Exercise 12-4

1. ear
2. ear
3. eye
4. eye
5. ear
6. ear
7. tongue

8. ear
9. eye
10. ear
11. ear
12. ear
13. ear
14. ear
15. between the nose and the mouth

Exercise 12-5
1. anisocoria
2. binocular
3. cataract
4. edema
5. fundus
6. <
7. mydriasis
8. obtundation
9. ophthalmoscopy
10. optic nerve
11. palpebral
12. PLR = pupillary light reflex
13. retina
14. splenomegaly
15. tapetum
16. vitreous humor

Chapter 13

The Endocrine System

Ah, hormones. You can tell a gelding; you can ask a mare; but you must discuss with a stallion.

Anonymous

WORD PARTS

| aden/o | **ahd**-ehn-ō | andr/o | **ahn**-drō | pseud/o | **soo**-dō | trop/o | **trō**-pō |
| adren/o | ahd-**rē**-nō | crin/o | **krihn**-ō | thyr/o | **thī**-rō | -trophy | **trō**-phē |

OUTLINE

THE ENDOCRINE SYSTEM
ENDOCRINE SYSTEM GLANDS

LEARNING OBJECTIVES

When you have completed this chapter, you will be able to:

1. Understand the components and functions of the endocrine system.

2. Identify and recognize the meanings of word parts related to the endocrine system, using them to build or analyze words.

3. Apply your new knowledge and understanding of clinical veterinary language in the context of medical reports.

CASE STUDY 13-1   2005-1374 THEUDIS

Signalment and History: A 6-year-old 2696-lb Percheron **gelding** named Theudis was evaluated at the Frisbee LA Clinic because of **bilateral blepharospasm** and head shaking. Theudis was current on his vaccinations and had no remarkable prior history. Theudis was admitted to the hospital for further diagnostic testing.

Physical Examination: Jess performed the initial physical examination and discovered that Theudis was overweight (he should have weighed about 2100 pounds) and had a marked **adipose** deposit over the crest of his neck. The **TPR** was within the expected reference range. Theudis displayed some abnormal behaviors, including mild repetitive vertical movement of the head, snorting, and **flehmen response**—all indicative of head-shaking syndrome. Jess drew blood samples for a CBC, serum biochemical testing, and a serum thyroxine level. Dr. Murdoch discovered bilateral **paresthesia** and **dysesthesia** with **nasolabial** muscle **hypertrophy** during his examination of Theudis's nostrils and face.

Dr. Beauregard was called in to perform a complete **ophthalmologic** examination that included direct and indirect **ophthalmoscopy**, slit-lamp **biomicroscopy**, and cranial nerve examination. He found moderate bilateral blepharospasm, and the **conjunctivas** of both eyes were **hyperemic** and **edematous**. The **corneas** were dull. Theudis's **nasal** mucosa was dry. The cranial nerve examination revealed no other abnormalities. **Hemogram** results were within expected reference ranges. According to the lab results, the serum **thyroxine** concentration was low, and the results of **thyrotropin-releasing hormone** and **thyroid-stimulating hormone** stimulation tests were negative, indicating that Theudis had developed **hypothyroidism**.

(See the rest of the story later in the chapter.)

THE ENDOCRINE SYSTEM

Your prototype animal has come a long way from his original bag of bones. Thanks to his nervous system, the faster processes he needs to survive are controlled. He breathes, his heart beats, he eats, he thinks, and he can respond to just about any sensory input or emergency. However, what about other processes? How does he grow and mature? Do his bones contain enough calcium? How is the level of glucose in his blood controlled? Will he be able to reproduce? These functions are just as important as breathing and eating.

The animal's body produces chemicals called **hormones** and uses them to control certain functions such as body growth, metabolism, and sexual development. The endocrine system is responsible for the production and release of hormones to control these processes that happen slowly.

BOX 13-1   Terms That Defy Word Analysis

- antagonistic—acting in opposition
- circadian rhythm—biological cycles that occur at approximately 24-hour intervals
- endorphin—a compound produced in the brain and in other body tissues that reduces the sensation of pain; the body's natural painkiller
- gland—a group of specialized cells in the body that produce and secrete a specific substance, such as a hormone
- hormone—a substance produced by one tissue or by one group of cells that is carried by the bloodstream to another tissue or organ to affect its physiological functions such as metabolism or growth
- receptor—a protein molecule on a cell wall with a unique shape that will allow only one type of molecule, such as a hormone, to attach to it
- target cells—cells that have appropriate receptors on their cell walls to allow attachment of a specific molecule

TABLE 13-1   Word Parts Associated with the Endocrine System

Word Part	Meaning	Example and Definition	Word Parts	
crin/o	secrete	**endocrinology** branch of biology that deals with the study of hormones and their receptors, and the diseases and conditions associated with them	endo- = within, inner crin/o = secrete -logy = to study, or to have knowledge of	crin/o
trop/o	affinity to, turn to, respond to a stimulus	**aerotropism** turning toward or away from a supply of air; response to a gaseous stimulus	aer/o = air, gas trop/o = affinity to, turn to, respond to a stimulus -ism = state, condition, action, process, or result	trop/o
		⚠ *Do not confuse this* trop/o *with* -trophy, *meaning "growth."* **amyotrophy** muscular degeneration; wasting away of the muscles	a- = without, no, not my/o = muscle -trophy = growth	-trophy
aden/o	gland	**adenopathy** a disease of a gland	aden/o = gland -pathy = disease	aden/o
adren/o	adrenal gland	**adrenomegaly** enlargement of the adrenal gland	adren/o = adrenal gland megal/o = large or enlarged -y = made up of, characterized by	adren/o
thyr/o	thyroid gland	**thyroidectomy** surgery to remove all or part of the thyroid gland 💡 *The thyroid gland is small and lies in the neck ventral to the trachea. It gets its name because to the early Greeks it resembled a shield* (thyreos).	thyr/o = thyroid -oid = resembling -ectomy = surgical removal	thyr/o
andr/o	male, masculine	**androgen** general term for a hormone (e.g., testosterone) that regulates body changes associated with male sexual development	andr/o = male, masculine gen/o = formation or beginning	andr/o
pseudo/o	false, deception	**pseudoanorexia** a condition in which an individual claims to have no appetite and is unable to eat, yet eats secretly	pseud/o = false, deception an- = without, no, not orexia = appetite, desire	pseud/o

The endocrine system is made up of endocrine **glands** that are located all over the body (Table 13-1). Each endocrine gland is composed of a group of specialized cells that produce one or more hormones. The glands of the endocrine system are ductless glands. This means that their hormones are absorbed into capillaries and are carried throughout the body by the bloodstream. Compare this with **exocrine glands,** which have ducts to carry their glandular secretions onto an epithelial surface (e.g., sweat glands and the glands that produce digestive enzymes).

Each **hormone** is a unique chemical messenger that delivers a signal to cells. Tiny amounts of hormones have a powerful effect on the body. They affect growth, the shape of the body, and the way the body uses food, and they allow the body to make the proper adjustments to changes in the outside world. Pheromones are also chemical messengers, but they are secreted externally to affect other animals. A hormone works internally only on the animal that produces it. And a hormone acts only on the cells that have **receptors** for it on their cell walls. These cells are called **target cells.** The receptor on a target cell wall is uniquely shaped so that only one type of hormone molecule will fit. Think of a receptor as a lock into which only specific keys (hormones) will fit. Not every cell in the body has a receptor for every hormone, and a hormone can attach itself only to cells that have its unique receptor. So when the hormone attaches itself to the receptor, the hormone–receptor combination transmits a chemical instruction to working structures inside the cell.

Many hormones come in **antagonistic pairs** (i.e., when one hormone tells a cell to do one thing, the antagonistic hormone will tell the cell to do the opposite thing). This is called a **feedback system,** and it works much like the thermostat on a heater that is controlling the temperature in a room.

EXERCISE 13-1   *Pseudo-Spelling!*

By now you should be aware that wherever you see a word part in clinical veterinary language, it will ALWAYS be spelled the same—no matter how the word is pronounced. The following list of words is filled with "pseudo-spellings," but not all of the words are misspelled. Correct the misspelled words.

1. _____correct_____ ankylosis

2. _____ante_____ antibrachium

3. _____correct_____ arthritis

4. _____megaly_____ cardiomegalie

5. _____chondro_____ chrondoplasty

6. _____dermopathy_____ dermopathey

7. _____dystrophy_____ distrophe

8. _____erythro_____ erithrocyte

9. _____correct_____ hemoptysis

10. _____larynx_____ larnix

11. _____correct_____ milligram

12. _____necroscopy_____ neckroscopy

13. _____correct_____ purpura

14. _____correct_____ pyrogen

15. _____Splenopexy_____ splenopeksy

Check your answers at the end of the chapter, Answers to Exercises.

ENDOCRINE SYSTEM GLANDS

This chapter will introduce you to the hormones produced by the major glands of the endocrine system. (You will study them in greater detail during your endocrinology coursework.) The major glands of the endocrine system are as follows:

- anterior pituitary
- posterior pituitary
- thyroid
- parathyroid
- adrenal cortex
- adrenal medulla
- pancreas
- gonads

Figure 13-1 shows the locations of major endocrine glands in a cat.

The **hypothalamus** is located in the center of the brain, just above the pituitary gland. Its most important function is to act as the link between the nervous system and the endocrine system by way of the pituitary gland. Nerve cells in the hypothalamus control the pituitary gland by producing chemicals (releasing and inhibiting hormones) that stimulate or stop pituitary gland hormone production. The rate at which the releasing hormones are produced can be affected by environmental temperature and by light exposure patterns. Four important releasing hormones produced by the hypothalamus are:

- growth hormone–releasing hormone (GHRH)
- thyrotropin-releasing hormone (TRH)
- corticotropin-releasing hormone (CRH)
- gonadotropin-releasing hormone (GnRH)

The **pituitary gland** is located at the base of the brain. It is sometimes referred to as the *master endocrine gland* because it has great influence over other endocrine glands. It is divided into two sections that produce two different sets of hormones. The **anterior pituitary gland** produces:

- prolactin (PRL)
  - This stimulates milk production in the dam after she has given birth.
- growth hormone (GH)
  - This stimulates growth in young animals and helps maintain muscle mass, bone mass, and fat distribution in adults.
  - Its release is controlled by GHRH from the hypothalamus.

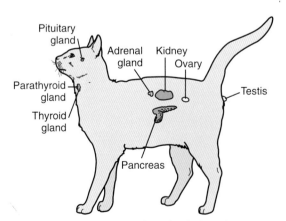

FIGURE 13-1 **Relative locations of major endocrine glands in cat.** (Modified from McBride DF: *Learning Veterinary Terminology,* ed 2, St Louis, 2002, Mosby. Also in Colville TP: *Clinical Anatomy and Physiology for Veterinary Technicians,* ed 2, St Louis, 2009, Mosby.)

- adrenocorticotropic hormone (ACTH)
  - This stimulates the adrenal gland cortex to produce hormones.
- thyroid-stimulating hormone (TSH)
  - This stimulates the thyroid gland to make thyroid hormones that will help regulate the animal's metabolism, energy, growth, development, and nervous system activity.
- luteinizing hormone (LH)
  - This regulates testosterone production in males and estrogen production and ovulation in females.
- follicle-stimulating hormone (FSH)
  - This regulates sperm production in males and stimulates the female's ovaries to produce eggs.
  - LH and FSH work together for normal male and female sex hormone production.
- endorphins
  - These are the animal's natural painkillers that reduce the nervous system's sensitivity to pain signals.

The **posterior pituitary** releases two hormones:
- oxytocin
  - This causes the uterus to contract during the birthing process and milk letdown (as opposed to production) in lactating females.
- antidiuretic hormone (ADH)
  - This hormone is also called *vasopressin*.
  - It regulates water balance in the animal's body.

The **thyroid gland** is a small gland located in the animal's neck region in front of the trachea, and just below the larynx. The function of the thyroid is to act as kind of a regulator to speed up or slow down the rate at which the body uses food and oxygen. It does its job by trapping the iodine in food and combining it with other chemicals to make its hormones. The thyroid produces three hormones:
- triiodothyronine (T3)
  - This helps control the animal's metabolic rate or the rate at which the cells burn fuel from food to produce energy.
- thyroxine (T4)
  - T4 is converted to T3 in the body: T3 + T4 = Thyroid hormone
- calcitonin
  - This helps maintain homeostasis of blood calcium levels by preventing **hypercalcemia.**

The thyroid gets its instructions for T3 and T4 hormone production from the pituitary gland via the thyroid-stimulating hormone (TSH). If insufficient amounts of TSH, or thyroid hormone, are being produced, the animal may develop **hypothyroidism.** If too much TSH, or thyroid hormone, is produced, **hyperthyroidism** may result.

The **parathyroid glands** are small glands located in, on, and around the thyroid gland. They secrete one hormone, parathyroid hormone (parathormone) (PTH), which is the antagonist to calcitonin. It maintains homeostasis of blood calcium by preventing **hypocalcemia.**

CASE STUDY 13-1 2005-1374 THEUDIS

Signalment and History: A 6-year-old 2696-lb Percheron **gelding** named Theudis was evaluated at the Frisbee LA Clinic because of **bilateral blepharospasm** and head shaking. Theudis was current on his vaccinations and had no remarkable prior history. Theudis was admitted to the hospital for further diagnostic testing.

Physical Examination: Jess performed the initial physical examination and discovered that Theudis was overweight (he should have weighed about 2100 pounds) and had a marked **adipose** deposit over the crest of his neck. The **TPR** was within the expected reference range. Theudis displayed some abnormal behaviors, including mild repetitive vertical movement of the head, snorting, and **flehmen response**—all indicative of head-shaking syndrome. Jess drew blood samples for a CBC, serum biochemical testing, and a serum thyroxine level. Dr. Murdoch discovered bilateral **paresthesia** and **dysesthesia** with **nasolabial** muscle **hypertrophy** during his examination of Theudis's nostrils and face.

Dr. Beauregard was called in to perform a complete **ophthalmologic** examination that included direct and indirect **ophthalmoscopy,** slit-lamp **biomicroscopy,** and cranial nerve examination. He found moderate bilateral blepharospasm, and the **conjunctivas** of both eyes were **hyperemic** and **edematous.** The **corneas** were dull. Theudis's **nasal** mucosa was dry. The cranial nerve examination revealed no other abnormalities. **Hemogram** results were within expected reference ranges. According to the lab results, the serum **thyroxine** concentration was low, and the results of **thyrotropin-releasing hormone** and **thyroid-stimulating hormone** stimulation tests were negative, indicating that Theudis had developed **hypothyroidism.**

Diagnosis: Dr. Murdoch and Dr. Beauregard agreed that Theudis's primary diagnosis was hypothyroidism. Secondary peripheral **neuropathies** included **keratoconjunctivitis sicca** and dry nares caused by **parasympathetic** facial nerve **dysfunction,** and head-shaking **syndrome** with paresthesia and dysesthesia of the face caused by **sensory** trigeminal nerve disorder. Dr. Murdoch noted that both secondary neuropathies were most likely a result of the hypothyroidism.

Treatment and Outcome: Dr. Murdoch put Theudis on thyroid medication for his hypothyroidism, and ophthalmic drops and ointments for his eyes. Dr. Beauregard prepared a **subconjunctival** injection of a long-lasting, **anti-inflammatory** medication for Dr. Murdoch to administer. Five weeks later, while Dr. Murdoch and Jess were making farm calls in the area, they stopped and visited Theudis, who had undergone a significant weight loss and an obvious change in behavior. The episodes of snorting and flehmen display had all but disappeared; however, the blepharospasm was still evident. The owner reported later that the blepharospasm did not resolve until after 5 months of treatment. Dr. Murdoch had a telephone conversation with the owner 6 months after Theudis's **diagnosis,** and he reported that Theudis had only an occasional **serous** discharge from his eyes. Dr. Murdoch told the owner to watch the serous discharge, and if it turned to a **mucopurulent** discharge, he should put ophthalmic antibiotic ointment in the affected eye. A year after Theudis started his thyroid treatment, all of his clinical signs had been resolved.

EXERCISE 13-2 *Case It!*

Read Case Study 13-1 again. Then write words in the blanks to complete the definitions. Underlined portions of the clinical terms will give you clues to the answers to write in the blanks.

1. Another name for keratoconjunctivitis sicca is <u>xero</u>phthalmia,

    or _____ eye.

2. Paresthesia is a _____feeling_____ of numbness or tingling on the skin.

3. Bilateral blepharospasm involves intermittent involuntary abnormal muscle contractions of _____Both eyelids_____.

4. Biomicroscopy involves examination of _____small_____ living tissues in the body.

5. Ophthalmoscopy is the examination of the _____eye_____.

6. Hyperemia refers to having a large volume of _____Blood_____ in any given place in the body.

7. The nasolabial muscle is in the area of the _____Nose_____ and _____lips_____.

8. A muscle showing hypertrophy has greater than normal _____Growth_____.

9. The hormone thyroxine is secreted by the _____thyroid_____ gland.

10. The conjunctiva is located _____lining eyelids_____.

11. A neuropathy is a _____Disease_____ of nerves.

12. The serous discharge contained _____Serum_____.

13. The mucopurulent discharge contained _____mucus_____ and pus.

14. The action of the thyroid is _____less than normal_____ in hypothyroidism.

15. Dysfunction is _____bad or defect_____ ability of a body, organ, or organ system to perform normally.

Check your answers at the end of the chapter, Answers to Exercises.

The **adrenal glands** are located near the cranial ends of the kidneys. They are composed of two distinct glands: the adrenal cortex and the adrenal medulla. The **adrenal cortex** creates the outer layer of the adrenal gland. It produces three groups of hormones:

- glucocorticoids
  - These include cortisone, cortisol, and corticosterone. Together, they cause the blood glucose level to rise, help maintain blood pressure, and help the animal cope with stress.
  - Their production is under the influence of ACTH from the pituitary gland.
  - Too much glucocorticoid production (hyperadrenocorticism) leads to a condition known as **Cushing's syndrome.**

- **Addison's disease** (hypoadrenocorticism) is caused by insufficient production of glucocorticoid hormones produced by the adrenal cortex.
- mineralocorticoids
  - The primary hormone produced in the adrenal cortex is aldosterone. It helps to regulate the sodium, potassium, and hydrogen levels in the animal. Its target cells are in the kidney, where it affects the composition of urine to maintain the animal's homeostasis. (See Chapter 14.)
- sex hormones
  - Very small amounts are produced in both males and females. Their effects are usually minimal.
  - The male sex hormones are the **androgens.**
  - The female sex hormones are the **estrogens.**

The **adrenal medulla** is located in the center of the adrenal gland. Its hormone-secreting cells are actually modified neurons that secrete their hormones directly into the bloodstream. The hormones are **epinephrine** (sometimes called *adrenaline*) and **norepinephrine.** Together, these two hormones, along with the sympathetic nervous system, are responsible for the "fight-or-flight" response to a threat.

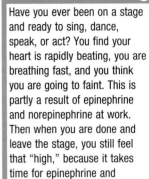

Have you ever been on a stage and ready to sing, dance, speak, or act? You find your heart is rapidly beating, you are breathing fast, and you think you are going to faint. This is partly a result of epinephrine and norepinephrine at work. Then when you are done and leave the stage, you still feel that "high," because it takes time for epinephrine and norepinephrine to be metabolized.

CASE STUDY 13-2 #2007-2243 MACKERS

Signalment and History: A 33-year-old intact **F** Palm cockatoo named Mackers was brought to the Frisbee SA Clinic because her owner noticed a coelomic (body cavity) distention. Mackers had recently gained weight and exhibited **polyuria** and **poly-dipsia.** She was admitted to the hospital for further diagnostic workup.

Physical Examination: Veterinary technician, Lou Sandness, performed the initial physical exam on Mackers, and held her while Dr. Nesheim drew blood samples for a CBC and **plasma** chemistry tests. Mackers appeared mildly depressed. Her respirations and heartbeat were **auscultated** and sounded normal. Her plumage was normal. Dr. Nesheim indicated that the coelomic distention might be secondary to an **abdominal hernia,** so he performed an **ultrasonography** on Mackers. He discovered a **pseudohernia** that appeared to contain her **jejunum, ileum, pancreas,** and reproductive tract. **Hemogram** results showed a **heterophilia, lymphopenia,** and mild **monocytosis.** Results of plasma biochemical analysis showed **hyperglycemia** and **hypophosphatemia.** Dr. Nesheim collected a bx sample of the liver and submitted it for **histological** evaluation. The pathologist found evidence of **chronic hepatic lipidosis.** On the basis of the clinical signs, Dr. Nesheim had a strong clinical suspicion of **hyperadrenocorticism,** but **ACTH** stimulation test results were not conclusive.

Diagnosis: Mackers had a pseudohernia and possible hyperadrenocorticism, most likely caused by a **pituitary gland** neoplasm that was releasing ACTH. The increased amount of ACTH would be stimulating the adrenal gland to produce excessive amounts of **glucocorticoids.**

Treatment and Outcome: Mackers was anesthetized, and the body wall in the area of the pseudohernia was strengthened with a piece of sterile mesh. **Postsurgical** recovery was uneventful. Mackers continued to be mildly depressed and exhibited polyuria and polydipsia. Despite ongoing **palliative** care, Mackers developed complications associated with the **herniorrhaphy,** and the owner elected to have her euthanatized. A **necropsy** was performed. Dr. Nesheim's suspicion of **hyperadrenocorticism** was confirmed by **histological** evaluation of the **pituitary gland,** where an **ACTH**-producing **neoplasm** was discovered.

EXERCISE 13-3 *Case It!*

Several of the bolded words in Case Study 13-2 are found in the following questions. Circle the correct word or phrase in the parentheses that makes each statement true.

1. Herniorrhaphy refers to a procedure where the hernia was (removed), (attached to the ribs), or (sutured).

2. Histological evaluation is examination of a (tissue), (bone), or (gland).

3. A condition that has a slow onset with a long duration is known as (chronic), (acute), or (hormone).

4. Plasma is the (cellular portion of blood), (the liquid portion of blood without the clotting proteins), or (the liquid portion of blood with the clotting proteins).

5. Ultrasonography is a procedure that uses (high heat), (sound), or (electricity).

6. Hepatic lipidosis is a condition affecting the (liver), (blood), or (hernia).

7. Lipidosis refers to the presence of an (abnormally large amount of fat), (abnormally small amount of fat), or (enlargement of the lips).

8. Heterophilia refers to the presence in the blood of (an increased number of white blood cells), (an increased number of red blood cells), or (a decreased number of red blood cells).

9. Hyperadrenocorticism is an (exocrinopathy) or (endocrinopathy).

10. In a lymphopenia, the cells are (of unequal size), (increased in number), or (decreased in number).

11. Hyperglycemia involves an increase in (sugar in the body), (sugar in the blood), or (sugar in the urine).

12. The ileum is a section of the (pelvis), (large intestine), or (small intestine).

13. Diagnosis of a pseudohernia meant the presence of (an inflamed sac simulating a strangulated hernia) or (a bulge or protrusion of organs through the muscle wall that usually contains it).

14. Another term for polydipsia might be (dysdipsia), (hyperdipsia), or (oligodipsia).

Check your answers at the end of the chapter, Answers to Exercises.

The **pancreas** is both an exocrine and an endocrine gland. Digestive enzymes produced by the pancreas and released into ducts that carry them to the gastrointestinal (GI) tract make the pancreas an exocrine gland. The endocrine portion of the pancreas produces two important hormones:
- insulin
  - Insulin helps blood sugar move from the blood into the cells, where it is converted to energy.
  - Without insulin, the blood sugar would rise, resulting in **hyperglycemia.**

- glucagon
    - It has the opposite effect of insulin.
    - Glucagon stimulates the liver to convert the glycogen that it is storing into glucose, and then to send the glucose into the bloodstream.
    - Without glucagon, the blood sugar would fall, resulting in **hypoglycemia.**

Insulin and glucagon are antagonistic to each other; but the animal needs both hormones to maintain blood sugar homeostasis.

Diabetes mellitus is a disease that results if the animal's pancreas is not producing enough insulin (type 1), or if the insulin that is produced cannot attach to the receptors of its target cells (type 2). In either case, the blood sugar becomes very high, and the animal must start to break down its own fat and proteins as a source of energy.

CASE STUDY 13-3 #2008-4808 MYSHKIN

Signalment and History: An 11-year-old obese **M(C)** DSH cat named Myshkin was brought to the Frisbee SA Clinic because his owner claimed he was losing weight but was mystified because he was eating as if he was starving. She noted that Myshkin was also drinking a lot of water, and that his litter box was soaked with urine every day. Myshkin was current on his vaccinations.

Physical Examination: On the initial physical exam, Jess found that Myshkin was **lethargic** and wanted to lie down all the time. His **TPR** was within the expected reference range. He weighed 19.7 pounds. Myshkin's owner claimed that he had lost at least 5 pounds in the last couple of weeks. Jess drew blood samples for a **CBC** and **serum** chemistry tests. Dr. Frisbee had Jess put a **STAT** on the chemistry tests, especially the glucose. On abdominal **palpation,** Dr. Frisbee felt **hepatomegaly.** With gentle pressure on Myshkin's urinary bladder, Dr. Frisbee was able to get him to give up a urine sample. He used a urine dipstick in the urine and found that large quantities of glucose and **ketones** were present in the urine. The urine sample was taken to the lab for further analysis, also STAT. The urine analysis confirmed the high levels of glucose and ketones that Dr. Frisbee had found in the urine using the dipstick. Numerous bacteria were present in the urine sample, but because the sample was not collected under sterile conditions, Dr. Frisbee said their relevance was questionable. **Hemogram** results showed mild **leukocytosis, neutrophilia,** and **lymphopenia. RBCs** appeared normal. The serum glucose level was more than three times the expected reference norm, signifying **hyperglycemia.** A note indicated that the serum was **lipemic.**

Diagnosis: Myshkin was diagnosed with **diabetes mellitus** with possible secondary **hepatopathy** and urinary tract infection. The owner agreed to admit Myshkin to the hospital so the staff could regulate his insulin injections and control his diet to a point where the owner could maintain him at home.

Treatment and Outcome: Myshkin received **bid** insulin injections **SQ** at gradually increasing doses until the ideal dose that could control the hyperglycemia was reached. He was also put on a high-fiber, high-complex-carbohydrate diet that would encourage him to lose weight at a healthy rate. Seven days after he was admitted to the hospital, Myshkin went home, where his owner faithfully kept up his insulin injections and kept him on his diet. Myshkin returned for blood glucose monitoring on a regular basis as he lost weight. And as he lost weight, the amount of insulin that he needed decreased. This pointed to a good **prognosis** for Myshkin. Two years after his initial diagnosis, Myshkin weighed a healthy 9.3 pounds, had become very active, and was completely off his insulin injections.

EXERCISE 13-4 *Case It!*

The following list includes words from Case Study 13-3, and makes reference to words that you probably remember from previous case studies. Match the words with their descriptions.

1. *hypoglycemia* high amount of sugar (glucose) in the blood

2. *polydipsia* extreme thirst

3. *polyphagia* increased appetite

4. *parathyroid* enlargement of the liver

5. *thymus* gland that produces insulin

6. *Anterior pitu* hormone necessary to move sugar from the blood into the cells

7. *Pancreas* state of being sluggish and listless

8. *hypothalamus* increase in the number of white blood cells in the blood

9. *Pineal Gland* set of values used to interpret test results from blood samples

10. *Adrenal cortex* excessive amount of fat in the blood

11. *Posterior pit* immediately; urgently

12. *hypothalamus* disease of the liver

13. *testes* reduction in the number of lymphocytes in the blood

14. *ovaries* disease that results if not enough insulin is produced

15. *Pancreas* situated or lying underneath the skin

diabetes mellitus

hepatomegaly

hepatopathy

~~hyperglycemia~~

insulin

lethargy

leukocytosis

lymphopenia

pancreas

polydipsia

polyphagia

reference range

SQ

STAT

Check your answers at the end of the chapter, Answers to Exercises.

The **gonads** are the primary source of sex hormones in an animal. They are under the control of the pituitary gland via the gonadotropin-releasing hormone (GnRH). In males, the gonads are the **testes** (*singular* = testicle). The testes secrete a number of hormones called **androgens,** which regulate body changes associated with male sexual development. The most important androgen is **testosterone.** It is testosterone that promotes sperm production.

In females, the gonads are the **ovaries** (*singular* = ovary). The ovaries produce eggs and secrete **estrogen** and **progestins.** Estrogen is associated with female sexual development. The progestins are a group of related hormones, of which **progesterone** is the most important. Progesterone and estrogen together are involved in the breeding cycles of animals (estrogen) and support pregnancy (progesterone).

The **pineal gland** is a small gland located in the middle of the brain. This gland is not fully understood, but it is known to secrete a hormone-like substance, **melatonin,** which appears to control the **circadian rhythm** (the body's internal 24-hour clock) in animals. Production of melatonin is greater at night than during the day. For this reason, it is thought that melatonin may regulate the sleep/wake cycle in animals. Melatonin also helps to control the release of the female sex hormones that play a part in the breeding cycle.

The **thymus** is a large gland in young animals, located near the base of the neck. The thymus shrinks as the animal grows, so that by the time the animal reaches adulthood, it is nearly impossible to find any remnant of the thymus. It secretes hormones called **humoral factors,** which play a crucial role in the development of an animal's immunity when it is young. With the help of humoral factors, the lymphoid tissue throughout the body will develop the ability to provide immunity against invading antigens.

"Sweetbreads" is the culinary name for the thymus, usually taken from a calf. Other glands that are sometimes eaten are the pancreas and the salivary glands. They are also called *sweetbreads*. Testes from lambs and calves are called "Rocky Mountain oysters."

EXERCISE 13-5   *Who Am I?*

Endocrine glands are situated in various parts of the body; they control organs from a distance by producing hormones. Name the endocrine gland involved in each of the various functions listed.

1. _parathyroid_ maintains homeostasis of calcium

2. _thyroid_ controls the metabolic rate

3. _pituitary_ is the master gland

4. _parathyroid_ is located in and around the thyroid gland

5. _thymus_ plays a role in providing immunity

6. _Anterior Pituitary_ growth hormone is produced here

7. _Pancreas_ helps move sugar from the blood into the cells

8. _Hypothalamus_ link between nervous system and pituitary gland

9. _Pineal Gland_ controls the body's internal 24-hour clock

10. _Adrenal cortex_ maintains blood pressure and helps cope with stress

11. _Posterior Pit_ regulates water balance in the animal's body

12. _Hypothalmus_ produces the "releasing" hormones

13. _testes_ primary source for the male sex hormones

14. _ovaries_ primary source for the female sex hormones

15. _pancreas_ both an endocrine gland and an exocrine gland

Check your answers at the end of the chapter, Answers to Exercises.

ANSWERS TO EXERCISES

Exercise 13-1
1. -correct-
2. antebrachium
3. -correct-
4. cardiomegaly
5. chondroplasty
6. dermopathy
7. dystrophy
8. erythrocyte
9. -correct-
10. larynx
11. -correct-
12. necroscopy
13. -correct-
14. -correct-
15. splenopexy

Exercise 13-2
1. dry
2. feeling or sensation
3. both (two sides) eyelids
4. small
5. eye
6. blood
7. nose and lips
8. growth
9. thyroid
10. lining the eyelids and covering the sclera
11. disease
12. serum
13. mucus
14. less than normal
15. bad or defective

Exercise 13-3
1. sutured
2. tissue
3. chronic
4. the liquid portion of blood with the clotting proteins
5. sound
6. liver
7. an abnormally large amount of fat
8. an increased number of white blood cells
9. endocrinopathy
10. decreased in number
11. sugar in the blood
12. small intestine
13. an inflamed sac simulating a strangulated hernia
14. hyperdipsia

Exercise 13-4
1. hyperglycemia
2. polydipsia
3. polyphagia
4. hepatomegaly
5. pancreas
6. insulin
7. lethargy
8. leukocytosis
9. reference range
10. lipemia
11. STAT
12. hepatopathy
13. lymphopenia
14. diabetes mellitus
15. SQ

Exercise 13-5
1. parathyroid
2. thyroid
3. pituitary
4. parathyroid
5. thymus
6. anterior pituitary
7. pancreas
8. hypothalamus
9. pineal gland
10. adrenal cortex
11. posterior pituitary
12. hypothalamus
13. testes
14. ovaries
15. pancreas

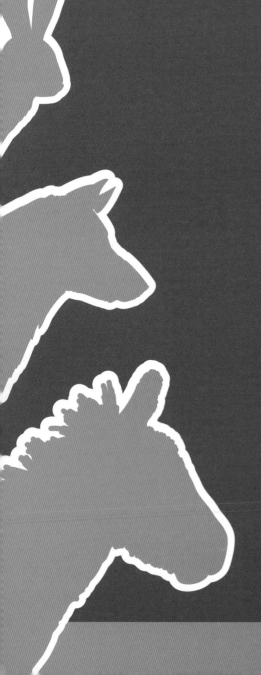

Chapter 14

The Urinary System

This too shall pass … just like a kidney stone.

Hunter Madsen

WORD PARTS

albumin/o	ahl-**bū**-mihn-ō	kali/o	**kā**-lē-ō	nephr/o	**nehf**-rō	-tripsy	**trihp**-sē
azot/o	**āz**-oht-ō	ket/o	**kē**-tō	olig/o	**ohl**-ih-gō	tub-	toob
bacteri/o	bachk-**tehr**-ē-ō	keton/o	**kē**-tōn-ō	-ptosis	pah-**tō**-sihs	ur/o	**ū**-rō
bilirubin/o	**bihl**-ē-**roo**-bihn-ō	lith/o	**lihth**-ō	py/o	**pī**-ō	ureter/o	ū-**rē**-tər-ō
cyst/o	**sihs**-tō	natr/i	**nā**-trē	pyel/o	**pī**-eh-lō	urethr/o	ū-**rē**-thrō
hydr/o	**hī**-drō	natr/o	**nā**-trō	ren/o	**rē**-nō	-uria	**uhr**-ē-ah

OUTLINE

THE URINARY SYSTEM

ANATOMY OF THE URINARY SYSTEM
    The Upper Urinary Tract
    The Lower Urinary Tract

URINALYSIS (UA)

LEARNING OBJECTIVES

When you have completed this chapter, you will be able to:

1 Understand the components and functions of the urinary system.

2 Identify and recognize the meanings of word parts related to the urinary system, using them to build or analyze words.

3 Apply your new knowledge and understanding of clinical veterinary language in the context of medical reports.

CASE STUDY 14-1 #2010-1010 BILLY

Signalment and History: A 4-year-old Pygmy goat **buck** named Billy was brought to the Frisbee LA Clinic because the owner noticed that he was "acting strange." When questioned further, the owner said that Billy was standing with his back legs stretched out and was vocalizing more than usual. He seemed restless and anxious, looking back at his abdomen frequently. And his tail was twitching. The owner also thought that maybe Billy was a little **anorexic**.

Physical Examination: When Billy was brought into the exam area, Pat noticed a few drops of blood on the floor. He examined Billy and found a few blood drops dripping from Billy's **urethra** and confirmed with Dr. Murdoch that Billy had **dysuria** with **hematuria**. Pat proceeded with the exam and found that Billy weighed 79 pounds and was in good physical condition. He exhibited **tachycardia, tachypnea,** and **pyrexia**. His mental condition seemed to be depressed. Billy's prepuce was swollen and **hypothermic** to the touch. Pat drew blood samples from Billy for a **CBC** and **serum** chemistry tests. Dr. Murdoch performed a **rectal** examination and found an enlarged **urinary bladder** and a distended urethra. He also did a **transabdominal palpation** and confirmed the presence of an enlarged bladder accompanied by **cystoplegia** and most likely **cystitis**. When palpating along the penis on Billy's **ventral** surface, Dr. Murdoch thought he could feel a **calculus** near the **distal** end of the urethral **sigmoid flexure**. **Ultrasonography** showed an extended bladder and a distended urethra that could be followed to the single, large calculus. **Hemogram** results showed a normal **RBC** component and a **leukocytosis** with a **neutrophilia** and **lymphocytopenia**. The serum chemistry results were consistent with a **uremia**: elevated **BUN, hyperkalemia, hyponatremia, hypochloremia,** elevated muscle enzymes, and **acidemia**.

Diagnosis: Billy had a case of obstructive, **post-renal urolithiasis**. Dr. Murdoch identified the results of the WBC evaluation as a stress **leukogram** brought on by the urolithiasis.

(See the rest of the story later in the chapter.)

THE URINARY SYSTEM

It has taken a while, but you have created an almost complete animal. From a bag of bones, you have watched your animal grow, system by system, to where it is today. You have learned of the many processes that must take place to put your animal in a homeostatic state. But what you have learned so far will not quite lead to homeostasis. There are still waste materials in your animal that must be eliminated. Some of the waste materials produced by living cells find their way out of the body through the respiratory system, and some, but very few, leave through the skin, as in sweat. By far, the greatest proportion of unwanted material leaves the body in a solution that has been filtered by the kidneys. This is the main function of the urinary system (Table 14-1).

The urinary system removes waste materials primarily from two sources:
- products of cellular metabolism
  - These are produced when cells break down nutrients to create energy.
- fluids and minerals
  - The body needs to be rid of these substances when too great an amount in the body would be harmful.

In both cases, the waste materials are dumped into the blood and are carried to their disposal site, the urinary system. If the kidneys were to fail, these waste materials would build up in the blood, eventually causing death.

TABLE 14-1	Word Parts Associated with the Urinary System		
Word Part	**Meaning**	**Example and Definition**	**Word Parts**
ren/o nephr/o	kidney	**renogram** record made of the kidney, e.g., an X-ray or a record of the excretion of a radioactive substance that has been injected into the renal system	ren/o = kidney -gram = written record produced, something recorded or written
		nephroblastoma rapidly developing tumor of the kidneys, made up of embryonic elements; most often malignant	nephr/o = kidney blast/o- = bud, seed, formative cell -oma = tumor or abnormal new growth, a swelling
ur/o -uria	urine	**uremia** literally, "urine constituents are found in blood"; poisonous waste products build up in blood because of insufficient secretion in urine or kidney disease	ur/o = urine -emia = blood condition (usually abnormal)
		dysuria painful urination of any etiology	dys- = bad, defective, painful, difficult -uria = urine
pyel/o	kidney pelvis	**pyeloplasty** surgical repair of the kidney pelvis	pyel/o = kidney pelvis -plasty = surgical repair
tub-	pipe	**tubule** a small tube, e.g., the proximal convoluted tubule of a nephron	tub- = pipe -ule = indicating something small
ureter/o	ureter	**ureteralgia** pain in the ureter	ureter/o = ureter -algia = pain
cyst/o	bladder, a sac containing fluid	**cystitis** inflammation of the bladder *Be careful!* cyst/o *may refer to the urinary bladder or to one of several other sacs in the body that contain a fluid, e.g., the keratin cyst of skin or the fluid-filled gall bladder.*	cyst/o = bladder, a sac containing fluid -itis = inflammation
urethr/o	urethra	**urethroscope** apparatus for observing the urethra	urethr/o = urethra -scope = instrument for examining or viewing
-tripsy	crushing, grinding	**lithotripsy** crushing of a stone	lith/o = stone -tripsy = crushing, grinding
-ptosis	drooping or sagging	**nephroptosis** downward displacement of the kidney; prolapse of the kidney	nephr/o = kidney -ptosis = drooping or sagging

ren/o

nephr/o

ur/o

-uria

pyel/o

tub-

ureter/o

cyst/o

urethr/o

-tripsy

-ptosis

BOX 14-1   Terms That Defy Word Analysis

- calculus (*plural* = calculi)—a stone
  - Large urinary stones are typically concretions.
  - Some calculi may be microscopic crystals, not concretions.
- catheter—tube for injecting or removing fluids
- concretion—a solid or calcified mass formed by disease and found in a body cavity or tissue
  - It is built up layer by layer.
  - A concretion in the urinary system is called a **urolith.**
- creatinine—the end-product of muscle metabolism; waste product excreted in urine
- denude—loss of epidermis, caused by exposure to urine, feces, body fluids, wound drainage, or friction; not associated with necrosis of the tissue
- electrolyte—chemical element (e.g., potassium, sodium) that carries an electrical charge when dissolved in water; proper balance in blood is maintained by the kidneys
- filtration—process in the kidney whereby blood pressure forces materials through a filter (the glomerulus)
- micturition—urination; also called *voiding*
- parenchyma—the functional tissue of an organ, as opposed to supporting tissue
- slough—a mass or layer of necrotic tissue that separates from the underlying healthy tissue
- solute—a substance dissolved in a solution (e.g., glucose in blood)
- stranguria—painful urination due to muscle spasms in the urinary bladder and urethra
- urea—a water-soluble, nitrogen-based compound that is the waste material of protein metabolism by the body's cells; a major component of mammalian urine

---

EXERCISE 14-1   *Recall It!*

Repetitive use of terms that defy word analysis will help you commit them to memory. Define the following clinical veterinary language terms. You will find terms here that were introduced in previous chapters.

1. aberrant _____

2. aorta _____

3. ascites _____

4. denude _____

5. ecchymosis _____

6. enzyme _____

7. fossa _____

8. impulse _____

9. infarct _____

10. insufficiency _____

11. lavage _____

12. nocturnal _____

13. pastern _____

14. peristalsis _____

15. recumbency _____

16. signalment _____

17. solute _____

18. subluxation _____

19. topical _____

20. urea _____

Check your answers at the end of the chapter, Answers to Exercises.

CASE STUDY 14-2 #2001-5299 ANNABELLE

Signalment and History: A 3-year-old 10-lb Burmese **F(S) queen** named Annabelle was brought to the Frisbee SA Clinic because of a 3-day history of **emesis, lethargy,** and **anorexia.** Five days before her visit, another veterinary clinic had performed a **hysterectomy** and a right **ovariectomy** through a **ventral midline abdominal incision** along the **linea alba.** The surgery had been performed because Annabelle continued to display signs of heat a year after an ovariectomy through a **flank** incision, which had been performed at this same veterinary clinic.

Physical Examination: On physical examination at the clinic, Jess found that Annabelle was **listless,** had pale mucous membranes, and was **hypothermic. Auscultation** of the **thorax** revealed crackles in all lung fields, muffled **cardiac** sounds, **tachypnea,** and **tachycardia.** Jess drew blood samples for a **CBC** and **serum** chemistry tests. **Abdominal palpation** by Dr. Frisbee revealed a distended abdomen and **bilateral renomegaly.** An **electrocardiography** was performed and showed a **ventricular arrhythmia** with wide **QRS complexes** and high **T waves.** Urine for a **urinalysis** could not be obtained by gently trying to express the urinary bladder. Results of the CBC were within reference limits. Serum biochemical abnormalities included **azotemia** or **uremia** (elevated **blood urea nitrogen [BUN]**) and **hyperkalemia.** Excretory **urography** that had been performed at the referring veterinary clinic the day before revealed **bilateral hydronephrosis** and dilation of the **proximal half** of each **ureter.**

Dr. Frisbee performed an **abdominocentesis** and withdrew 75 **mL** of a **serosanguineous** fluid that was determined not to be urine.

Diagnosis: Dr. Frisbee made a diagnosis of ureter obstruction based on results of the **diagnostic** tests.

Treatment: Dr. Frisbee explained to Annabelle's owner that treatment for bilateral ureteral obstruction is **ureteral anastomosis** or implantation of the more **proximal** healthy portion of the ureters directly into the urinary bladder after removal of the damaged portions. Annabelle's status made her a poor risk for **anesthesia,** so Dr. Frisbee, with the owner's consent, decided that the best course of action was to place temporary bilateral **nephrostomy** catheters. This approach would provide urine drainage while allowing time for the uremia to be corrected and giving Annabelle the chance to become rehydrated. Annabelle would then be a better candidate for ureteral anastomosis surgery.

On the second day after placement of the nephrostomy catheters, Annabelle was ready for surgery. A ventral midline abdominal incision was made, and approximately

100 mL of serosanguineous fluid was aspirated from the abdominal cavity. The anastomosis surgery was uneventful. One week after surgery, Annabelle was discharged from the hospital. Two weeks after surgery, results of a urinalysis on a sample obtained by means of **cystocentesis** were within expected reference ranges and there was no evidence of **cystitis** that might have been accompanied by a **bacteriuria** or **pyuria.** Results of CBC and serum chemistry tests performed 2 weeks and 5 months **post surgery** were within expected reference ranges. Six months post surgery, an **aerobic** bacterial culture of a urine sample collected by cystocentesis did not yield any growth, and an excretory **urogram** indicated that both ureters were open and were passing urine from the kidneys to the urinary bladder. Annabelle's owner was contacted by telephone 8 months after surgery; she reported that Annabelle's activity level and appetite were normal.

EXERCISE 14-2 *Case It!*

Read Case Study 14-2. Match words found in the Case Study, and listed in the right column, with their definitions.

1. _Cystocentesis_ surgical puncture of the bladder

2. _nephrostomy_ surgical creation of a new permanent opening into the kidney

3. _catheter_ tube for injecting or removing fluids

4. _hyperectomy_ surgical removal of the uterus

5. _Ausculation_ act of listening to body sounds through an instrument

6. _serosanguineas_ consisting of serum and blood

7. _aerobic_ living organism that needs air to live

8. _anastomosis_ opening between two organs in a place not normally connected

9. _arrhythmia_ irregular heartbeat

10. _tachypnea_ fast breathing

11. _anesthesia_ loss of feeling or sensation

12. _renomegaly_ enlarged kidney

13. _pyuria_ presence of pus in the urine

14. _emesis_ vomiting

15. _flank_ the side of an animal between the ribs and the rear legs

aerobic

anastomosis

anesthesia

arrhythmia

auscultation

catheter

cystocentesis

emesis

flank

hysterectomy

nephrostomy

pyuria

renomegaly

serosanguineous

tachypnea

Check your answers at the end of the chapter, Answers to Exercises.

ANATOMY OF THE URINARY SYSTEM

The urinary system (Figure 14-1) is divided into two separate systems:
- the upper urinary tract
  - This is composed of the two kidneys and the two ureters.
  - The primary function of the kidneys is to filter blood to remove waste materials and produce urine.
  - The ureters are muscular tubes that carry urine from the kidneys to the urinary bladder.

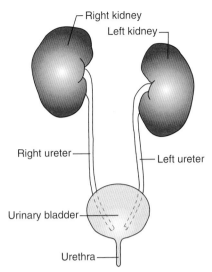

FIGURE 14-1 **The components of the urinary system.** (From Colville TP: *Clinical Anatomy and Physiology for Veterinary Technicians,* ed 2, St Louis, 2009, Mosby.)

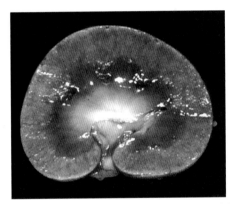

FIGURE 14-2 **A normal dog kidney showing the outer renal cortex (light color) and the inner renal medulla (darker red color).** The capsule has been removed. The renal pelvis is continuous with the ureter that is entering the kidney at the hilus. (Courtesy of Dr. B. Weeks, College of Veterinary Medicine, Texas A&M University; and Noah's Arkive, College of Veterinary Medicine, The University of Georgia. In McGavin MD: *Pathologic Basis of Veterinary Disease,* ed 4, St Louis, 2007, Mosby.)

- the lower urinary tract
  - This is composed of urinary bladder, urethra, and urethral sphincters.
  - The bladder collects and stores urine until it is released.
  - The urethra carries urine from the bladder to be passed out of the body.

The Upper Urinary Tract

The two **kidneys** are the major filtering organs of the urinary system. They are reddish-brown. The outer surface of the kidneys is smooth, except for bovine kidneys. In the bovine, the kidneys have a lobulated appearance (Figure 14-3, *B*). The medial surface of each kidney is indented by an opening called the **hilus** (Figure 14-2). This is where the renal artery and vein, ureters, lymph vessels, and nerves enter and leave the kidney.

The kidneys lie against the muscles on either side of the lumbar vertebrae. The kidneys are located in the dorsal part of the abdominal cavity, just ventral to the most cranial lumbar vertebrae. They are positioned very close to the aorta, the main artery leaving the heart. High pressure from contraction of the heart forces blood through the filtering structure in the kidney. The right kidney sits more cranial than the left kidney, except in the pig, where they are at the same level. There is no anatomical reason why the kidneys sit at different levels.

Kidney beans get their name from their shape and color, which resemble the shape and color of real kidneys.

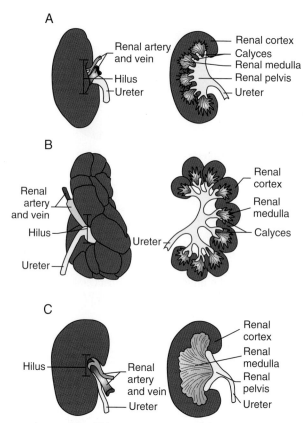

FIGURE 14-3 **Gross anatomy of the kidneys. A,** Pig. **B,** Cow. **C,** Cat/dog. (From Colville TP: *Clinical Anatomy and Physiology for Veterinary Technicians,* ed 2, St Louis, 2009, Mosby.)

The location of the kidneys is **retroperitoneal,** that is, they are located outside the peritoneum that lines the abdominal cavity. To demonstrate the kidney's retroperitoneal location between the abdominal cavity and the body wall, lay a kidney bean (to represent a kidney) on a hard surface that will represent the body wall. Place a tissue to correspond to the peritoneum over the kidney bean. Your side of the tissue represents the abdominal cavity with all its viscera. Under the tissue lies the kidney bean—retroperitoneal.

The kidneys are covered with a fibrous tissue capsule. Below the capsule is the outer renal cortex, and beneath the cortex is the inner renal medulla. Grossly visible in a kidney cut lengthwise are the capsule, cortex, and medulla (see Figure 14-2). The inner cavity of the kidney is the **renal pelvis.** Urine is collected here before it enters the ureters to travel to the urinary bladder (Figure 14-3).

In addition to filtering waste products from the body, the kidney has other functions:
* clears drugs from the body
* balances the conservation or elimination of body fluids through tubular reabsorption and the influence of antidiuretic hormone (ADH) from the pituitary gland
* releases the hormones **renin** and **angiotensin,** which help to regulate blood pressure
* promotes calcium absorption from the intestines through the release of **calcitriol** (vitamin D)
* controls the production of red blood cells (RBCs) through production of the hormone **erythropoietin,** which will be transported to the bone marrow, where it will stimulate RBC production

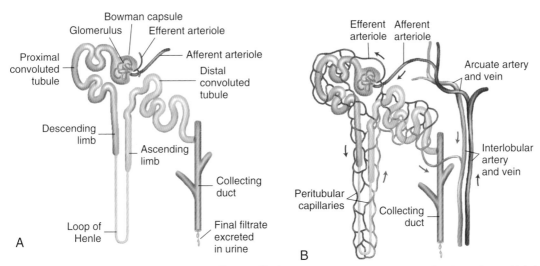

FIGURE 14-4 **A,** Nephron and **(B)** nephron with surrounding capillaries. **A,** The nephron is composed of a glomerulus and tubules. **B,** As the filtrate passes through the tubular portion of the nephron, reabsorption of variable quantities of water, electrolytes, and other substances occurs across the tubule walls into nearby blood capillaries. (From Leonard PC: *Quick and Easy Medical Terminology,* ed 6, St Louis, 2011, Saunders.)

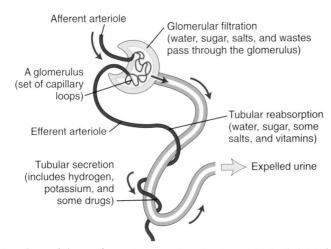

FIGURE 14-5 **Functions of the nephron.** Glomerular filtration *(upper right),* tubular reabsorption *(center),* and tubular secretion *(lower left).* (From Leonard PC: *Quick and Easy Medical Terminology,* ed 6, St Louis, 2011, Saunders.)

Microscopically, a kidney is made up of hundreds of thousands of individual filtering units. Each unit is called a **nephron** (Figure 14-4, *A*). It resembles a microscopic funnel with a long stem and tubular sections. The **glomerulus** is a cluster of blood vessels surrounded by a structure called the *glomerular capsule* (or *Bowman's capsule*). As you follow the long, twisting nephron tubule, you will see that it consists of the proximal convoluted tubule, the loop of Henle, and the distal convoluted tubule, which opens into a collecting duct.

The nephrons constantly filter the blood. All blood in the body passes through the kidneys many times a day. Some substances are reabsorbed across the tubular walls into nearby blood capillaries. Waste substances are secreted into the tubule, where urine carries them into the collecting duct (see Figure 14-4, *B*).

Urine production can be described in three steps: glomerular filtration, tubular reabsorption, and tubular secretion (Figure 14-5). The blood enters each nephron through a tiny arteriole branch of the **renal artery.** The arteriole carrying blood into the glomerulus is the **afferent arteriole,** which becomes the glomerulus (i.e., that cluster of blood vessels that sits in the glomerular capsule). Blood leaving the glomerulus is carried in the **efferent arteriole,** which carries blood to the capillary network surrounding the tubules. The capillaries from all networks eventually converge until they become the **renal vein,** which carries purified blood out of the kidney.

Large quantities of water and solutes (salts, glucose, and urea, but not large protein molecules) diffuse out of the blood in the glomerular capillaries and into the space made between the two layers of the glomerular capsule, where they becomes known as the **glomerular filtrate.** The glomerular filtrate passes from the glomerular capsule into the proximal convoluted tubule, where reabsorption begins.

Tubular reabsorption involves taking back into the body substances that were filtered out by the glomerulus but are still needed by the body. This means that most of the water and solutes are taken back into the body. However, if the body has more water (or any solute, e.g., glucose) than it needs to maintain homeostasis, not all of it will be reabsorbed, and it will stay in the filtrate to be eliminated in the urine.

Tubular secretion is a process that involves substances being added to the filtrate, rather than being taken out. It occurs when excess amounts of substances in the body need to be eliminated to maintain normal homeostasis. These are substances in the blood that were not sufficiently removed by glomerular filtration. They are secreted from the capillaries surrounding the tubules, through the tubular epithelium, and into the tubule. Potassium ions, hydrogen ions, ammonium ions, urea, certain hormones, and drugs are examples of substances eliminated from the body by tubular secretion. Different parts of the nephron are more or less permeable to water and solutes.

Damage to any part of the nephron can affect the ability of the nephron to reabsorb water or certain solutes. Under normal conditions, only about 1% of the original glomerular filtrate reaches the collecting duct as urine; the rest is reabsorbed back into the body. The thousands of collecting ducts deposit the urine in the renal pelvis, where the urine is moved to the renal pelvis and enters the ureters, which will move it to the urinary bladder.

The **ureters** continually move urine from the kidneys to the urinary bladder because the kidneys are continually making urine. The muscle layer of the ureters propels the urine by peristaltic action, much in the way that food is moved through the intestinal tract.

CASE STUDY 14-3 #2011-374 BO

Signalment and History: A 2-year-old M mixed-breed dog named Bo was brought to the Frisbee SA Clinic because of signs of severe lethargy and occasional **emesis.** Bo had **anorexia** of 3 days' duration and a 1-month history of **melena.** His vaccination status was current, and he had no other notable medical history.

Physical Examination: Jess found that Bo was very **lethargic,** with signs of depressed mentation. He exhibited **tachypnea** and **tachycardia,** and he was **hypothermic.** When he entered the exam room, Bo had **defecated** soft **feces** mixed with mucus and blood. During blood sample collection, Jess noted that excessive bleeding had occurred at the **venipuncture** site. The **CBC** revealed no abnormalities other than mild **neutrophilia** and **thrombocytopenia,** but platelet clumps were present so the estimated platelet count was considered adequate. Serum chemistry results showed signs of **uremia,** including **azotemia** (elevated **blood urea nitrogen [BUN]**), **hypercalcemia,** and **hyperphosphatemia.** Urine specific gravity on a sample collected by cystocentesis was low, but urinalysis findings otherwise were within expected reference ranges.

Abdominal X-rays and **ultrasonography** showed **bilateral renomegaly** and enlargement of regional lymph nodes. Aspirates of the lymph nodes, spleen, and liver were collected for **cytological** examination. The pathologist found **extramedullary hematopoiesis** in samples from the spleen, but no other abnormal cell populations were detected in the other tissue samples.

Outcome: Because Bo's condition was rapidly deteriorating, leading to a poor **prognosis** for recovery, Bo's owner elected to have him humanely **euthanatized.** A **necropsy** was performed. Grossly, both kidneys were distorted by variably sized pale tan nodules.

Diagnosis: After reading the necropsy report, Dr. Frisbee presented a diagnosis of **lymphoma** of the kidneys, liver, and bone marrow. The pathologist had noted widespread soft tissue mineralization of the lung, stomach (with **gastric** mucosal destruction and **myonecrosis**), and kidneys.

EXERCISE 14-3 *Case It!*

In Case Study 14-3, you learned of the tentative diagnosis of uremia: poisonous waste materials build up in blood because of their insufficient secretion in urine. Signs of advanced cases of uremia may include those in the following list. Write a term for each of the signs. Have fun while you are at it. Make up your own clinical veterinary language! Your term may not be found in any dictionary, but others could deconstruct your word to determine its meaning.

1. abdominal pain _____
2. breath that smells like urine _____
3. frequent and fluid elimination from the bowels _____
4. dizziness _____
5. drowsiness _____
6. headache _____
7. hiccups _____
8. itchy yellowish skin _____
9. lack of appetite _____
10. vomiting _____
11. convulsions _____
12. mental disturbances _____
13. muscle twitching _____
14. unconsciousness _____
15. death _____

Check your answers at the end of the chapter, Answers to Exercises.

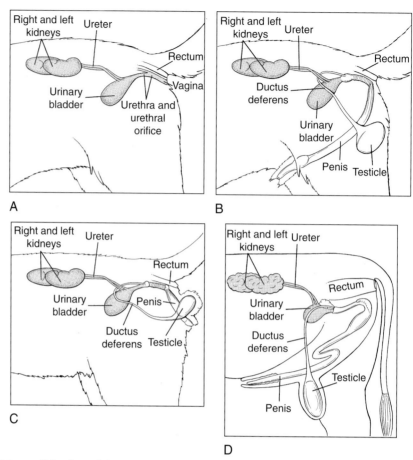

FIGURE 14-6 Side view of the male and female urinary system. A, Female dog. **B,** Male dog. **C,** Male cat. **D,** Bull. (From Wanamaker BP: *Applied Pharmacology for Veterinary Technicians,* ed 4, St Louis, 2009, Saunders.)

The Lower Urinary Tract

Thanks to peristalsis, urine enters the urinary bladder from the two ureters in spurts (rather than by a continuous flow) on the average of every 10 to 30 seconds, depending on the species. The urinary bladder is the storage tank for urine before it is released to outside the body. It has two parts: the sac and the neck. The sac is extremely elastic and varies in size and position, depending on how much urine it contains. As the sac fills with urine, its walls stretch. As the sac gets larger, gravity pulls it ventrally. The amount of urine that a urinary bladder holds varies among species and with water intake. When the urinary bladder is about one-half full, stretch receptors send a message that the bladder should be emptied.

The release of urine from the urinary bladder involves muscle contractions. In the wall of the bladder are three layers of muscles, each running in a different direction. When all three layers contract at the same time, the sac is emptied, much in the way that a water balloon would be emptied if you wrapped your hands around it and squeezed.

The neck extends caudally from the sac and into the pelvic canal, where it joins the urethra. The neck has a circular sphincter of skeletal muscle surrounding it. The sphincter is under voluntary control to release the urine from the sac. This is how urination (also known as *micturition* or *uresis*) is controlled.

The urethra is a continuation of the neck of the urinary bladder. It runs through the pelvic canal and carries urine to the outside environment. In all animals, the kidneys, ureters, and urinary bladder are located in approximately the same position. Differences arise from the anatomical location where the urethra discharges the urine (Figure 14-6). In males, the urethra is narrower and longer, runs down the center of the penis, and also has a reproductive function. The urethra in females is shorter and straighter and has only a urinary function. The female reproductive system has a separate opening.

EXERCISE 14-4 *How Do They Do It?*

The process of forming urine and expelling it from the body involves many steps and several structures. List the structures in order of their use, starting with the bloodstream.

1. _bloodstream_   (waste products build up here)

2. *Renal Artery*   (blood flows to the kidney through this vessel)

3. *Glomerulus*   (a cluster of blood vessels in the nephron)

4. *glomerual filtrate*   (this solution contains water, sugar, salts, urea, and other wastes)

5. *Bowmans capsule*   (structure that surrounds the cluster of blood vessels)

6. *Renal tubules*   (water and solutes are reabsorbed; other substances such as urea, drugs, and ions are secreted into the urine)

7. *Renal pelvis*   (urine is collected in this area of the kidney)

8. *ureters*   (tubes that move urine away from the kidney)

9. *bladder*   (storage tank for urine)

10. *Urethra*   (tube that carries urine to the outside of the body)

11. *sphincter muscle* (voluntary muscle control for urine release)

Check your answers at the end of the chapter, Answers to Exercises.

TABLE 14-2	Clinical Terms Commonly Associated with the Urinary System	
Term	**Meaning**	**Example**
diuresis	increased *production* of urine	Too much fluid intake by an animal can result in diuresis.
polyuria	increased *passage* of urine	Diuresis will result in polyuria in an animal with healthy kidneys.
oliguria	decreased passage of urine	A dehydrated animal usually will try to maintain its body fluid balance through oliguria.
anuria	lack of urine passage	One of the reasons an animal would be suffering from anuria is that it is reabsorbing all the water that is being filtered through the nephron to conserve water to maintain body fluid balance.

Continued

TABLE 14-2	Clinical Terms Commonly Associated with the Urinary System—cont'd	
Term	**Meaning**	**Example**
renal threshold	the amount of a solute (e.g., glucose) that can be reabsorbed from the glomerular filtrate	If the renal threshold of glucose is surpassed, the excess glucose will be excreted in urine and reported as glucosuria. This is what happens with diabetes mellitus.
diabetes insipidus	decreased amounts of antidiuretic hormone (ADH) from the pituitary gland prevent water from being reabsorbed from the collecting ducts, resulting in loss of water from the body	Diabetes insipidus is also associated with polyuria/polydipsia (PU/PD) and must be differentiated from diabetes mellitus. *Urine from an animal with diabetes mellitus contains a high concentration of sugar and therefore would taste sweet.* Insipid *means "tasteless," so this would indicate that the urine from an animal with diabetes insipidus is tasteless, because a high concentration of glucose is not present. The problem is water reabsorption, not a high concentration of glucose. Do you wonder who first tasted the urine to find this out?*
uremia, azotemia (azot/o = nitrogen)	a buildup of nitrogenous waste material (urea) in the blood	Uremia can be prerenal (decreased blood flow to the kidney), renal (nephron damage), or post-renal (obstruction). All types can lead to kidney dysfunction.
struvite	the primary component of struvite uroliths	Struvite stones are composed of magnesium, ammonium, and phosphate. They are sometimes called *triple phosphate crystals.*
urolithiasis	presence of urinary calculi anywhere in the urinary system	Urolithiasis occurs when a solute in urine precipitates, interacts with other particles, and forms aggregates. The pH and concentration of urine are important factors in urolithiasis. Horses rarely develop urolithiasis.
incontinence	lack of voluntary control of urination or defecation	Urinary incontinence can be a problem in older, spayed, female dogs.

TABLE 14-3	Word Parts Associated with Urinary Substances		
Word Part	**Meaning**	**Example and Definition**	**Word Parts**
hydr/o	water	**hydruria** excessive dilution of urine so that it has a low specific gravity	hydr/o = water -uria = urine
olig/o	scanty, small	**oliguresis** excretion of an abnormally small amount of urine	olig/o = little, few, small ur/o = urine -esis = process of an action
albumin/o	albumin (a protein in blood)	**albuminuria** presence of albumin in urine, indicating a malfunction of the kidneys	albumin/o = albumin -uria = urine
natr/i natr/o	sodium or natrium, chemical symbol Na$^+$	**natriuresis** excretion of an abnormal amount of sodium in the urine	natr/i = sodium ur/o = urine -esis = process of an action
		hypernatremia presence of an excess amount of sodium in the blood	hyper- = above, over, or excess natr/o = sodium -emia = blood condition (usually abnormal)

hydr/o

olig/o

albumin/o

natr/i

natr/o

TABLE 14-3	Word Parts Associated with Urinary Substances—cont'd		
Word Part	**Meaning**	**Example and Definition**	**Word Parts**
kali/o	potassium or kalium; chemical symbol K⁺	**kaliopenia** less than the normal amount of potassium; a hypokalemia	kali/o = potassium -penia = lack, deficiency
azot/o	nitrogen	**azotemia** higher than normal blood level of nitrogen-containing compounds (e.g., urea) in the blood; usually caused by the inability of the kidney to excrete these compounds	azot/o = nitrogen -emia = blood condition (usually diseased)
bilirubin/o	bilirubin, the orange-yellow pigment in bile produced primarily from the breakdown of hemoglobin in red blood cells	**bilirubinuria** presence of bilirubin in urine; not normally found in the horse, sheep, pig, and cat; indicative of liver disease when found at high levels *To break down this combining form even further, you will find bil/o = bile and rubri- = red.*	bilirubin/o = bilirubin -uria = urine
ket/o keton/o	ketones, ketone bodies; the by-products of fat metabolism	**ketosis** amount of glycogen in liver is depleted, causing formation of an elevated number of ketone bodies *Low-carb diets can cause a body to go into a dangerous metabolic state called ketosis, because the body burns fat instead of glucose for energy. The body forms substances known as ketones, which can cause organs to fail and can result in gout, kidney stone formation, or kidney failure. Ketones can also cause anorexia, nausea, and breath with a "fruity" odor.*	ket/o = ketone bodies -osis = disease or abnormal condition
		ketonuria presence of ketone bodies in the urine	keton/o = ketone bodies -uria = urine
py/o	pus	**ureteropyosis** diseased condition of pus within a ureter	ureter/o = ureter py/o = pus -osis = disease or abnormal condition
bacteri/o	bacteria	**bacterium** one single-cell microorganism that can exist independently or as a parasite	bacteri/o = bacteria -ium = structure, thing
lith/o	stone	**nephrolithotomy** incision into the kidney to remove a stone	nephr/o = kidney lith/o = stone -tomy = surgical incision

kali/o

azot/o

bilirubin/o

ket/o

keton/o

py/o

bacteri/o

lith/o

URINALYSIS (UA)

The examination of urine, along with CBC and blood analyses, is a common laboratory test that can be readily performed in a veterinary practice. The condition of urine is often an index to an animal's health. This is the reasoning behind the urinalysis. A finding of abnormal conditions in the urine is indicative of various diseases (Table 14-2). Test results may provide information regarding the status of carbohydrate metabolism, kidney and liver function, and the presence of bacteria (Table 14-3).

Urinalysis begins with the collection of a urine sample. The easiest (?) way to collect urine is to catch the animal during the act of voiding, and to fill a clean container with 3 to 5 mL of midstream urine. The next least invasive way to collect urine is to manually express the urinary bladder. This works only in small animals. However, care must be taken to avoid trauma, especially in cases of suspected urethral obstruction or bladder stones. Catheterization and cystocentesis are the preferred methods for urine collection in many veterinary practices. Properly done, they yield a sample free of contaminants.

Once the sample is obtained, it should be examined within 30 minutes, or refrigerated. Normal urine in most species is transparent and pale amber in color. However, horses, rabbits, hamsters, and a few other animals have normally cloudy urine because of substances that are suspended, but not dissolved, in the urine. The specific gravity is determined by using a special instrument called a *refractometer*. Specific gravity reflects the ability of the kidneys to concentrate or dilute urine.

A sample of the urine should also be examined microscopically to determine the presence of bacteria, inflammatory cells, crystals, and any other components of the urine sediment. Urine is approximately 95% water, but many substances are dissolved in it. "Dipsticks" are firm, plastic sticks to which several different reagent-saturated pads are affixed. They are commercially available and, when dipped into urine, provide important information about pH, urine glucose, urine protein content, blood, bilirubin, and ketones.

> Over the years, some innovative people have devised urine collection methods that make you scratch your head and wonder. For instance, if you hold the nostrils of a sheep closed for up to 45 seconds, it will urinate if the bladder was not already empty. And then there is the cow. If you gently massage the skin under her vulva, she will urinate within a minute.

EXERCISE 14-5 *Test It!*

The following would be considered normal results for a urinalysis:

Test	Normal Results
Color	amber-yellow
Appearance	clear or cloudy (depending on species)
pH	4.6-8.0 (depending on diet)
Protein	none or small amount
Glucose	none
Ketones	none
Bilirubin	none
Specific gravity	1.010 (pig)-1.060 (dog)
Sediment	none to scant

Name the appropriate test for detecting or evaluating each of the following:

1. dilution or concentration of urine _____

2. albumin in urine _____

3. hematuria _____

4. sugar in urine _____

5. pus in urine _____

6. bacteria in urine _____

7. amount of bile pigment in urine _____

8. degree of acidity or alkalinity of urine _____

9. fat, rather than sugar, is being burned _____

Check your answers at the end of the chapter, Answers to Exercises.

TABLE 14-4	Abbreviations	
Abbreviation	**Meaning**	**Example**
cath	catheter, catheterization	A urinary cath was sutured in place to prevent the tom cat from developing a plugged urethra again.
cysto	cystocentesis	In veterinary medicine *cysto* most often refers to collection of urine directly from the bladder through a surgical puncture of the bladder.
GFR	glomerular filtration rate; the rate at which blood is filtered in the glomerulus	GFR is a mathematical estimation of the amount of kidney function an animal has. It is based on the amount of creatinine in the blood.
K^+	potassium; from the Latin *kalium*	Hypokalemia is described as a low K^+ concentration in blood.
Na^+	sodium; from the Latin *natrium*	Hypernatremia is described as a high Na^+ level in the blood.
pH	potential hydrogen; scale to indicate degree of acidity or alkalinity	The pH of dairy cow urine is normally around 8.0.
UA	urinalysis	UA performed on a fresh urine sample will include gross examination, biochemical evaluation, specific gravity, and microscopic examination of the sediment from a centrifuged sample.
sp gr SG	specific gravity; a measure of the concentration of urine	The sp gr of the urine sample was 1.005, indicating that the urine was very dilute. *Kidneys must be able to concentrate and dilute urine, depending on the body's needs. A fixed SG of 1.008 to 1.010 indicates that the kidneys can do neither.*
BUN	blood urea nitrogen	BUN is a biochemical test that measures the amount of urea *in blood* to help determine kidney function, diagnose disease, or monitor chronic and acute kidney disease.
UTI	urinary tract infection	UTI involves the presence of a pathological microorganism in the urine. Urine is normally sterile.
FLUTD	feline lower urinary tract disease	FLUTD is a group of diseases that affect the lower urinary tract in cats. These diseases include feline interstitial cystitis (FIC), urolithiasis, and urethral obstruction.
PU/PD	polyuria/polydipsia	PU/PD is one of the classic signs of diabetes mellitus, but it is seen with other diseases as well.

cath

cysto

GFR

K^+

Na^+

pH

UA

sp gr *or* SG

BUN

UTI

FLUTD

PU/PD

EXERCISE 14-6 *Case It!*

Read Case Study 14-1. Circle the best answer to complete each of the statements following the case study.

CASE STUDY 14-1 #2010-1010 BILLY

Signalment and History: A 4-year-old Pygmy goat **buck** named Billy was brought to the Frisbee LA Clinic because the owner noticed that he was "acting strange." When questioned further, the owner said that Billy was standing with his back legs stretched out and was vocalizing more than usual. He seemed restless and anxious, looking back at his abdomen frequently. And his tail was twitching. The owner also thought that maybe Billy was a little **anorexic.**

Physical Examination: When Billy was brought into the exam area, Pat noticed a few drops of blood on the floor. He examined Billy and found a few blood drops dripping from Billy's **urethra** and confirmed with Dr. Murdoch that Billy had **dysuria** with **hematuria.** Pat proceeded with the exam and found that Billy weighed 79 pounds and was in good physical condition. He exhibited **tachycardia, tachypnea,** and **pyrexia.** His mental condition seemed to be depressed. Billy's **prepuce** was swollen and **hypothermic** to the touch. Pat drew blood samples from Billy for a **CBC** and **serum** chemistry tests. Dr. Murdoch performed a **rectal** examination and found an enlarged **urinary bladder** and a distended urethra. He also did a **transabdominal palpation** and confirmed the presence of an enlarged bladder accompanied by **cystoplegia** and most likely **cystitis.** When palpating along the penis on Billy's **ventral** surface, Dr. Murdoch thought he could feel a **calculus** near the **distal** end of the urethral **sigmoid flexure. Ultrasonography** showed an extended bladder and a distended urethra that could be followed to the single, large calculus. **Hemogram** results showed a normal **RBC** component and a **leukocytosis** with a **neutrophilia** and **lymphocytopenia.** The serum chemistry results were consistent with a **uremia:** elevated **BUN, hyperkalemia, hyponatremia, hypochloremia,** elevated muscle enzymes, and **acidemia.**

Diagnosis: Billy had a case of obstructive, **post-renal urolithiasis.** Dr. Murdoch identified the results of the WBC evaluation as a stress **leukogram** brought on by the urolithiasis.

Treatment and Outcome: Billy was admitted to the hospital and immediately started on **IV** fluids to correct his acidemia and **electrolyte** imbalance. Dr. Murdoch tried to pass a urinary **catheter** to flush the calculus out of the urethra. The calculus was nearly completely blocking the urethra and did not move when normal saline was pushed through the catheter. Dr. Murdoch then tried urethral **endoscopy** to visualize the calculus. After seeing the calculus and talking over surgical options with the owner, he decided to try endoscopically guided laser **lithotripsy** to break down the calculus in lieu of a **urethrostomy.** This more economical treatment was successful, and urine started to flow as soon as the calculus was destroyed.

There is a high rate of recurrence of urolithiasis if nothing besides destroying the calculus is done. Dr. Murdoch went over Billy's diet with his owner and came up with a feeding program that he hoped would lower the chances of recurrence. Six months after the lithotripsy, Billy was doing well, with no more signs of dysuria or hematuria. On a 1-year recheck, Dr. Murdoch concluded that Billy had not developed any mucosal **necrosis** at the site of the lithotripsy and told the owner that Billy's future had a good **prognosis.**

1. Dysuria is a term for (painful urination), (scanty urination), or (increased production of urine).

2. A calculus refers to a (bladder), (crystal), or (stone).

3. The prepuce is (a fold of skin that covers the head of the penis), (a tube that carries urine), or (an abscess).

4. Hypothermic would refer to something that is (wet), (cold), or (dry) to the touch.

5. Ultrasonography is a procedure that involves (high frequencies of sound), (large electrical impulses), or (passage of a dye through the ureters).

6. Urolithiasis is a pathological condition that results from (a urinary infection), (the production of urine), or (a stone in the urinary tract).

7. Cystoplegia is (an infection), (a paralysis), or (a diseased condition).

8. The reported hyperkalemia, hyponatremia, and hypochloremia are indications of (an electrolyte imbalance), (a sigmoid flexure), or (hematuria).

9. Lithotripsy is (a surgical fixation), (a surgical removal), or (a surgical crushing or grinding).

10. The distally located stone was (still in the bladder), (in the urethra near to the neck of the bladder), or (in the urethra, in the pelvic cavity).

Check your answers at the end of the chapter, Answers to Exercises.

ANSWERS TO EXERCISES

Exercise 14-1

1. abnormal, deviating from the usual or ordinary
2. the largest blood vessel in the body
3. accumulation of fluid in the abdominal cavity
4. loss of epidermis, caused by exposure to urine, feces, body fluids, wound drainage, or friction
5. blood leaking from a ruptured blood vessel into subcutaneous tissue; a bruise
6. protein produced by living cells that initiates a chemical reaction (e.g., digestion) but is not affected by the reaction
7. depression, trench, or hollow area
8. electrical signal that travels along the axon of a neuron
9. localized area of tissue that is dying or dead because of lack of a blood supply
10. condition that results when the heart valves do not completely close, allowing some blood to backflow
11. washing out a hollow organ by rinsing with fluid that has been introduced into the organ and suctioned out
12. active at night
13. area where the leg angles forward; located between the fetlock and the hoof
14. progressive wave of contraction and relaxation of muscles that moves food along in the digestive tract
15. lying down
16. detailed description, including distinctive features, of an animal
17. substance dissolved in a solution (e.g., glucose in blood)
18. partial dislocation of a joint
19. applied to, or an action on the surface of the body
20. water-soluble, nitrogen-based compound that is the waste material of protein

Exercise 14-2

1. cystocentesis
2. nephrostomy
3. catheter
4. hysterectomy
5. auscultation
6. serosanguineous
7. aerobic
8. anastomosis
9. arrhythmia
10. tachypnea
11. anesthesia
12. renomegaly
13. pyuria
14. emesis
15. flank

Exercise 14-3

(Your answers are correct. These are just some thoughts.)

1. vicerodynia, ventralgia
2. malodorourospiration, osmouresis
3. diarrhea, rectorrhage, fecal rhinoacousia
4. vertigo, kinesioid, kinesiophilia
5. blepharoptosis, palpebroparesis
6. cephalodynia, cranialgia
7. diaphragmospasm, tachyaeroglottis
8. xanthodermatosis, xerocutaneous
9. anorexia, contravore, hypophagy
10. emesis, gastroptysis
11. myospasm, hyperneural
12. multiphobias
13. musculokinesiosis
14. hypognosis, catesthesia, ipsidysesthesia
15. necrosis, asystemobiosis

Exercise 14-4

1. bloodstream
2. renal artery
3. glomerulus
4. glomerular filtrate
5. Bowman's capsule
6. renal tubules
7. renal pelvis
8. ureters
9. bladder
10. urethra
11. sphincter muscle

Exercise 14-5

1. specific gravity
2. protein
3. color
4. glucose
5. appearance
6. sediment
7. bilirubin
8. pH
9. ketones

Exercise 14-6

1. painful urination
2. stone
3. a fold of skin that covers the head of the penis
4. cold
5. high frequencies of sound
6. a stone in the urinary tract
7. a paralysis
8. electrolyte imbalance
9. a surgical crushing or grinding
10. in the urethra, in the pelvic cavity

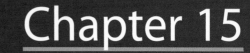

Chapter 15

The Reproductive System

A rooster might do all the crowing, but it's the hen that lays the eggs.

Anonymous

WORD PARTS

cervic/o	**sihr**-vih-cō	gravida	**grahv**-ihd-ah	ovari/o	ō-**vahr**-ē-ō	sperm/o	**spər**-mō
coit/o	**kō**-ih-tō	hyster/o	**hihs**-tehr-ō	ovul/o	**ōhv**-yoo-lō	spermat/o	**spər**-mah-tō
colp/o	**kohl**-pō	mamm/o	**mahm**-mō	par-	pahr	test/o	**tehs**-tō
copul/o	**kohp**-ū-lō	mast/o	**mahs**-tō	para	**pahr**-ah	theri/o	**thēr**-ē-ō
crypt/o	**krihp**-tō	metr/o	**meh**-trō	partum	**pahr**-tuhm	urethr/o	ū-**rē**-thrō
-cyesis	**sī**-ē-sihs	nulli-	**nuhl**-lih	parturi/o	pahr-**tuhr**-ē-ō	uter/o	**ū**-tər-ō
ejacul/o	ē-**jahck**-yoo-lō	o/o	**ō**-ō	pen/i	**pē**-nih	vagin/o	vah-**jī**-nō
embry/o	**ehm**-brē-ō	oophor/o	ō-**ohff**-ohr-ō	pregn/o	**prehg**-nō	vulv/o	**vuhl**-vō
epididym/o	ehp-ih-**dihd**-ih-mō	orch/o	**ohr**-kō	priap/o	**prī**-ah-pō	zo/o	**zō**-oh
episi/o	uh-**pē-zē**-ō	orchi/o	**ohr**-kē-ō	prim/i	**prī**-mah		
genit/o	**jehn**-eh-tō	orchid/o	**ohr**-kih-dō	pseud/o	**soo**-dō		
gest/o	**jehs**-tō	ov/o	**ō**-vō	salping/o	sahl-**ping**-ō		

OUTLINE

THE REPRODUCTIVE SYSTEM

REPRODUCTION
    The Male Reproductive System
    The Female Reproductive System

LEARNING OBJECTIVES

When you have completed this chapter, you will be able to:

1. Understand the components and functions of the reproductive system.

2. Identify and recognize the meanings of word parts related to the reproductive system, using them to build or analyze words.

3. Apply your new knowledge and understanding of clinical veterinary language in the context of medical reports.

CASE STUDY 15-1 **#2003-2015 SADIE**

Signalment and History: A 5-year-old Golden Retriever **multiparous bitch** named Sadie was brought to the Frisbee SA Clinic 2 days after **parturition,** along with her eight **neonate** puppies. The owner was concerned because Sadie had a **malodorous serosanguineous vaginal** discharge, and was **anorexic** and **lethargic.** Sadie had an episode of **emesis** that morning. Sadie was current on all vaccinations and was receiving regular heartworm **prophylaxis.** Sadie had a medical history of **chronic otitis externa,** but no **otic** treatments or other medications had been administered during her pregnancy.

Sadie whelped at 65 days' **gestation.** One week before whelping, Sadie had been brought to the clinic, and eight **fetal** skeletons were identified on **abdominal** X-rays. During a 15-hour period, Sadie gave birth to her eight puppies. Because of a dystocia, manual assistance through the **vagina** was required for delivery of all puppies. The owner reported that she had seen only two placentas being passed; the remaining six fetal membranes presumably were **retained** in the uterus.

(See the rest of the story later in the chapter.)

THE REPRODUCTIVE SYSTEM

Congratulations! Your prototype animal is complete. He can do everything he needs to do to grow, thrive, and survive. Or is it a she? Up to this point, it did not really matter whether you were putting together a male or a female animal. But now you are going to need other animals to perpetuate the species. You see, the animal you just created is only one-half of the entire reproductive system. To produce an offspring, a male reproductive system and a female reproductive system work together.

REPRODUCTION

Animals come and animals go; but species survive because of the production of offspring. Through sexual reproduction, two animals produce an offspring with the genetic characteristics of both parents. And yet this offspring is unique, because half of its genetic code is determined by the sire and half by the dam.

Sexual reproduction in animals is quite straightforward. Two animals mate when the female is ready to accept the male. Through copulation, the male delivers mature sexual cells **(gametes)** to the female. She gets pregnant, and a baby is born. The mother feeds the baby until it is ready to live on its own. Is that all there is to it? Maybe in a nutshell. You need to know a lot more before you fully understand how reproduction works, and how sometimes it does not work.

The rest of this chapter will be devoted to **theriogenology.** You will learn about the male reproductive system, the female reproductive system, and what happens when they work together to produce offspring.

TABLE 15-1		Word Parts Associated with the Male Reproductive System	
Word Part	**Meaning**	**Example and Definition**	**Word Parts**
theri/o	animal, wild beast	**theriogenology** the branch of veterinary medicine that deals with all aspects of the reproductive system	theri/o = animal, wild beast gen/o = formation or beginning -logy = to study, or to have knowledge of
genit/o	reproduction; sex organs	**genitalia** the organs of reproduction, especially the external organs	genit/o = reproduction; sex organs -al = pertaining to -ia = pertaining to

theri/o

genit/o

TABLE 15-1	Word Parts Associated with the Male Reproductive System—cont'd		
Word Part	**Meaning**	**Example and Definition**	**Word Parts**
orch/o orchi/o orchid/o test/o	testicle (*plural =* testes)	**orchectomy** or **orchiectomy** surgical removal of a testicle (or testes)	orch/o = testicle orchi/o = testicle -ectomy = surgical removal
		orchialgia pain in the testicle (or testes)	orchi/o = testicle -algia = pain
		orchidotomy a surgical incision into a testicle	orchid/o = testicle -tomy = surgical incision
		testicular artery small blood vessel that carries blood to a testicle	test/o = testicle -ic = pertaining to -ul(e) = indicating something small -ar = pertaining to arter/o = artery -y = made up of, characterized by
crypt/o	hidden	**cryptorchidism** condition of failure of one or both of the testes to descend into the scrotum	crypt/o = hidden orchid/o = testes -ism = state, condition, action, process, or result
sperm/o spermat/o	spermatozoa; male reproductive cell	**spermous** pertaining to sperm, the male reproductive cell	sperm/o = spermatozoa; male reproductive cell -ous = pertaining to
		spermaturia presence of sperm in urine	spermat/o = spermatozoa; male reproductive cell -uria = urine
epididym/o	epididymis	**epididymoplasty** surgical repair of the epididymis	epididym/o = epididymis -plasty = surgical repair
urethr/o	urethra	**urethrocele** protrusion of the urethra	urethr/o = urethra -cele = protrusion, hernia
pen/i priap/o	penis; male organ of copulation	**penectomy** surgical or traumatic removal of the penis *The word* penis *is taken from the* *Latin word for "tail," and the original* *meaning of the word* pencil *is "little* *penis." Small brushes were used for* *writing before modern lead pencils.* *An artist's brush made of fine camel* *hairs was known as a "little tail."*	pen/i = penis -ectomy = surgical removal
		priapitis inflammation of the penis *To the Greeks, he was* Priap**os**. *To the* *Latins, he was* Priap**us**. *Anyway, he* *was the god of procreation, shown* *with a large* peni**s**.	priap/o = penis -itis = inflammation
ejacul/o	eject, discharge, to throw out	**ejaculation** to eject or discharge fluids from the body	ejacul/o = eject, discharge -ation = state, condition, action, process, or result

orch/o

orchi/o

orchid/o

test/o

crypt/o

sperm/o

spermat/o

epididym/o

urethr/o

pen/i

priap/o

ejacul/o

CASE STUDY 15-2 #2006-5209 BLACK HAWK

Signalment and History: A 2-year-old Morgan **stallion** named Black Hawk was brought to the Frisbee LA Clinic for evaluation of **penile** swelling. On the previous day, three **mares** had gained access to Black Hawk's pasture, and he had bred or attempted to breed at least two of them. After the mares were removed from the pasture, the owner noticed that Black Hawk had a severe penile swelling. On Dr. Murdoch's advice, Black Hawk received an **anti-inflammatory** drug (2.2 **mg/kg PO q12h**), and the penis received cold **hydrotherapy** by means of a hose. During hydrotherapy, Black Hawk was observed urinating normally.

Physical Examination: Pat found Black Hawk **BAR** when the physical exam was begun. The **TPR** was within expected reference ranges. He looked to be in good physical condition. Black Hawk's penis was **flaccid** and **edematous;** approximately 9 inches of the **penis** and **prepuce** was prolapsed through the **preputial orifice.** Dr. Murdoch noted multiple **superficial lacerations** and **bruises** on the penis and prepuce, as well as a cuff of edema **distal** to the preputial ring. A **hematoma** was present on the left **dorsolateral** aspect of the penis. The penis could not be retracted into the preputial cavity. The **testes** appeared unaffected.

Diagnosis: On the basis of Black Hawk's extracurricular activities of the previous day, Dr. Murdoch diagnosed trauma-induced **paraphimosis.**

Treatment: Black Hawk was restrained and **sedated** with a **sedative/analgesic IV.** The penis and prepuce were initially treated with cold hydrotherapy, **topical** application of glycerol for lubrication, and vigorous massage to decrease edema. An attempt to replace the penis within the preputial cavity was unsuccessful. Black Hawk was hospitalized. The treatment regimen was repeated **bid** for the next 96 **h.** At the end of each treatment, an **antimicrobial** cream was applied **topically** to the penis and prepuce. Between treatments, the penis and the prepuce were covered with a nonadherent dressing, wrapped with an elastic bandage material, and supported against Black Hawk's **ventral abdomen** with a mesh sling. The bandage and sling provided steady pressure to prevent formation of additional edema. Black Hawk was also walked for 20 minutes bid. Dr. Murdoch prescribed **antibiotic** tablets (**30 mg/kg PO q12h for 14 days**) and an **analgesic (1.1 mg/kg IV q24h for 1 day, then 0.5 mg/kg IV q12h for 6 days).**

On the fifth day of treatment, the edema had decreased slightly, but the hematoma on the left dorsal aspect of the penis had enlarged. Dr. Murdoch performed **ultrasonography** and found no communication between the hematoma and the **erectile tissue** of the penis. Therefore, Black Hawk was sedated, and the hematoma was **incised,** resulting in approximately 200 mL of **clotted** blood being removed. The area was flushed with a dilute **topical antiseptic solution.** The penis was then coated with the antimicrobial cream, and a rubber compression bandage was tightly wrapped on the penis and prepuce, beginning **distally** and proceeding **proximally.** The compression bandage was allowed to remain in place for 5-minute intervals. After the compression bandage had been repositioned in this manner for 1 hour, the penis was substantially less edematous. Complete reduction and retraction into the prepuce and preputial cavity were then possible. A purse-string suture was placed around the distal edge of the sheath and was tightened to keep the penis within the preputial cavity. Over the next 5 days, the suture was released twice a day to allow Dr. Murdoch to examine the penis and prepuce.

Outcome: Ten days after admission, Black Hawk was discharged from the hospital. The owner was instructed to continue the antibiotic and analgesic treatments at home. The penile and preputial edema decreased substantially over the next 4 weeks. Black Hawk was able to extend and retract his penis through the preputial ring and sheath on his own approximately 2 to 3 weeks after discharge. At 6 weeks after the injury, Black Hawk's penis and prepuce appeared grossly normal, except for a 3-cm **erythematous** area where the hematoma had been located. At 8 weeks after the injury, Black Hawk escaped from his pasture and bred a mare.

EXERCISE 15-1 *Case It!*

In Case Study 15-2, you read of various medications that were prescribed for Black Hawk. Reword each prescription in everyday language that you could use to report to Black Hawk's owner.

1. sedative/analgesic IV _____

2. anti-inflammatory drug 2.2 mg/kg (1 mg/lb) PO q12h _____

3. topical application repeated bid for 96 h _____

4. antibiotic tablets (30 mg/kg PO q12h for 14 days) _____

5. analgesic (1.1 mg/kg IV q24h for 1 day, then 0.5 mg/kg IV q12h for 6 days) _____

Check your answers at the end of the chapter, Answers to Exercises.

The Male Reproductive System

The male reproductive system (Table 15-1; Figure 15-1) is responsible for creating the male gametes and delivering them to a receptive female. It all begins in the testicle and involves **spermatogenesis,** the production of male gametes called *spermatozoa* or, more commonly, **sperm.** Each sperm has a head (its nucleus) and a long, thread-like tail. (Sperm can wriggle their tails to move.) Before the sperm can be delivered to the female, fluid must be added for nutritional and delivery purposes. This fluid is called **seminal fluid. Semen** is the term used for the combination of sperm cells and seminal fluid.

The male sex organs are outside of the abdominal cavity. Behind the penis (or beneath it in cats) hangs a small sac of skin called the **scrotum.** This is part of the external genitalia of a male. This sac of skin houses the testes.

There are two **testes** (*singular* = testicle). They are the male sex glands **(gonads)** in which the gametes are produced, that is, they produce sperm. Actual sperm production takes place in canals within the testes called the **seminiferous tubules.** Located between these tubules are **interstitial cells.** Their function, under the influence of luteinizing hormone (LH), is to produce the male sex hormones (androgens), primarily testosterone. Testosterone stimulates spermatogenesis and the development of **secondary sex characteristics.** (Think of the mane in lions, horns on goats, racks on moose, peacock feathers, and deep voices.) A third hormone regulates the male reproductive system. Follicle-stimulating hormone (FSH) also stimulates spermatogenesis.

A complex system of ducts, called the **efferent ducts,** carries the sperm out of each of the testes and into the **epididymis.** This flat structure lies on top of the testicle and acts as a maturation and storage area for sperm until it is needed. The **vas deferens** is a continuation of the epididymis. A vas deferens leaves each testicle to carry sperm from the epididymis to the urethra. In addition to its urinary function, the urethra has a reproductive function—to carry sperm during **ejaculation.**

The link between the scrotum (which lies outside the body) and the urethra (which lies inside the body in the pelvic canal) is the **spermatic cord.** This cord contains the vas deferens plus blood vessels, nerves, and lymphatic vessels. One spermatic cord comes from each testicle.

Several accessory reproductive glands provide seminal fluid secretions that make up most of the volume of semen. **Seminal vesicles (vesicular glands)** have ducts that enter the urethra near where the vas deferens enters the urethra. (Seminal vesicles are not present in dogs or cats.) The **prostate gland** is a singular gland that is wrapped around the urethra; it has many ducts that enter the urethra. All domestic animals possess a prostate gland. It is the only accessory reproductive gland in dogs.

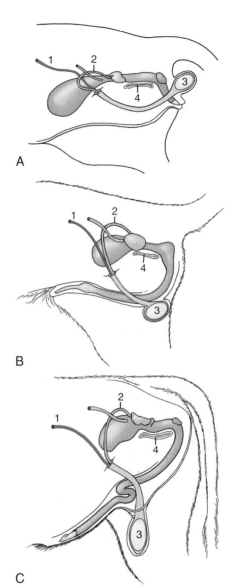

FIGURE 15-1 The male reproductive system exhibited by the tomcat (A), dog (B), and bull (C). *1,* Testicular artery; *2,* vas deferens; *3,* testis; *4,* pelvic symphysis. (From Dyce K, Sack W, Wensing CJG: *Textbook of Veterinary Anatomy,* ed 4, St Louis, 2010, Saunders.)

Bulbourethral glands are the most caudal of the accessory reproductive glands. Just before ejaculation, they secrete a mucus-containing **(mucinous)** fluid that clears and cleans the urethra before the semen passes through. All common domestic animals, except for the dog, have bulbourethral glands.

The **penis** is the male breeding organ that carries urinary and reproductive products out of the body. Two cords **(roots)** attach the penis to the pelvis. The penis is composed of muscle, connective tissue, and erectile tissue. The body of the penis is composed primarily of **erectile tissue.** This spongy tissue containing many sinuses can become engorged with blood, causing the tissue to swell, which results in an **erection.** When the penis is not erect, a protective **sheath** of skin **(prepuce)** covers the end of the penis. The **glans** is the distal tip of the penis; it is rich in sensory nerve endings and is sensitive to physical stimulation.

Two types of penises may be seen in male domestic animals. A **fibroelastic** penis is seen in bulls, rams, billy goats, and boars. This type is characterized by small sinuses in its erectile tissue. The penis does not get larger in diameter during erection, it gets longer. When the penis is not erect, it is pulled back into the prepuce by the **retractor penis muscle** to form an S-shaped **sigmoid flexure** (see Figure 15-1, *C*). A **musculo-cavernous** penis is seen in the stallion. It is characterized by large sinus spaces. The penis grows in diameter and length when it is erect; it does not form a sigmoid flexure when it is not erect.

The penis of the dog is unusual in that it has two specialized structures that are absent in other species. It includes a bone called the *os penis*, which holds the shape and direction of the penis during mating. The other unique structure is the bulb of the glans, which becomes engorged with blood after the penis has entered the female's vagina. This locks the penis in place during mating, thus **tying** the two animals together for a time.

The penis of the tom cat has **penile spines** on its glans. The spines are evident in the presence of testosterone but disappear in the absence of testosterone, as is seen in a neutered male. The urethra of a tom is short, so that the external opening of the penis is in the perineum (see Figure 15-1, *A*); when erect, the penis elongates and curves forward.

Some of the more common **anatomical abnormalities** of the male reproductive system include the following:

- cryptorchidism—failure of one or both testes to descend into the scrotum after birth, from the abdominal cavity where they develop; also known as *retained testicles*
- micropenis—hypoplasia of the penis
- megalopenis—hypertrophy of the penis
- hypospadiasis—occurs when the urethra opens on the ventral surface of the penis or in the perineum

Functional abnormalities of the penis include those listed here:

- phimosis—inability to extend the penis, most often caused by stenosis of the urethral opening
- paraphimosis—idiopathic (in most cases) protrusion of the nonerect penis with the inability to retract it
- priapism—persistent erection of the penis, possibly caused by increased arterial blood flow and/or decreased venous drainage

TABLE 15-2	Word Parts Associated with the Female Reproductive System		
Word Part	**Meaning**	**Example and Definition**	**Word Parts**
o/o ov/o ovul/o	ovum, egg (*plural* = ova)	**oocyte** a developing egg inside an ovarian follicle	o/o = egg -cyte = cell
		ovum a mature female gamete cell that has been released from its ovarian follicle (*plural* = ova)	ov/o = egg -um = structure, thing
		ovulation release of an egg from the ovary	ovul/o = egg -ation = state, condition, action, process, or result

Continued

ovari/o

oophor/o

salping/o

uter/o

hyster/o

metr/o

cervic/o

TABLE 15-2	Word Parts Associated with the Female Reproductive System—cont'd		
Word Part	**Meaning**	**Example and Definition**	**Word Parts**
ovari/o oophor/o	ovary	**ovariectomy** surgical removal of an ovary	ovari/o = ovary -ectomy = surgical removal
		oophorrhagia bleeding from the ovary *Did you see the combining form for "eggs" within the combining forms for the "ovary"?*	oophor/o = ovary -rrhag(e) = excessive flow -ia = pertaining to
salping/o	salpinx; a trumpet-shaped tube; oviduct in the reproductive system	**salpingotomy** surgical incision into the salpinx (oviduct); incision into a trumpet-shaped tube	salping/o = salpinx; a trumpet-shaped tube; oviduct in the reproductive system -tomy = surgical incision
		*The combining form of salping/o may also be used in words referring to other tubes in the body, e.g., the eustachian tube in the ear. An example would be **rhinosalpingitis**: inflammation of the mucous membrane of the nose and eustachian tube. Common sense tells you that this is not an inflammation of the nose and the oviduct.*	rhin/o = nose salping/o = salphinx; a trumpet-shaped tube -itis = inflammation
uter/o hyster/o metr/o	uterus	**uterocystostomy** surgical creation of a new permanent opening between the uterus and the bladder	uter/o = uterus cyst/o = sac containing fluid, a bladder -stomy = surgical creation of a new permanent opening
		hysterectomy surgical removal of the uterus *Just because "hysteric disturbances" most frequently occurred in women, the ancient Greeks erroneously credited the womb as its cause. Hysteria was known as a "disease of the womb."*	hyster/o = uterus -ectomy = surgical removal
		metrorrhagia bleeding from the uterus, at irregular and unexpected intervals *Watch out! This combining form metr/o also means "measure."*	metr/o = uterus -rrhag(e) = excessive flow -ia = pertaining to
cervic/o	neck; cervix (neck of the uterus)	**cervicoplasty** surgical repair of the neck of the uterus; surgical repair of the neck	cervic/o = neck; cervix (neck of the uterus) -plasty = surgical repair

TABLE 15-2	Word Parts Associated with the Female Reproductive System—cont'd		

Word Part	Meaning	Example and Definition	Word Parts
		⚠ The neck is any constricted portion. The uterus has a neck, called the cervix. A neck holds up the head. A **cervicectomy** would certainly be performed only on the neck of the uterus unless you were living in France during the French Revolution and met up with a guillotine.	cervic/o = neck; cervix (neck of the uterus) -ectomy = surgical removal
vagin/o colp/o	vagina	**vaginodynia** pain in the vagina	vagin/o = vagina -dynia = pain
		colpocentesis surgical puncture of the vagina	colp/o = vagina -centesis = surgical puncture
vulv/o episi/o	vulva	**vulvitis** inflammation of the vulva	vulv/o = vulva -itis = inflammation
		episiorrhaphy suturing of the vulva	episi/o = vulva -rrhaphy = suturing
mamm/o mast/o	breast, mammary gland	**mammogram** written record that is produced of the breast by the procedure *mammography*	mamm/o = breast, mammary gland -gram = written record produced, something recorded or written
		mastopathy disease of the breast	mast/o = breast, mammary gland -pathy = disease

vagin/o

colp/o

vulv/o

episi/o

mamm/o

mast/o

BOX 15-1	Terms That Defy Word Analysis

- clitoris—a sensitive female external organ homologous to the penis; an erectile body
- cornus—horn
- corpus—body
- fimbria—a fringe-like structure, found in the infundibulum of the oviduct
- follicle—a small cavity or sac
- infundibulum—the flared end of a funnel-shaped duct or passageway such as the oviduct

The Female Reproductive System

The female part of the reproductive system is much more complex than the male part—it has more jobs to do (Table 15-2). Not only is the female reproductive system responsible for producing the female gamete (the egg or ovum), it delivers it to the oviduct, where it can be fertilized by the male gamete (the sperm). Then it provides a protective environment for the embryo to grow until it is fully developed. After the offspring is pushed out into the world, mammary glands provide nutrition to the newborn.

Nearly all of the female reproductive system is internal and is located within the abdominal and pelvic cavities. The organs and structures (Figure 15-2) that are involved in ova production, mating, and pregnancy are these:

- paired **ovaries**
  - These are the female gonads responsible for oogenesis.
  - They are located in the dorsal part of the abdomen.
  - They have both gametogenic and endocrine functions.
- numerous **follicles**
  - They are little sacs found in the parenchyma (cortex) of the ovary.
  - Each follicle contains one oocyte in some stage of development.
- paired **oviducts,** also called **uterine tubes**
  - They catch the ova as they are released from their follicles.
- infundibulum
  - This is the flared end of the oviduct.

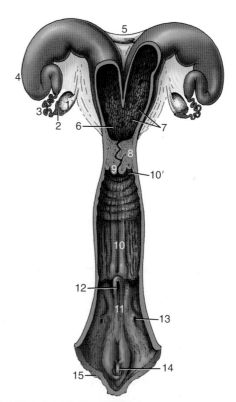

FIGURE 15-2 **The reproductive tract of a cow, opened dorsally.** *1,* Ovary; *2,* infundibulum; *3,* uterine tube; *4,* horn of uterus; *5,* intercornual ligaments; *6,* body of uterus; *7,* caruncles; *8,* cervix; *9,* vaginal part of cervix; *10,* vagina; *10′,* fornix; *11,* vestibule; *12,* external urethral opening; *13,* opening of major vestibular gland; *14,* clitoris; *15,* vulva. (From Dyce K, Sack W, Wensing CJG: *Textbook of Veterinary Anatomy,* ed 4, St Louis, 2010, Saunders.)

- fimbriae
  - They make up the finger-like fringe border of the infundibulum.
  - They help sweep the ova into the oviduct.
- **uterus** (the womb)
  - An embryo comes here to rest and grow into a fetus, ready to be born. The embryo/fetus is nourished and protected here during pregnancy.
  - The **body** of the uterus lies just cranial to the cervix. In common domestic animals (including dogs and cats), it is **bicornuate.** This means that it splits into two **horns,** much like the arms of a **Y.** The oviducts extend from the cranial end of each horn.
  - The wall of the uterus has three layers. The **endometrium** is the inner epithelial layer that contains mucus and other types of glands. In ruminants, numerous permanently raised areas are called **caruncles,** which are the areas where a developing embryo will attach to the uterus.
  - The **myometrium** is the thickest layer of the uterine wall and is made up of smooth muscle cells. The **perimetrium,** the outer layer, is covered by the visceral layer of the peritoneum.
- cervix
  - This is the narrow, caudal neck of the uterus.
  - It is a sphincter that controls access between the vagina and the uterus.
- vagina
  - Its cranial portion from the cervix to the urethral opening on the floor of the vagina has only a reproductive function.
  - Beyond the urethral opening, the vagina is called the *vestibule,* which has **urogenital** functions.
- vestibule
  - It opens to the exterior at the **vulva.**
- clitoris
  - It lies on the floor of the vestibule, caudal to the urethral opening.
- labia
  - They form the external boundary of the vulva.

The Ovarian Cycle

Ova production takes place in the ovaries. However, the female reproductive system works on a cycle, so oocytes are not constantly maturing. Under the influence of FSH, estrogen is produced in many of the developing ovarian follicles. Estrogen stimulates the physical and behavioral changes that prepare an animal for breeding. As the level of estrogen rises, the level of FSH falls and the level of luteinizing hormone (LH) rises. When the level of LH reaches its critical level, an ovum is released from one or more of the follicles, and production of the hormone progestin begins. The remaining follicles that had started to develop stop growing, degenerate, and are reabsorbed into the ovary.

Even though there are many follicles in an ovary, only a few are chosen to begin developing at the beginning of each cycle. Why certain follicles are picked while others are not seems to be one of the mysteries of the universe. The number of follicles that complete maturation and release ova depends on the species. Some species normally release only one ovum during a cycle. These animals are **uniparous** because they will normally give birth to only one offspring per pregnancy. Mares, cows, and humans are examples of uniparous animals. Animals that normally give birth to more than one offspring per pregnancy (litters) are called **multiparous** animals. In these animals, a varying number of follicles will release mature ova. Bitches, queens, and sows are examples of multiparous animals.

A follicle with a mature ovum is sometimes called a **graafian follicle,** or a **vesicular ovarian follicle.** When the mature follicle ruptures, the ovum is released **(ovulation)** into the peritoneal cavity, along with the fluid that was contained in the follicle. Once released, the ovum is gathered into the oviduct, helped in part by the action of the fimbriae. The empty follicle left behind fills with blood that rapidly clots. The follicle is now called the **corpus hemorrhagicum** (bloody body). The cells that line the follicle begin to multiply and gradually replace the clotted blood. The now-solid former follicle is called the **corpus luteum (CL)** (yellow body). It is the corpus luteum that produces progestin hormones (mainly progesterone) under the influence of LH after the ovum has left, and if the animal becomes pregnant. The progestins prepare the uterus for, and help sustain, pregnancy. If no pregnancy occurs, the corpus luteum degenerates.

BOX 15-2 **Terms That Defy Word Analysis**

- congenital—pertaining to a condition existing at birth or dating from birth
- DNA (deoxyribonucleic acid)—the molecule that carries the genetic information (genetic code) that is the basis of heredity
- fecund—fertile; capable of producing offspring
- fetus—an animal in later stages of development within the womb
- gamete—a mature sexual reproduction cell; a sperm or an ovum
- mutant—the result of altered DNA; a genetic abnormality
- natal—birth
- perineum—the region between the scrotum and the anus in males; also the region between the vulva and the anus in females
- placenta—a vascular, membranous organ between a mother and her offspring in the womb, formed by membranes from the mother and the embryo, providing nourishment to and taking waste products away from the embryo/fetus during the entire pregnancy
- teat—nipple of the breast or mammary gland
- zygote—a cell produced by the union of two gametes

TABLE 15-3 **Word Parts Associated with Breeding, Pregnancy, and the Neonatal Period**

Word Part	Meaning	Example and Definition	Word Parts
copul/o coit/o	coming together; to fasten together; sexual intercourse	**copulation** a joining together or coupling; sexual intercourse	copul/o = coming together; to fasten together; sexual intercourse -ation = state, condition, action, process, or result
		coitophobia intense or abnormal fear of sexual intercourse	coit/o = coming together; to fasten together; sexual intercourse -phobia = intense or abnormal fear
embry/o	animal in the very early stages of development within the womb; an embryo	**embryectomy** surgical removal of an animal in the very early stages of development within the womb; surgical removal of an embryo	embry/o = embryo; animal in the very early stages of development within the womb -ectomy = surgical removal
prim/i	first	**primary** belonging to the first stage of any process, as in the primary grades	prim/i = first -ar = pertaining to -y = made up of, characterized by

copul/o

coit/o

embry/o

prim/i

TABLE 15-3	Word Parts Associated with Breeding, Pregnancy, and the Neonatal Period—cont'd		
Word Part	**Meaning**	**Example and Definition**	**Word Parts**
pseud/o	false, deception	**pseudoarthrosis** joint formed in an old fracture by fibrous tissue between two pieces of bone that have not grown together	pseud/o = false, deception arthr/o = joint -osis = disease or abnormal condition
-cyesis pregn/o	pregnancy; having offspring developing in the body	**pseudocyesis** false pregnancy	pseudo/o = false -cyesis = pregnancy; having offspring developing in the body
		pregnant carrying developing offspring within the body	pregn/o = pregnancy; having offspring developing in the body -ant = a person who does, or things which do, something specified
gravida	pregnant female	**primigravida** a female pregnant for the first time *Compare* gravida *with* gravity, *i.e., something heavy.*	prim/i = first gravida = pregnant female
gest/o	carry, produce	**gestation** to carry an offspring from conception to delivery *Other words using this combining form that would be familiar to you are* digestion, indigestion, *and* congestion.	gest/o = carry, produce -ation = state, condition, action, process, or result
par- para parturi/o partum	giving birth to a live fetus	**uniparous** giving birth to only one offspring at a time	uni- = one, single par- = giving birth to a live fetus -ous = pertaining to
		bipara a female that has given birth twice, in separate pregnancies *Did you remember* para- *from previous clinical veterinary language terms? This prefix means "near, beside, abnormal, apart from." You could almost say that the live fetus was "near, beside, or apart from," just hopefully not "abnormal."*	bi- = two para = giving birth to a live fetus
		parturiometer device used to measure the strength of uterine contractions during the birthing process	parturi/o = giving birth to a live fetus -meter = measure, a device to measure
		postpartum the period of time just after the birth of offspring	post- = after, behind, later partum = giving birth to a live fetus
nulli-	none, zero	**nulliparous** a female who has never borne an offspring	nulli- = none, zero par(a)- = giving birth to a live fetus -ous = pertaining to

pseud/o

-cyesis

pregn/o

gravida

gest/o

par-

para

parturi/o

partum

nulli-

> **BOX 15-3**   **Terms Associated with Estrous Cycles in Animals**
>
> - artificial insemination (AI)—injecting semen into the vagina or uterus by use of a special syringe rather than by natural copulation
> - diestrous animals—species that have two estrous cycles per year; dogs
> - estrous—an adjective used to describe events associated with the breeding cycle
> - estrus—a noun; the period when the female accepts the male
> - heat—a common name for estrus; "My dog is in heat."
> - induced ovulator—species that must be bred before they ovulate; cats
> - monestrous animals—animals that cycle only one time per year; wolves, foxes, bears
> - polyestrous animals—species that have estrous cycles throughout the year; humans, cattle, pigs
> - presentation—the orientation of the fetus when parturition begins
> - seasonally polyestrous animals—species that have more than one estrous cycle per year, but only during certain times of the year (e.g., spring, fall); cats, horses, sheep, goats, hamsters
> - synchronized estrus—the use of hormones to create a group of females that will come into estrus at the same time; used with artificial insemination procedures so many females can be inseminated at the same time

The Estrous Cycle

The estrous cycle is sometimes referred to as the "heat period." Estrous cycles begin at the start of an animal's puberty and continue throughout the animal's life. Mother Nature, in her infinite wisdom, has devised a way for the females of a species to develop mature ova only during certain times of a year, so that offspring are born at a time when the environment is most favorable for survival of the newborn. This ingenious process is called the *estrous cycle*, of which the ovarian cycle is only a part.

In the time it takes the earth to make one trip around the sun (1 year), every species wants to generate offspring, or **procreate.** To this end, the female of the species goes through a cyclical process that will prepare her to become pregnant at that optimum time during the year. The periods during this process will vary in length, depending on the species, but all females of a species will go through the same periods to create the right window, or windows, of opportunity for successful breeding (Table 15-3).

Although the estrous cycle is a nonstop process, it can be divided into a series of distinctive stages. **Anestrus** is a period when there is no ovarian activity. This could be the result of pregnancy, nursing, the season of the year, poor nutrition, or even disease. **Proestrus** is the period of follicular/oocyte development in the ovary. In some species (e.g., dogs), a bloody discharge from the vagina may be noticed; ovulation has not yet taken place. Estrogen levels are rising. The male is getting interested in the female, but the female is not yet interested in the male.

Estrus is the period of breeding. There is mutual attraction between the male and the female. The female accepts the male. Ovulation occurs in some species. **Metestrus** is the period of ovulation in some species (or right after ovulation in species that ovulate during estrus). The corpus luteum develops, and the uterus prepares to accept an embryo and go through pregnancy.

Diestrus is the active luteal stage; the CL has reached its maximum size. If pregnancy occurs, the CL will be retained to help support pregnancy through hormone release. If no pregnancy occurs, the CL will degenerate. After the CL has disappeared, the female will go into anestrus or will go back into proestrus for another cycle (i.e., in polyestrous animals). The period between estrous cycles in polyestrous animals is **interestrus.**

The **follicular stage** is the time during the proestrus and estrus stages when rising levels of estrogen are responsible for reproductive changes. Together, the metestrus and diestrus stages are known as the **luteal stage.** Ovulation has taken place, and rising levels of progesterone provide the prevailing hormonal influence.

Pregnancy

If a female is bred during estrus, the hopeful outcome is a pregnant female. The mother-to-be has gone through all sorts of hormonal changes and has prepared her uterus for an embryo. The ovum, once released from the follicle, does not travel far from home into the oviduct, where it waits for a sperm to arrive. For fertilization between the ovum and the sperm to take place, a pretty remarkable journey has to be completed by the sperm. The sperm must get deposited in the female's vagina or uterus (depending on the species), swim up the uterus with the help of uterine and oviduct contractions, and pass through a uterine horn into the oviduct, where it will meet the ovum of its dreams.

There is a lot of competition for these ova. For example, a single ejaculate from a rabbit contains about 280 million sperm. One from a boar contains about 8 billion sperm.

Fertilization (Figure 15-3) takes place when one sperm penetrates the wall of the ovum and deposits its genetic material. It takes only one sperm to fertilize an ovum. Do the math. Eight billion sperm are delivered by a boar, and only one sperm will successfully penetrate the wall of each ovum that a sow has released. Even if 8 to 12 ova were released, the odds are not so good. Sperm that swim the fastest and are the strongest get the ova. The rest of the sperm are sorry-out-of-luck and will die.

Each sperm has a little cap on its head called the **acrosome,** which contains digestive enzymes. When the sperm reaches the ovum, the acrosome releases these enzymes to help the sperm penetrate the wall of the ovum. Once one sperm has penetrated the wall and delivered its genetic material, no other sperm can penetrate the same ovum.

The genetic materials from each parent join together, and the fertilized ovum quickly begins dividing. The **zygote** is the name given to a fertilized ovum. As the zygote travels down the oviduct into the uterus, it continues to divide and goes through more stages of development until it reaches the **blastocyst** stage. Then it is ready to implant itself into the wall of the uterus.

Implantation (see Figure 15-3) results when the blastocyst attaches itself into the endometrium of the uterus. It is now called an **embryo** and must find a method of surviving the period of the pregnancy. Enter Mama. A fluid-filled **placenta** is formed around the embryo, which joins the embryo to its mother. In this way, she can supply the oxygen and nutrients that the fetus needs and can carry away the waste materials that it does not need.

The placenta connects to the embryo via the **umbilical cord.** The placenta attaches to the uterine wall by way of one of four general types of attachments (Figure 15-4). Mares and sows have a *diffuse* attachment, that is, the areas of attachment are spread all over the surface of the placenta and the uterine wall. Ruminants have a *cotyledonary* attachment. Here small separate areas of attachment are formed from raised areas on the uterine wall (caruncles) attaching to a corresponding area on the placenta **(cotyledons).** The entire attachment area is called a **placentome.** In a *zonary* attachment, the area of attachment is belt-shaped and encircles the entire placenta. This type of attachment is seen in bitches and queens. If the attachment is a single disk-shaped area, it is referred to as *discoid* attachment. The placentas of humans and of other primates have this type of attachment.

The length of a pregnancy is called the **gestation period.** It varies among species from an average of 336 days in the mare, to 63 days in dogs and cats, to 16 days in hamsters. Gestation periods are usually divided into three unequal **trimesters,** each indicating a period of growth and development for the embryo/fetus.

Parturition (labor) is the birthing process, the long- (or short-) awaited arrival of a live baby. The exact stimulus to begin parturition is unknown, but the eventual outcome of a multitude of hormonal interactions is the beginning of uterine wall contractions under the influence of **oxytocin** released from the posterior pituitary gland. Parturition is divided into three **stages of labor:**

The longest gestation of any mammal is an average of 624 days for an elephant. Camels and giraffes cannot even compete, at 410 days and 460 days, respectively. Imagine what would happen to the world's human population if women had to carry babies for nearly 2 years before delivery!

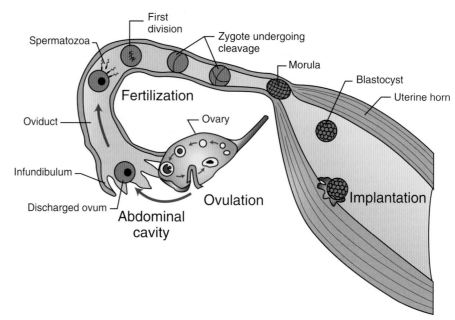

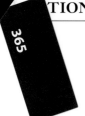

FIGURE 15-3 Fertilization and implantation. (From Colville TP: *Clinical Anatomy and Physiology for Veterinary Technicians,* ed 2, St Louis, 2009, Mosby.)

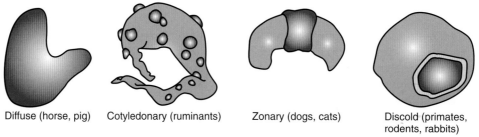

Diffuse (horse, pig)   Cotyledonary (ruminants)   Zonary (dogs, cats)   Discold (primates, rodents, rabbits)

FIGURE 15-4 Placenta structural attachments in mammals. (From Colville TP: *Clinical Anatomy and Physiology for Veterinary Technicians,* ed 2, St Louis, 2009, Mosby.)

- uterine contraction causing the cervix to dilate
- delivery of the newborn
  - The fetus will be in anterior presentation (head or front feet first), posterior presentation or breech (hind legs first), or something in-between.
- delivery of the placenta **(afterbirth)** after separation from the uterine wall

After parturition, many dams will eat the placenta. The uterus will gradually return to its nonpregnant resting state through a process called **involution.** During this time, there will be a bloody discharge from the uterus from where the placenta pulled away. This will gradually stop as the uterus heals.

Now that there is a new baby on the scene, the dam must continue to provide it with nourishment. She does this through the milk she produces in her **mammary glands.** These glands are specialized skin glands and are not really part of the reproductive system. The number of mammary glands and their locations differ among species. A dairy cow has four mammary glands contained in a structure called an **udder.** It is located in the groin area. A bitch has 10 mammary glands, five on each side of the ventral midline that runs the length of the ventrum.

Milk production is called **lactation.** The mammary gland will continue to produce milk as long as it is emptied on a regular basis, either by nursing or by milking. Once the stimulus to produce milk is gone, the mammary gland undergoes involution to its nonlactating state.

Right before a baby is born, the dam starts to produce a pre-milk called **colostrum.** The highly nutritious colostrum is an important first meal for the newborn. It contains high levels of antibodies from the mother, which will provide immunity during the first few weeks to months of life. Colostrum also acts as a **laxative** to help the newborn pass its first bowel movement—the dark, sticky material in its intestinal tract called **meconium.**

When a newborn is ready to support itself nutritionally, it is gradually **weaned** off its mother's milk. The age at which weaning begins varies with the species. Calves are usually weaned when they are 6 to 7 months old. Foals are completely weaned by the time they are 4 to 6 months old. Kittens and puppies begin the weaning process sometime between the ages of 4 and 6 weeks. Weaning has to be a gradual process to give the young animal's digestive system a chance to adapt to a new diet. If the food is switched too rapidly, diarrhea can develop.

EXERCISE 15-2 *Recall it!*

For fertilization between the ovum and the sperm to take place, a pretty remarkable journey has to be completed by the sperm. Track the journey of a sperm from its formation in a testicle until it meets the ovum.

testicle → _____ → _____ →

_____ → _____ → _____ →

_____ → _____ → _____

Check your answers at the end of the chapter, Answers to Exercises.

BOX 15-4 **Terms Associated with Pregnancy, Parturition, and the Uterus**

- abortion—removal of an embryo or fetus from the uterus to end a pregnancy; a miscarriage is a spontaneous abortion
- Cesarean section (C-section)—surgical delivery of a fetus through an incision in the dam's abdominal wall
- dystocia—abnormally slow, difficult birth
- ectopic pregnancy—abnormal development of an embryo occurring somewhere other than inside the lumen of the uterus, usually in the oviduct; also known as *eccyesis*
- hermaphroditism—a condition whereby an animal has both male and female reproductive organs
- pseudocyesis—false pregnancy; the physical symptoms of pregnancy develop without conception
- pyometra—an accumulation of pus in the uterus
    - If the cervix is open (open pyometra), the pus will drain. If the cervix is closed (closed pyometra), the pus will continue to accumulate in the uterus.
    - Etiology is not fully understood, but prolonged progesterone stimulation and bacterial invasion of the uterus play a part.
    - A closed pyometra is considered an emergency situation.
- retained placenta—all or part of the placenta is left in the uterus after the third stage of labor
- sterile—not able to produce offspring; can affect both males and females
- stillborn—born dead

Many people mispronounce "pyometra" by saying "pyometra." Do not be one of them!

CASE STUDY 15-1 #2003-2015 SADIE

Signalment and History: A 5-year-old Golden Retriever **multiparous bitch** named Sadie was brought to the Frisbee SA Clinic 2 days after **parturition,** along with her eight **neonate** puppies. The owner was concerned because Sadie had a **malodorous serosanguineous vaginal** discharge, and was **anorexic** and **lethargic.** Sadie had an episode of **emesis** that morning. Sadie was current on all vaccinations and was receiving regular heartworm **prophylaxis.** Sadie had a medical history of **chronic otitis externa,** but no **otic** treatments or other medications had been administered during her pregnancy.

Sadie's reproductive history included two prior pregnancies at 2 and 3 years of age. For her first pregnancy, Sadie **whelped** prematurely at 60 days' **gestation.** At 59 days' gestation, a green vaginal discharge (i.e., **uteroverdin**) was detected. Sadie gave birth to 11 puppies, 8 of which were **stillborn.** A **nonenteric** bacteria was cultured from one of the placentas. The premature labor was thought to be a result of bacterial **placentitis** and subsequent **metritis.**

For her second pregnancy, Sadie whelped at 65 days' gestation. During a 5-hour period, Sadie gave birth to eight puppies, the last two of which were stillborn. Repeated uterine and fetal heart rate monitoring was used to follow the progression of labor, to evaluate fetal distress, and to assess the possibility of **dystocia.** Parturition was medically assisted with **SubQ** administration of two units of **oxytocin,** which stimulated uterine contractions.

For this pregnancy, Sadie whelped at 65 days' **gestation.** One week before whelping, Sadie had been brought to the clinic, and eight **fetal** skeletons were identified on **abdominal** X-rays. During a 15-hour period, Sadie gave birth to her eight puppies. Because of a dystocia, manual assistance through the **vagina** was required for delivery of all puppies. The owner reported that she had seen only two placentas being passed; the remaining six fetal membranes presumably were **retained** in the uterus.

Physical Examination: Jess examined Sadie and her puppies. The abnormal clinical findings for Sadie were **pyrexia, lethargy,** and a moderate amount of malodorous serosanguineous vaginal discharge. Her respiration rate and heart rate were within expected reference ranges upon **auscultation.** Sadie's **mammary glands** and milk appeared normal. All her puppies appeared to be clinically normal. Jess drew blood samples from Sadie for a CBC and serum chemistry tests.

Dr. Frisbee performed an **abdominal ultrasonography,** which revealed that both uterine horns were beginning to **involute,** and it was surprising to note that a single fetus was located in the body of the uterus **cranial** to the pelvic brim. In the jumble of skeletons visible on Sadie's X-ray, everyone had missed one skeleton. No fetal heartbeat was detected. No evidence of **peritonitis** was noted.

The hemogram revealed **anemia** and **leukopenia** with **granulocytopenia.** Serum chemistry test results showed **hypoalbuminemia, hypoproteinemia,** and a decreased **BUN** concentration.

Diagnosis: At this point, Dr. Frisbee noted that her **ddx** for Sadie's **febrile** condition included infection, **hypocalcemia, neoplasia,** or an excessively hot ambient temperature. Her ddx for the vaginal discharge included retained **placentas,** metritis, and a retained fetus. Sadie's lethargy was considered to be a nonspecific **clinical sign** of a systemic illness.

Treatment and Outcome: Sadie and her puppies were hospitalized. **IV** fluid administration was begun at the rate of **6 mL/kg/h** for 24 hours. The low BUN concentration detected on serum chemistry analysis may have been caused by **nephrogenic diabetes insipidus** as a result of bacterial **endotoxins.** The mild anemia was considered to be a normal physiological condition for a **postparturient** bitch, and treatment for that condition was not considered necessary. Two antibiotics, one delivered at **22 mg/kg IV q8h** and one at **10 mg/kg PO q12h,** were started because of the leukopenia and granulocytopenia, which Dr. Frisbee thought might be caused by an infection and uterine **sequestration** of **WBCs.** A uterine muscle stimulant was scheduled to be administered **tid** during working hours for several days in an attempt to induce fetal **expulsion** by stimulating uterine contractions.

A CBC and serum chemistry tests performed after two doses of the stimulant showed anemia and leukopenia, **lymphopenia,** and **monocytopenia.** The serum chemistry results showed continued hypoalbuminemia, hypoproteinemia, and a low BUN concentration. The retained fetus was expelled after the fifth injection of the stimulant, 30 hours after initiation of treatment. The CBC was repeated 12 hours after fetal expulsion, and **Hct** and WBC counts were within expected reference ranges. Serum chemistry tests repeated at that time showed mild hypoalbuminemia with total protein and BUN concentrations within expected reference ranges.

All Sadie's puppies remained healthy during her treatment and were weaned 5 weeks later.

EXERCISE 15-3 *Case It!*

In Case Study 15-1, you read about Sadie's pregnancies. Dr. Frisbee wants to make sure you were paying attention to what was going on. So write your answers, in everyday language, to the following questions in the space provided.

1. Describe Sadie's vaginal discharge at the time of admission.

2. The report says that Sadie had a fever. What were some of the differential diagnoses that Dr. Frisbee considered as possible etiologies?

3. What is secondary nephrogenic diabetes insipidus? Is it contagious to Sadie's pups?

4. What was the state of Sadie's red blood cell and white blood cell numbers when she was admitted?

5. In your nonprofessional, but educated, opinion, do you think Sadie is a good candidate to be sold as a breeding bitch? Why or why not?

Check your answers at the end of the chapter, Answers to Exercises.

TABLE 15-4	Abbreviations	
Abbreviation	**Meaning**	**Example**
AI	artificial insemination	AI is an invaluable resource for breeding dams when the sire is not close enough for a personal visit.
C-section	Cesarean section	It was a relief that Sadie didn't need a C-section to deliver her puppies.
DNA	deoxyribonucleic acid	DNA testing is being used in dogs to determine the breed makeup of mixed breed dogs.

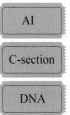

AI

C-section

DNA

EXERCISE 15-4 *Use It!*

Over-the-counter (OTC) drugs are medicines that may be sold directly to a customer without a prescription from a healthcare professional, whereas prescription drugs require written authorization under direct supervision by a doctor before the drugs can be purchased.

Following is a list of some of the OTC drugs that you might find at your nearby pharmacy. Decide which of the systems of the body would be affected by each of these drugs. Then write the part of the word that gave you the clue. The first drug is given as an example.

1. Aerolate®	respiratory system	aer/o = air
2. Amerituss®		
3. Anusol®		
4. Boniva®		
5. Bronkaid®		
6. Cortizone®		
7. Dentek®		
8. Dermacin®		
9. Dermarest®		
10. Donatussin®		
11. Emetrol®		
12. Estroven®		
13. Exelderm®		
14. Flexall®		
15. Flonase®		
16. Gas-X®		
17. Giltuss®		
18. Glucophage®		
19. Glucotrol®		
20. Glytuss®		
21. JointFlex®		
22. Joint-Ritis®		
23. Liposyn®		
24. Micardis®		
25. Micronase®		
26. Mucinex®		
27. Ocuhist®		
28. Orabase®		
29. Orajel®		
30. Pepcid®		
31. Robitussin®		
32. Rhythmol®		
33. Theraflu®		
34. Vaginex®		

Check your answers at the end of the chapter, Answers to Exercises.

EXERCISE 15-5 *Use It!*

Just because you have reached this last exercise, you have by no means finished learning. There are many more word parts waiting to be discovered by you. However, you have mastered a method for analyzing words. Clinical veterinary language has become understandable, as well as easy—even fun—to learn.

So to send you on your way, here is one last combining form to add to your list. The combining form for animals or living beings is **zo/o.** Had you ever wondered why the park-like area in which live animals are kept in cages or large enclosures for public viewing is called a zoo (which is short for *zoological garden*)? It is because of the animals! This exercise will give you a chance to dissect and define "new-to-you" clinical veterinary language terms about animals, as you match them to their definitions.

zo/o

1. _____ an animal living on fecal material

2. _____ one animal living within another animal

3. _____ a large animal

4. _____ a very small animal

5. _____ pertaining to the skin of animals

6. _____ the red pigment in bird feathers

7. _____ animals that reproduce sexually

8. _____ of animal origin

9. _____ one who describes or depicts animals

10. _____ an animal hormone

11. _____ resembling an animal

12. _____ animal rock; a fossil

13. _____ a person who specializes in the study of animals

14. _____ the black pigment in bird feathers

15. _____ measurement of the proportionate lengths or sizes of the parts of animals

16. _____ having the form of an animal

17. _____ any human disease transmitted from an animal

18. _____ feeding on animals

19. _____ a lover of animals

20. _____ an irrational fear of animals

21. _____ surgical repair of an animal organ

22. _____ a hallucination in which a person believes he sees animals

23. _____ dissection of animals, not humans

24. _____ pertaining to or providing nutrition to animals for growth

zootomy

zoonosis

zoodermic

zoogenous

zooid

zoologist

zoomorphic

zoophile

zooscopy

coprozoite

zoometry

zoohormone

zootrophic

zooplasty

zoogamous

zoographer

zoolith

zoomelanin

zoophagy

zoophobia

microzoon

megazoid

endozoic

zooerythrine

Check your answers at the end of the chapter, Answers to Exercises.

ANSWERS TO EXERCISES

Exercise 15-1

1. Drugs were administered intravenously to calm and soothe Black Hawk, and to relieve pain.
2. This drug was administered to relieve the symptoms of inflammation such as swelling, tenderness, fever, and pain. The dose was 2.2 milligrams per kilogram (or 1 milligram per pound weight of Black Hawk), given by mouth every 12 hours.
3. The cream was applied to the surface of the penis, twice a day for 4 days.
4. The purpose of the pills was to fight a bacterial infection. The pills were given by mouth 30 milligrams per kilogram weight of Black Hawk, every 12 hours (twice a day) for 14 days.
5. This drug was used to relieve pain. The dose was administered intravenously at 1.1 milligrams per kilogram weight of Black Hawk, once a day for 1 day. Then the intravenous dose was cut to 0.5 milligram per kilogram, given every 12 hours (twice a day) for 6 days.

Exercise 15-2

testicle → efferent duct → epididymis → vas deferens → urethra → vagina → cervix → uterus → oviduct

Exercise 15-3

1. Sadie's vaginal discharge smelled bad and was composed of a combination of serous fluid and blood.
2. The differential diagnoses included infection (bacterial, fungal, viral, protozoal, or rickettsial), inflammation or immune-mediated disease, low calcium blood levels, formation of a tumor, and an excessively hot environment.
3. *Secondary* means it is not Sadie's primary problem. *Nephrogenic* means it was formed or produced in the kidney/nephron. *Diabetes insipidus* is a condition of either a lack of ADH (antidiuretic hormone) that encourages collecting ducts to reabsorb water, or the inability of the collecting ducts to respond to the ADH stimulus. In either case, excessive amounts of water are lost in the urine. It is not contagious to Sadie's pups.
4. Sadie had fewer than normal numbers of both red blood cells and white blood cells. The low white blood cell count looks as though it was due to a low granulocyte count, probably the neutrophils.
5. Sadie probably wouldn't make a good breeding bitch because she has had problems with stillborn (dead) fetuses with all of her three pregnancies. She has had to have manual and medical help with her last two pregnancies. Sadie would be a good candidate for an ovariohysterectomy—or a hysterosalpingo-oophorectomy. (Remember that word?)

Exercise 15-4

1. respiratory system; aer/o = air
2. respiratory system; tuss/o = cough
3. digestive system; anus
4. skeletal system/reproductive system; bon(e)
5. respiratory system; bronch/o = bronchus
6. endocrine system; corti(sone)
7. digestive system; dent/o = teeth
8. integumentary system; derm/o = skin
9. integumentary system; derm/o = skin
10. respiratory system; tuss/o = cough
11. digestive system; eme(sis) = vomiting
12. reproductive system; estro(gen)
13. integumentary system; derm/o = skin
14. muscular system; flex
15. respiratory system; nas/o = nose
16. digestive system; gas
17. respiratory system; tuss/o = cough
18. digestive system; gluc/o = sugar and phag/o = eat
19. digestive system; gluc/o = sugar
20. respiratory system; tuss/o = cough
21. skeletal system/muscular system; joint and flex
22. skeletal system/muscular system; joint
23. digestive system; lip/o = fat
24. cardiovascular system; cardi/o = heart
25. endocrine system; -ase = enzyme (not micro/nase but micron/ase, a small enzyme)
26. respiratory system; muc/o = mucus
27. sensory system; ocu(l)/o = eye
28. digestive system; or/o = mouth
29. digestive system; or/o = mouth
30. digestive system; pep(s)/o = digestion
31. respiratory system; tuss/o = cough
32. cardiovascular system; rhythm/o = rhythm
33. respiratory system; flu
34. reproductive system; vagin/o = vagina

Exercise 15-5

1. coprozoite = an animal living on fecal material
2. endozoic = one animal living within another animal
3. megazoid = a large animal
4. microzoon = a very small animal
5. zoodermic = pertaining to the skin of animals
6. zooerythrine = the red pigment in bird feathers
7. zoogamous = animals that reproduce sexually
8. zoogenous = of animal origin
9. zoographer = one who describes or depicts animals
10. zoohormone = an animal hormone
11. zooid = resembling an animal
12. zoolith = animal rock; a fossil
13. zoologist = a person who specializes in the study of animals
14. zoomelanin = the black pigment in bird feathers
15. zoometry = measurement of the proportionate lengths or sizes of the parts of animals
16. zoomorphic = having the form of an animal
17. zoonosis = any human disease transmitted from an animal
18. zoophagy = feeding on animals
19. zoophile = a lover of animals
20. zoophobia = an irrational fear of animals
21. zooplasty = surgical repair of an animal organ
22. zooscopy = a hallucination where a person believes he sees animals
23. zootomy = dissection of animals, not humans
24. zootrophic = pertaining to or providing nutrition to animals for growth

Combining Forms, Prefixes, and Suffixes Alphabetized According to Word Part

Word Part	Definition of Word Part	Pronunciation	Example Word	Chapter
Combining Forms				
abdomin/o	abdomen	ahb-**dah**-mehn-ō	abdominohysteric	3
abomas/o	stomach in ruminants	ahb-ō-**mā**-sō	abomasopexy	10
acous/o	hearing, listening	ah-**koo**-sō	acoustics	12
aden/o	gland	**ahd**-ehn-ō	adenopathy	13
adip/o	fat	**ahd**-ih-pō	adipocyte, adipose	3, 4
adren/o	adrenal gland	ahd-**rē**-nō	adrenomegaly	13
aer/o	air, gas	**ehr**-rō	aerobic	9
albin/o	no color	ahl-**bī**-nō	albinism	5
albumin/o	albumin	ahl-**bŭ**-mihn-ō	albuminuria	14
aliment/o	food	ahl-ih-**mehn**-tō	alimentary canal	10
alveol/o	alveolus	ahl-**vē**-ō-lō	alveolar dysplasia	9
amyl/o	starch	**ahm**-mehl-ō	amylodyspepsia	10
an/o	anus	**ā**-nō	anospasm	10
andr/o	male, masculine	**ahn**-drō	androgen	13
ang/o	vessel, often a blood vessel	**ahn**-jō	periangitis	7
angi/o	vessel, often a blood vessel	**ahn**-jē-ō	hemangioma	7
ankyl/o	stiff, not movable, bent, crooked	**ahng**-kih-lō	ankylosis	5
anter/o	front or before	ahn-**tər**-ō	anterior	3
aort/o	aorta	ā-**ohr**-tō	aortectomy	7
aque/o	water, watery solution	**ah**-kwē-ō	aqueous	12
arachn/o	spider, spider web	ah-**rahck**-nō	arachnoid	11
arter/o	artery	ahr-**tehr**-ō	panarteritis	7
arteri/o	artery	ahr-**tehr**-ē-ō	arteriospasm	7
arthr/o	joint	**arth**-rō	arthropathy, arthrodysplasia	2, 5
articul/o	joint	ahr-**tihck**-yoo-lō	articular	5
astr/o	star	**ahs**-trō	astrocyte	11
atel/o	incomplete, imperfect	aht-**ehl**-ō	atelectasis	9
atri/o	atrium (upper chamber of the heart)	**ā**-trē-ō	atriotomy	7
audi/o	sound	**ahw**-dē-ō	audiology	12
auricul/o	auricle of the heart, or the ear flap	aw-**rihck**-ū-lō	auricular hyperplasia, auricular mange	7
aut/o	self	**aw**-tō	autodermic	4
azot/o	nitrogen	**āz**-oht-ō	azotemia	14
bacteri/o	bacteria	bachk-**tehr**-ē-ō	bacterium	14

Continued

Word Part	Definition of Word Part	Pronunciation	Example Word	Chapter
bi/o	life	**bī**-ō	endobiosis, biology	4, 6
bilirubin/o	bilirubin	**bihl**-ē-**roo**-bihn-ō	bilirubinuria	14
blephar/o	eyelid	**blehf**-ər-ō	blepharospasm	12
brachi/o	brachium	**brā**-kē-ō	cervicobrachial	5
bronch/o	bronchus	**brohng**-kō	bronchospasm	9
bucc/o	cheek	**būk**-ō	buccal	10
capn/o	carbon dioxide	**kahp**-nō	hypercapnia	9
cardi/o	heart	**kahr**-dē-ō	cardiomyopathy, acardia	6, 7
carp/o	carpus	**karh**-pō	intercarpal	5
caud/o	tail	**kahw**-dō	caudal, caudectomy	3
cec/o	cecum	**sē**-cō	cecorrhaphy	10
cellul/o	cell	**sehl**-yoo-lō	cellulitis	3
cep	head, origin of a muscle	sehp	biceps	6
cephal/o	head, skull	**seh**-fahl-ō	cephalocaudal	6
cerebr/o	brain	sehr-**ē**-brō	cerebroatrophy	11
cervic/o	neck	**sihr**-vih-cō	cervicodorsal	5
cervic/o	neck; cervix (neck of the uterus)	**sihr**-vih-cō	cervicoplasty	15
cheil/o	lip	**kī**-lō	cheilophagia	10
chlor/o	green	**klohr**-ō	chlorosis	5
chol/e	bile, gall	**kō**-lē	cholangitis	10
choledoch/o	common bile duct	**kō**-lē-dō-kō	choledochohepatostomy	10
chondr/o	cartilage	**kohn**-drō	osteochondritis, chondrectomy	2, 3
chrom/o	color	**krō**-mō	achromodermic	5
chyl/o	chyle	**kī**-lō	chylorrhea	10
cirrh/o	orange-yellow	**sihr**-ō	cirrhosis	5
clast/o	break in pieces, crush	**klahs**-tō	karyoclastic	8
coagul/o	process of clotting	kō-**ahg**-ū-lō	coagulation	8
coccyg/o	tail	kohck-**sihd**-jō	coccygectomy	5
coit/o	coming together; to fasten together; sexual intercourse	**kō**-ih-tō	coitophobia	15
col/o	colon	**kō**-lō	colocentesis	10
colon/o	colon	**kō**-lohn-ō	colonoscopy	10
colp/o	vagina	**kohl**-pō	colpocentesis	15
copr/o	feces	**kohp**-rō	coprophagia	10
copul/o	coming together; to fasten together; sexual intercourse	**kohp**-ū-lō	copulation	15
cor/o	skin, pupil of the eye or heart	**kohr**-ō	corium, corectasis	4, 12
corne/o	cornea	**kohr**-nē-ō	corneitis	12
cornu/o	horn or structure that looks like a horn	**kohr**-nū-ō	cornual nerve block	4
coron/o	crown	**kohr**-ō-nō	coronary	7
corp/o	body	**kohr**-pō	corpus	11
cost/o	ribs	**kohs**-tō	costectomy, cervicocostal	2, 5
cox/o	hip	**kohx**-ō	coxofemoral	5

Word Part	Definition of Word Part	Pronunciation	Example Word	Chapter
crani/o	head, cranium, skull	**krā**-nē-ō	cranial, craniology, cranioplasty	3, 5
crin/o	secrete	**krihn**-ō	endocrinology	13
cry/o	freezing, icy-cold	**krī**-ō	cryotherapy	6
crypt/o	hidden	**krihp**-tō	cryptorchidism	15
cutane/o	skin	kyoo-**tā**-nē-ō	subcutaneous	4
cyan/o	blue	**sī**-ahn-ō	hypercyanosis	5
cyst/o	bladder, a sac containing fluid	**sihs**-tō	pilocystic, cystitis	4, 14
cyt/o	cell	**sī**-tō	chondrocytosis, polycythemia	3, 8
dacry/o	tears	**dahck**-rē-ō	dacryopyorrhea	12
dactyl/o	digit or toe or finger	**dahk**-tihl-ō	polydactyly	5
dendr/o	tree, dendrite	**dehn**-drō	dendroid	11
dent/o	teeth	**dehn**-tō	dentist	10
derm/o	skin	dər-**mō**	dermopathy, hypodermic	3, 4
dermat/o	skin	dər-mah-**tō**	dermatitis, dermatologist	3, 4
dextr/o	right or toward the right	**dehcks**-trō	dextroposition	3
digit/o	digit or toe or finger	**dihg**-iht-ō	interdigital	5
dips/o	thirst	**dihp**-sō	polydipsia	10
dist/o	remote, farther away from any point of reference	**dihs**-tō	distal	3
dont/o	teeth	**dohn**-tō	orthodontic	10
dors/o	back or top	**dohr**-sō	dorsal, dorsum	3
duoden/o	duodenum	**doo**-ō-də-nō	esophagoduodenostomy	10
dynam/o	force, energy	**dī**-nah-mō	dynamoscope, dynamogenesis	6, 9
edem/o	swelling	eh-**dē**-mō	dactyledema	7
ejacul/o	eject, discharge, to throw out	ē-**jahck**-yoo-lō	ejaculation	15
electr/o	electricity	ē-**lehck**-trō	electromyography, electrocardiograph	6, 7
embry/o	embryo	**ehm**-brē-ō	embryectomy	15
encephal/o	brain	ehn-**sehf**-ah-lō	electroencephalograph	11
enter/o	intestines in general	**ehn**-tehr-ō	enterokinesia	10
eosin/o	red	**ē**-ō-**sihn**-ō	eosinophil	8
epididym/o	epididymis	ehp-ih-**dihd**-ih-mō	epididymoplasty	15
episi/o	vulva	uh-**pē**-**zē**-ō	episiorrhaphy	15
erg/o	work	ər-**gō**	ergometer	6
erythemat/o	red	ehr-ih-**thēm**-ah-tō	erythematous	8
erythr/o	red	eh-**rihth**-rō	erythrocyanosis, erythrocyte	5, 8
esophag/o	esophagus	ē-**sohf**-ah-gō	esophagoplegia	10
esthesi/o	feeling, experience, sensation	ehs-**thē**-zē-ō	esthesiogenesis	12
eti/o	cause	**ē**-tē-ō	etiopathology	2
femor/o	femur	**fehm**-ohr-ō	pubofemoral	5
fibr/o	fiber	**fīb**-rō	myofibrosis, diacutaneous fibrolysis	6, 8
fibrin/o	fibrin	**fī**-brihn-ō	fibrinolysis	8
fibul/o	fibula	**fihb**-yoo-lō	tibiofibular	5
follicul/o	follicle	fohl-**lihck**-kuhl-ō	folliculitis	4

Continued

Word Part	Definition of Word Part	Pronunciation	Example Word	Chapter
gastr/o	stomach in simple-stomached animals	**gahs**-trō	gastropexy	10
gen/o	formation or beginning	**jehn**-ō	pathogenic, hematogenous	2, 5
genit/o	reproduction; sex organs	**jehn**-eh-tō	genitalia	15
gest/o	carry, produce	**jehs**-tō	gestation	15
gingiv/o	gums, gingiva	**jihn**-jih-vō	gingivostomatitis	10
gli/o	glue, glial cells	**glē**-ō	glioma	11
gloss/o	tongue	**glohs**-ō	glossopalatolabial	10
glott/o	glottis	**gloh**-tō	glottitis	9
gluc/o	glucose	**gloo**-cō	cytoglucopenia	10
glyc/o	sugar	**glī**-co	hypoglycemia	10
gnath/o	jaw	**gnahth**-ō	prognathism	5
granul/o	granule, small grain	**grahn**-ū-lō	agranulocyte	8
gravida	pregnant female	**grahv**-ihd-ah	primigravida	15
gust/o	taste	**guh**-stō	gustation	12
hal/o	breathing	**hah**-lō	exhalation, inhalant	9
hem/o	blood	**hē**-mō	hemostasis, electrohemostasis	3, 8
hemat/o	blood	hē-**mah**-tō	hematothorax, hematology	3, 8
hepat/o	liver	heh-**paht**-ō	hepatocyte	10
herni/o	hernia	**hər**-nē-ō	herniorrhaphy	10
heter/o	different, other, unlike	**heht**-tər-ō	heterophil	8
hidr/o	sweat	**hī**-drō	hidrosis	4
hist/o	tissue	**hihs**-tō	histology	3
histi/o	tissue	**hihs**-tē-ō	histiocytosis	3
home/o	similar	**hō**-mē-ō	homeostasis	9
humer/o	humerus	**hū**-mər-ō	scapulohumeral	5
hydr/o	water	**hī**-drō	hydrant, hydruria	4, 14
hypo-	under, beneath, below	**hī**-pō	hypodermic	3
hyps/o	height, altitude	**hihps**-ō	hypsography	10
hyster/o	uterus	**hihs**-tehr-ō	hysterosalpingo-oophorectomy, hysterectomy	2, 15
iatr/o	physician, medicine	**ī**-aht-rō	iatrogenic	9
ile/o	ileum	**ihl**-ē-ō	ileostomy, ileopathy	5, 10
ili/o	ilium	**ihl**-ē-ō	iliocostal	5
immun/o	immunity, immune	ihm-**yoo**-nō	immunocyte	8
irid/o	iris	ihr-ih-**dō**	iridocele	12
is/o	equal	**ī**-sō	anisocytosis	8
isch/o	stop, keep back, suppress	**ihs**-kō	ischemia	7
ischi/o	ischium	**ihs**-kē-ō	ischiococcygeal	5
jejun/o	jejunum	jeh-**joo**-nō	esophagojejunoplasty	10
kali/o	potassium, kalium	**kā**-lē-ō	kaliopenia	14
kary/o	nucleus	**kehr**-ē-ō	karyogenic, karyorrhexis	3, 8
kerat/o	hard, horn-like tissue, or cornea	**kehr**-ah-tō	keratodermia, keratitis	4, 12
ket/o	ketone bodies	**kē**-tō	ketosis	14
keton/o	ketone bodies	**kē**-tōn-ō	ketonuria	14

Word Part	Definition of Word Part	Pronunciation	Example Word	Chapter
kinesi/o	movement	kih-**nē**-sē-ō	kinesiology	6
labi/o	lip	**lā**-bē-ō	labionasal	10
lacrim/o	tears	**lahck**-rih-mō	nasolacrimal duct	12
lapar/o	flank, loin	**lahp**-ah-rō	laparosplenotomy	10
laryng/o	larynx, voice box	lah-**rihng**-gō	laryngospasm	9
later/o	side	**laht**-ər-ō	lateral	3
lept/o	thin, fine, slender, small	**lehp**-tō	leptocephaly	11
leuc/o	white	**loo**-kō	leucocytometer	8
leuk/o	white	**loo**-kō	melanoleukoderma, leukocyte	5, 8
lingu/o	tongue	**lihng**-gwah-ō	lingual	10
lip/o	fat	**lī**-pō	lipectomy, lipoma, lipolysis	3, 4, 10
lith/o	stone	**lihth**-ō	lithogenesis, nephrolithotomy	10, 14
log/o	to study, or to have knowledge of	**lō**-gō	chondrology	2
lumb/o	loin	**luhm**-bō	lumbocostal	5
lymph/o	lymph	**lihm**-fō	lymphangitis	8
lys/o	destruction, dissolution, dissolving, breakage	**lī**-sō	rhabdomyolysis, hemolysis	6, 8
malac/o	soft, softening	mah-**lā**-shō	osteomalacia	5
mamm/o	mammary gland; breast	**mahm**-mō	mammogram	15
mandibul/o	mandible (lower jaw bone)	mahn-**dihb**-ū-lō	mandibulectomy	5
mast/o	mammary gland; breast	**mahs**-tō	mastopathy	15
maxill/o	maxilla (upper jaw of skull)	mahck-**sih**-lō	maxillotomy	5
medi/o	middle	**mē**-dē-ō	mediolateral	3
mediastin/o	space between the two lungs that contains all the thoracic viscera except the lungs	mē-dē-ah-**stī**-nō	mediastinoscopy	9
megal/o	large or enlarged	**mehg**-ah-lō	cardiomegaly	7
melan/o	black, dark	**mehl**-ah-nō	melanoma, melanocyte	4, 5
mening/o	meninges	meh-**nihng**-ō	meningocele	11
mes/o	middle	**mēs**-ō	mesoappendix	3
mesi/o	middle	**mēs**-ē-ō	mesial	3
metr/o	measure, uterus	meh-**trō**	metric system, metrorrhagia	6, 15
morph/o	structure, shape	**mohr**-fō	morphology	8
muc/o	mucus (noun) or mucous (adjective)	**myoo**-kō	mucogenesis, mucous cell	9
muscul/o	muscle	**muhs**-kyoo-lō	cervicomuscular	6
my/o	muscle	**mī**-ō	myodysplasia, myopathology, cardiomyopathy	3, 6, 7
myel/o	spinal cord, bone marrow	mī-**eh**-lō	myelitis, periosteomyelitis, neuromyelitis	5, 11
myring/o	eardrum	**mihr**-ihng-ō	myringectomy	12
nas/o	nose	**nā**-zō	nasology	9
natr/i	sodium	**nā**-trē	natriuresis	14
natr/o	sodium	**nā**-trō	hypernatremia	14
necr/o	death	neh-**krō**	necrobiosis, avascular necrosis	4, 7
nephr/o	kidney	**nehf**-rō	nephroblastoma	14
neur/o	nerve, nervous system	**nər**-ō	neuritis, neuropathy	3, 11

Continued

Word Part	Definition of Word Part	Pronunciation	Example Word	Chapter
neutr/o	neutral	**nū**-trō	neutrophil	8
nod/o	knot	**nohd**-ō	nodule	4
norm/o	normal	**nohr**-mō	normocytic	8
o/o	ovum, egg	**ō**-ō	oocyte	15
ocul/o	eye	**ohk**-ū-lō	oculocutaneous	12
odont/o	teeth	ō-**dohn**-tō	odondopathy	10
odor/o	smell	**ō**-dər-ō	malodorous	12
olfact/o	smell	ohl-**fahck**-tō	olfaction, olfactory nerve	9, 12
olig/o	little, few, small, scanty	**ohl**-ih-gō	oligodendroglia, oliguresis	11, 14
omas/o	omasum	ō-**mā**-sō	omasal stenosis	10
oment/o	omentum	ō-**mehn**-tō	omentopexy	10
onych/o	claw, nail	**ohn**-ih-kō	onychectomy	4
oophor/o	ovary	ō-**ohff**-ohr-ō	hysterosalpingo-oophorectomy, oophorrhagia	2, 15
ophthalm/o	eye	**ohf**-thahl-mō	ophthalmologist	12
opt/o	eye	**ohp**-tō	optometrist	12
or/o	mouth	**ohr**-ō	oral	10
orch/o	testicle	**ohr**-kō	orchectomy	15
orchi/o	testicle	**ohr**-kē-ō	orchiectomy, orchialgia	15
orchid/o	testicle	**ohr**-kih-dō	orchidotomy	15
organ/o	organ	ohr-**gahn**-ō	organectomy	3
orth/o	straight, normal, correct	**ohr**-thō	orthodigitia	5
os	bone	ohs	os penis, os cordis, os rostri	5
osm/o	smell	**ohz**-mō	aosmia	12
oss/o	bone	**ohs**-sō	ossicle	12
osse/o	bone	**ohs**-ē-ō	osseous tissues	5
oste/o	bone	**ohs**-tē-ō	osteochondritis, osteoliposarcoma, osteoarthritis	2, 3, 5
ot/o	ear	ō-**tō**	otorhinolaryngology	12
ov/o	ovum, egg	**ō**-vō	ovum	15
ovari/o	ovary	ō-**vahr**-ē-ō	ovariohysterectomy, ovariectomy	2, 15
ovul/o	ovum, egg	**ōhv**-yoo-lō	ovulation	15
ox/o	oxygen	**ohck**-sō	hypoxia	9
palat/o	palate, roof of mouth	**pahl**-ah-tō	palatorrhaphy	10
palm/o	back surface of the forelimb distal to the carpus	**pahl**-mō	palmar	3
palmar/o	back surface of the forelimb distal to the carpus	pahl-**mahr**-ō	palmarodorsal	3
palpebr/o	eyelid	**pahl**-peh-brō	palpebration	12
pancre/o	pancreas	**pahn**-krē-ō	pancreopathy	10
pancreat/o	pancreas	**pahn**-krē-aht-ō	pancreatitis	10
papul/o	pimple, solid lesion <1 cm	**pahp**-yool-ō	papular	4
para	giving birth to a live fetus	**pehr**-ah	bipara	15
partum	giving birth to a live fetus	**pahr**-tuhm	postpartum	15
parturi/o	giving birth to a live fetus	**pahr**-tuhr-ē-ō	parturiometer	15
patell/o	patella	pah-**tehl**-ō	patellectomy	5

Word Part	Definition of Word Part	Pronunciation	Example Word	Chapter
path/o	disease	**pahth**-ō	chondropathology, myopathologist	2, 6
pelv/i	pelvis	**pehl**-vī	pelviscope	5
pelvi/o	pelvis	**pehl**-vē-ō	pelvioplasty	5
pen/i	penis	**pē**-nih	penectomy	15
peps/o	digestion	**pehp**-sō	apepsia	10
pept/o	digestion	**pehp**-tō	bradypeptic	10
phag/o	eat	**fā**-gō	dysphagia, hyperphagia	8, 10
phalang/o	phalanges	fah-**lahn**-jō	metacarpophalangeal	5
pharyng/o	pharynx, throat	fah-**rihng**-gō	pharyngostomy	9
phil/o	loving, or more than normal	**fihl**-ō	ergophilous, hydrophilic	7, 8
phleb/o	vein	**flē**-bō	phlebotomy	7
physi/o	to make grow, to produce	**fihz**-ē-ō	physiology	5
pil/o	hair	**pī**-lō	piloerection	4
plant/o	back surface of the rear limb distal to the tarsus	**plahn**-tō	plantar	3
plantar/o	back surface of the rear limb distal to the tarsus	plahn-**tahr**-ō	plantarodorsal	3
plas/o	growth, development, or formation	**plā**-zō	osteochondroplasia, hypoplasia, erythroplasia, plasmodysplasia	2, 5, 6, 8
plasm/o	plasma or related to plasma	**plahz**-mō	plasmocytoma, neoplasm, plasmodysplasia	8
pleur/o	pleura, thin membrane with two layers that lines the lungs and the chest cavity	**ploor**-ō	pleuritis, pleurisy	9
plur/i	several, more than one	**ploor**-ē	pluripotent	8
pne/o	breath or respiration	**nē**-ō *or* pah-**nē**-ō	pneopneic	9
pneum/o	air, and sometimes the lung	**nū**-mō	pneumothorax, pneumocentesis	9
pneumon/o	lung	**nū**-mohn-ō	pneumonoultramicroscopic-silicovolcanoconiosis	9
pod/o	foot	**pō**-dō	pododerm	5
poli/o	gray	**pohl**-ē-ō	poliomyelitis	11
por/o	a pore, small opening, or cavity	**pohr**-ō	osteoporous	5
poster/o	rear, behind, after	pō-**stēr**-ō	posterior	3
prandi/o	meal	**prahn**-dē-ō	postprandial	10
pregn/o	pregnancy	**prehg**-nō	pregnant	15
priap/o	penis	**prī**-ah-pō	priapitis	15
prim/i	first	**prī**-mah	primary	15
proct/o	rectum	**prohck**-tō	proctologist	10
propri/o	self, one's own	**prō**-prē-ō	proprioception	12
proxim/o	nearest	**prohck**-sih-mō	proximal	3
pseud/o	false, deception	**soo**-dō	pseudoanorexia, pseudoarthrosis	13, 15
ptyal/o	saliva, salivary gland	**tī**-uh-lō	hypoptyalism	10
pub/o	pubis	**pehw**-bō	pubocaudal muscles	5
pulmon/o	lung	**puhl**-mohn-ō	pulmonologist	7
purpur/o	purple	pər-pər-ō	purpura	4, 5
py/o	pus	**pī**-ō	pyoarthrosis, ureteropyosis	4, 14
pyel/o	kidney pelvis	**pī**-eh-lō	pyeloplasty	14

Continued

Word Part	Definition of Word Part	Pronunciation	Example Word	Chapter
pylor/o	pylorus	pī-**lohr**-ō	pyloric sphincter	10
pyr/o	heat, high temperature	**pī**-rō	pyrogen	6
pyrex/o	heat, high temperature	pī-**rehx**-ō	pyrexia	6
radi/o	radiation, radius	**rā**-dē-ō	radiodermatitis, radiohumeral	5
rect/o	rectum	**rehck**-tō	rectalgia	10
ren/o	kidney	**rē**-nō	renogram	14
reticul/o	reticulum	reh-**tihck**-yoo-lō	reticulorumen	10
retin/o	retina	**reht**-ih-nō	neuroretinitis	12
rhabd/o	rod, cylinder	**rahb**-dō	rhabdomyoma	6
rhin/o	nose	**rī**-nō	rhinoplasty, rhinitis	9, 12
rhythm/o	rhythm, regularly occurring motion	**rihth**-mō	arrhythmia	7
rostr/o	nose	**rohs**-trō	rostral	3
rubr/o	red	**rū**-brō	rubricity, rubric	5, 8
rumen/o	rumen	**roo**-mehn-ō	rumenotomy	10
rumin/o	rumen	**roo**-mihn-ō	ruminant	10
sacchar/o	sugar	**sahck**-ahr-ō	monosaccharide	10
sacr/o	sacrum	**sā**-krō	sacrocaudal	5
salping/o	oviduct, salpinx, a trumpet-shaped tube	sahl-**ping**-ō	hysterosalpingo-oophorectomy, salpingotomy, rhinosalpingitis	2, 15
sanguin/o	blood	**sahng**-gwihn-ō	exsanguination	8
sarc/o	flesh	**sahr**-kō	rhabdomyosarcoma	6
scapul/o	scapula	**skahp**-yoo-lō	scapulopexy	5
scler/o	hard	**sklehr**-ō	arteriosclerosis	7
scop/o	examine, view	**skō**-pō	necroscopy	4
seb/o	oil, sebum	**seh**-bō *or* **sē**-bō	sebum	4
sebac/o	oil, sebum	seh-**bā**-shō	pilosebaceous	4
ser/o	serum	**sehr**-ō	serosanguineous	8
sial/o	saliva, salivary gland	sī-**ahl**-ō	sialectasis	10
sinistr/o	left	sihn-**ihs**-trō	sinistrodextral	3
skelet/o	skeleton	**skehl**-eh-tō	skeletal	5
somat/o	body	**sō**-mah-tō	somatology	2
spasm/o	spasm (intermittent involuntary abnormal muscle contractions)	**spahz**-mō	myospasm	6
sperm/o	spermatozoa; male productive cell	**spər**-mō	spermous	15
spermat/o	spermatozoa; male productive cell	**spər**-mah-tō	spermaturia	15
spin/o	spine	**spī**-nō	spinous	3
spir/o	breathing or coil or spiral	**spī**-rō	spirograph	9
spirat/o	breathing	**spī**-rah-tō	inspiration	9
splen/o	spleen	**splehn**-ō	splenomyelomalacia	8
spondyl/o	vertebral column, spine	spohn-**dih**-lō	spondylosis	5
steat/o	fat	stē-**aht**-ō	steatorrhea	10
sten/o	narrow	**stehn**-ō	arteriostenosis	7
stern/o	sternum, breastbone	**stər**-nō	costosternoplasty	5
steth/o	chest	**stehth**-ō	stethoscope	7

Word Part	Definition of Word Part	Pronunciation	Example Word	Chapter
stom/o	mouth	**stō**-mō	anastomosis	10
stomat/o	mouth	stō-**mah**-tō	stomatomalacia	10
sudor/o	sweat	**soo**-dohr-ō	sudoral	4
system/o	system	sihs-**tehm**-ō	systemic	3
tars/o	tarsus	**tahr**-sō	tibiotarsal	5
tax/o	order, coordinated movement	**tahck**-sō	ataxia	11
ten/o	tendon	**tehn**-ō	tenophyte, tenotomy	3, 6
tendin/o	tendon	**tehn**-dihn-ō	tendinitis, polytendinitis	3, 6
tendon/o	tendon	**tehn**-dohn-ō	tendonectomy, tendonitis	3, 6
tenont/o	tendon	**tehn**-ohnt-ō	tenontology, tenontomyoplasty	3, 6
test/o	testicle	**tehs**-tō	testicular artery	15
theri/o	animal, wild beast	**thēr**-ē-ō	theriogenology	15
therm/o	heat	thər-mō	catathermal	6
thorac/o	thorax	**thōr**-ah-cō	thoracopathy, thoracoscopy	3, 5
thromb/o	thrombus, clot	**throhm**-bō	thrombectomy	8
thyr/o	thyroid gland	**thī**-rō	thyroidectomy	13
tibi/o	tibia	**tihb**-ē-ō	femorotibial	5
ton/o	pressure, tension	**tō**-nō	myotonia	6
trache/o	trachea, windpipe	**trā**-kē-ō	tracheotomy, tracheostomy	9
trich/o	hair	**trī**-kō	melanotrichia	4
trop/o	affinity to, turn to, respond to a stimulus	**trō**-pō	aerotropism	13
tuber/o	rounded projection, knob	**too**-bər-ō	tuberous	5
tuss/o	cough	**tuhs**-sō	tussiculation, antitussive	9
tympan/o	eardrum	**tihm**-puh-nō	tympanocentesis	12
uln/o	ulna	**uhl**-nō	ulnar	5
ur/o	urine	**ū**-rō	uremia	14
ureter/o	ureter	ū-**rē**-tər-ō	ureteralgia	14
urethr/o	urethra	ū-**rē**-thrō	urethroscope, urethrocele	14, 15
uter/o	uterus	**ū**–tər-ō	uterocystostomy	15
vacu/o	to empty, emptiness	**vahck**-ū-ō	vacuole	8
vagin/o	vagina	vah-**jī**-nō	vaginodynia	15
valvul/o	valve	**vahl**-vū-lō	valvulosis	7
vas/o	vessel (for blood or other fluids)	**vahs**-ō	vasodilation	7
vascul/o	blood vessel	**vahsk**-yoo-lō	cardiovascular	7
ven/o	vein	**vē**-nō	intravenous	7
ventr/o	belly	**vehn**-trō	dorsoventral	3
ventricul/o	ventricle (lower chamber of the heart)	vehn-**trih**-kū-lō	atrioventricular	7
vertebr/o	vertebra	vehr-**tē**-brō	intervertebral	5
vesicul/o	blister, small sac	veh-**sihk**-ū-lō	vesiculectomy	4
vestibul/o	entrance, cavity, or channel that is an entrance to another cavity	veh-**stihb**-ū-lō	vestibular	9
viscer/o	viscera (internal organs)	**vihs**-ər-ō	viscerate	3
vulv/o	vulva	**vuhl**-vō	vulvitis	15

Continued

Word Part	Definition of Word Part	Pronunciation	Example Word	Chapter
xanth/o	yellow	**zahn**-thō	xanthoma	5
xer/o	dry	**zē**-rō	xeroderma	4
zo/o	animal, living being	**zō**-oh	zoology, etc.	15
Prefixes				
a-	without, no, not	ah *or* ā	acellular, amyoplasia	4, 6
ab-	away from	ahb	abnormal, abductor muscles	5, 6
ad-	toward	ahd	adneural, admaxillary, adductor muscles	5, 6
ambi-	both, on both sides	**ahm**-bē	ambidextrous	5
amphi-	both, on both sides	**ahm**-fih	amphicranitis	5
an-	without, no, not	ahn	anhidrosis, anerythroplasia	4, 6
ante-	before, in front of, prior to	**ahn**-tē	antebrachium, anterior, antechamber	5, 8
anti-	against, opposed to	**ahn**-tē	anticoagulant	8
aqua-	water, watery solution	**ah**-kwah	aquatic	12
baso-	chemically basic	**bā**-sō	basophil	8
bi-	two	bī	bicycle, bicaudal	4, 6
brachy-	short	**brahk**-ē	brachydactyly	10
brady-	slow	**brā**-dē	bradycardia	7
carni-	flesh, meat	**kahr**-nē	carnivore	10
cata-	down, reverse, backward, degenerative	**kaht**-ah	catabiosis	6
centi-	one-hundredth, or one hundred	**sehnt**-ah	centimeter	6
circum-	around	**sehr**-kuhm	circumflex	4
contra-	against, contrary, opposing	**kohn**-trah	contralateral	6
de-	removal, separation, reduction	dē	deoxygenation	6
deci-	one-tenth	**deh**-sih	decibel	6
di-	two, twice, double	dī	dichromic	6
dia-	through, between, apart, across, complete	**dī**-ah	dialog, diagnosis, diadermal, diadermic	2, 3, 5
dis-	apart, away from, separation	dihs	disease	7
dys-	bad, defective, painful, or difficult	dihs	dysplasia	2
echo-	returned sound	**ehck**-ō	echocardiogram	7
ect-	outside, external	ehct	ectosteal	3
ecto-	outside, external	**ehct**-tō	ectodermatosis	3
em-	in, into, inward	ehm	emphysema, embolus	11
en-	in, into, inward	ehn	enchondroma	11
end-	within, inner	ehnd	endosteitis, endosteoma	3, 5
endo-	within, inner	**ehn**-dō	endoarthritis, endopelvic	3, 5
epi-	on or upon	**ehp**-ih	epidermis, epibiosis	3, 5
eu-	good, well, normal	ū	eupepsia	12
ex-	out, outside, outer, away from	ehcks	exostosis, excise	3, 5
exo-	out, outside, outer, away from	**ehcks**-ō	exogenous, exoskeleton	3, 5
extra-	outside	**ehcks**-trah	extracellular	3
hemi-	half, partial	**hehm**-ih	hemialgia	6
herbi-	plant, green crop	**hərb**-ih	herbivore	10
hyper-	above, over, or excess	**hī**-pər	hyperplasia	3

Word Part	Definition of Word Part	Pronunciation	Example Word	Chapter
hypo-	under, beneath, below	**hī**-pō	hypodermic	3
in-	in, within, inward, into, not	ihn	inside, inbreeding, inappropriate, inapt	3
infra-	below, beneath	**ihn**-frah	infraspinous	3
inter-	between, among	**ihn**-tər	interchondral, intercostal, interphalangeal	3, 5
intra-	within, inside	**ihn**-trah	intracellular, intracranial	3, 5
ipsi-	same, self	**ihp**-sē	ipsilateral	6
kilo-	one thousand	**kihl**-ō	kilosecond	6
macro-	large, enlarged	**mahck**-rō	macrobiotic	8
mal-	diseased, bad, abnormal, defective	mahl	malformation, malodorous	5, 10
mega-	large or enlarged	**mehg**-ah	megagnathia	7
meta-	beyond, after, next	**meht**-ah	metastasis, metaplasm	3, 5
meta- + carp/o	metacarpal bones	**meht**-ah-**kahr**-pō	metacarpectomy	5
meta- + tars/o	metatarsal bones	**meht**-ah-**tahr**-sō	metatarsophalangeal	5
micro-	one-millionth or small, very small	**mī**-krō	microcurie, microbiologist, microscope	6
milli-	one-thousandth	**mihl**-ih	milligram	6
mono-	one, single	**mohn**-ō	mononeuropathy	6
multi-	much or many	**muhl**-tī	multiarticular	6
nano-	one-billionth or extremely small	**nah**-nō	nanosecond, nanocranous	6
neo-	new	**nē**-ō	neogenic	2
noci-	injury, pain, harm	**nō**-sē	nociperception	12
nulli-	none, zero	**nuhl**-lih	nulliparous	15
omni-	all, every	**ohm**-nē	omnivision	10
pachy-	thick	**pahck**-ē	pachyderma, pachydermia	4, 5
pan-	all	pahn	panosteitis	6
par-	other than, abnormal, giving birth to a live fetus	pehr	paresthesia, uniparous	6, 15
para-	near, beside, abnormal, apart from	**pehr**-ah	parabiosis, paranuclear	4, 6
peri-	around, surrounding	**pehr**-ih	endoperiarthritis, periosteotomy	3, 5
pico-	one-trillionth	**pī**-cō	picoliter	6
poly-	much or many	**pohl**-ē	polyarthritis, polypathia	2, 6
post-	after, behind, later	pōst	postinfection	5
pre-	before (in time and place)	prē	prefix	10
pro-	before, anterior, in front of	prō	prognosis	2, 5
quadri-	four	**kwohd**-rih	quadrilateral	6
re-	again, back	rē	respirator, review	9
rubri-	red	**rū**-brih	rubricyte	8
semi-	half, partial	**seh**-mē	semiconscious	6
sub-	below, decrease, under	suhb	subdorsal	3
super-	above, over, exceeding the norm, implying excess	**soo**-pər	superman	3
supra-	above, over, on top of	**soo**-prah	supracranial	3
syn-	together, joined	sihn	synchondrosis, synergic muscles	5, 6

Continued

Word Part	Definition of Word Part	Pronunciation	Example Word	Chapter
tachy-	fast	**tahck**-ē	tachyrhythmia	7
tact-	touch	tahckt	tactile agnosis	12
tetra-	four	**teht**-rah	tetradactyly	6
trans-	across, through	trahnz	transillumination	3
tri-	three	trī	triphalangia	6
tub-	pipe	toob	tubule	14
ultra-	beyond, excess, on the other side of	**uhl**-trah	ultrasound	3
uni-	one, single	**ū**-nah	unicellular	6
Suffixes				
-a	structure, thing	ah	aquaria	2
-ac	pertaining to	ahck	cardiac	2
-al	pertaining to	ahl	thermal	2
-algia	pain	**ahl**-jē-ah	analgia	5
-ant	a person or a thing that does something specified	ahnt	assistant	2
-ar	pertaining to	ahr	binocular	2
-ase	enzyme	ās	lipase	10
-ate	to do, to cause, to act upon	āt	medicate	2
-ation	state, condition, action, process, or result	**ā**-shun	retardation	2
-blast	bud, seed, formative cell	blahst	osteoblast, hematoblast	5, 8
-cele	protrusion, hernia	sēl	tracheoaerocele	10
-centesis	surgical puncture	sehn-**tē**-sihs	abdominocentesis, pericardiocentesis	4, 7
-clast	to break	klahst	osteoclast, chondroclast	5, 8
-cyesis	pregnancy	sī-**ē**-sihs	pseudocyesis	15
-cyte	cell	sīt	chondrocyte, osteocyte, plasmocyte	3, 5, 8
-dynia	pain	**dihn**-ē-ah	ischiodynia, craniodynia	5
-ectasis	expansion, dilation, distention	**ehck**-tah-sihs	cardiectasis	9
-ectomy	surgical removal	**ehck**-tō-mē	hysterectomy, onychectomy	2, 4
-emia	blood condition (usually abnormal)	**ē**-mē-ah	hydremia, anemia	7, 8
-esis	process of an action	**ē**-sihs	morphogenesis	8
-esthesia	feeling, experience, sensation	ehs-**thē**-zē-ah	anesthesia	12
-genesis	formation or beginning	**jehn**-eh-sihs	pathogenesis	5
-gnosis	knowledge	**nō**-sihs	diagnosis	2
-gram	written record produced, something recorded or written	grahm	myogram, arthrogram	4, 6
-graph	instrument used to write or record	grahf	myograph, polygraph	4, 6
-graphy	method of recording	**grahf**-ē	myography, autobiography	4, 6
-ia	pertaining to	**ē**-ah	hypothermia	2
-iasis	pathological condition that results from	**ī**-ah-sihs	lithiasis	10
-ic	pertaining to	ihck	microscopic	2
-ide	pertaining to	īd	carbon dioxide	2
-ile	capable of, pertaining to	īl	infantile	12
-ion	state, condition, action, process, or result	shun	vision	2
-is	structure, thing	ihs	analysis	2
-ism	state, condition, action, process, or result	ihsm	dwarfism	2

Word Part	Definition of Word Part	Pronunciation	Example Word	Chapter
-ist	a person or a thing that does something specified	ihst	pathologist	2
-itis	inflammation	ī-tihs	arthritis	2
-ity	capable of, pertaining to	ih-tē	abnormality	12
-ium	structure, thing	ē-uhm	bacterium	2
-ive	pertaining to	ihv	positive	2
-ize	to engage in a specific activity, to become like, to treat	īz	crystallize	2
-lith	stone	lihth	cholelith	10
-logy	to study, or to have knowledge of	lō-jē	chondrology	2
-lytic	destruction, dissolution, dissolving, breakage	liht-ihck	cellulolytic	8
-meter	measure, a device to measure	mē-tər	cytometer	6
-oid	resembling	oyd	osteoid, myoid	2, 6
-ole	indicating something small	ohl	ovariole	2
-oma	a tumor or abnormal new growth, a swelling	ō-mah	osteoma, multiple myeloma	2, 5
-or	a person or a thing that does something specified	ohr	injector	2
-orexia	appetite, desire	ō-rehck-sē-ah	anorexia	10
-ory	pertaining to	ohr-ē	inflammatory	2
-ose	made up of, characterized by	ōs	cellulose	2
-osis	condition, process, or action; disease or abnormal condition	ō-sihs	osteochondrosis	2
-ous	pertaining to	uhs	enormous	2
-paresis	partial paralysis, weakness	pah-rē-sihs	hemiparesis	6
-pathy	disease	pahth-ē	arthropathy, myopathy	2, 6
-penia	lack, deficiency	pē-nē-ah	leukopenia	8
-pexy	surgical fixation, stabilization	pehck-sē	hysteropexy	4
-philia	loving, or more than normal	fihl-ē-ah	thermophilia, hematophilia	7, 8
-phobia	intense or abnormal fear	fō-bē-ah	hydrophobia, hippopotomonstroses-quipedaliophobia	7, 8
-phyte	pathological growth.	fīte	chondrophyte, dermatophyte	2, 4
-plasm	formed material (as of a cell or tissue)	plahzm	neoplasm, cytoplasm, neoplasm	2, 5, 8
-plasty	surgical repair	plahs-tē	epidermatoplasty	4
-plegia	paralysis	plē-jē-ah	myoplegia	6
-pnea	breath or respiration	pah-nē-ah	apnea	9
-poiesis	making, producing	poy-ē-sihs	hematopoiesis	8
-ptosis	downward placement, drooping or sagging	pah-tō-sihs	enteroptosis, nephroptosis	10, 14
-ptysis	spitting	pah-tuh-sis	hemoptysis	10
-rrhage	excessive flow	rihdj	hemorrhage	7
-rrhaphy	suture	rahf-ē	dermorrhaphy	4
-rrhea	flow, flowing	rē-ah	diarrhea	10
-rrhexis	to break, rupture	rehx-sihs	arteriorrhexis	7
-sarcoma	a malignant neoplasm arising in bone, cartilage, or striated muscle that spreads into neighboring tissue or by way of the bloodstream	sahr-kō-mah	chondrosarcoma	2

Continued

Word Part	Definition of Word Part	Pronunciation	Example Word	Chapter
-scope	instrument for examining or viewing	skōp	endoarthroscope	4
-sion	state, condition, action, process, or result	shuhn	exclusion	2
-sis	state, condition, action, process, or result	sihs	thesis	2
-stasis	stopping, slowing, or a stable state	**stā**-sihs	diastasis, venostasis, arteriostasis	2, 7
-staxis	bleeding	**stahck**-sihs	epistaxis	9
-stomy	surgical creation of a new permanent opening	**stō**-mē	hysterosalpingostomy	4
-(t)ic	pertaining to	tihck *or* ihck	asthmatic	2
-tion	state, condition, action, process, or result	shuhn	absorption	2
-tomy	surgical incision	**tō**-mē	craniotomy	4
-tripsy	crushing, grinding	**trihp**-sē	lithotripsy	14
-trophy	growth	**trō**-phē	hypertrophy, amyotrophy	6, 13
-ule	indicating something small	ūhl	glandule	2
-um	structure, thing	uhm	aquarium	2
-uria	urine	**uhr**-rē-ah	dysuria	14
-vore	eat, devour, swallow	vohr	omnivore	10
-y	made up of, characterized by	ē	fruity	2

Combining Forms, Prefixes, and Suffixes Alphabetized According to Definition

Definition of Word Part	Word Part	Pronunciation	Example Word	Chapter
abdomen	abdomin/o	ahb-**dah**-mehn-ō	abdominohysteric	3
above, over, exceeding the norm, implying excess	super-	**soo**-pər	superman	3
above, over, on top of	supra-	**soo**-prah	supracranial	3
above, over, or excess	hyper-	**hī**-pər	hyperplasia	3
across, through	dia-	**dī**-ah	diadermic	5
across, through	trans-	trahnz	transillumination	3
adrenal gland	adren/o	ahd-**rē**-nō	adrenomegaly	13
affinity to, turn to, respond to a stimulus	trop/o	**trō**-pō	aerotropism	13
after, behind, later	post-	pōst	postinfection	5
again, back	re-	rē	respirator, review	9
against, contrary, opposing	contra-	**kohn**-trah	contralateral	6
against, opposed to	anti-	**ahn**-tē	anticoagulant	8
air, and sometimes the lung	pneum/o	**nū**-mō	pneumothorax, pneumocentesis	9
air, gas	aer/o	**ehr**-rō	aerobic	9
albumin	albumin/o	ahl-**bū**-mihn-ō	albuminuria	14
all	pan-	pahn	panosteitis	6
all, every	omni-	**ohm**-nē	omnivision	10
alveolus	alveol/o	ahl-**vē**-ō-lō	alveolar dysplasia	9
animal, living being	zo/o	zō-oh	zoology	15
animal, wild beast	theri/o	**thēr**-ē-ō	theriogenology	15
anus	an/o	**ā**-nō	anospasm	10
aorta	aort/o	ā-**ohr**-tō	aortectomy	7
apart, away from, separation	dis-	dihs	disease	7
appetite, desire	-orexia	ō-**rehck**-sē-ah	anorexia	10
around	circum-	**sehr**-kuhm	circumflex	4
around, surrounding	peri-	**pehr**-ih	endoperiarthritis, periosteotomy	3, 5
artery	arteri/o	ahr-**tehr**-ē-ō	arteriospasm	7
artery	arter/o	ahr-**tehr**-ō	panarteritis	7
atrium (upper chamber of the heart)	atri/o	**ā**-trē-ō	atriotomy	7
auricle of the heart, or the ear flap	auricul/o	aw-**rihck**-ū-lō	auricular hyperplasia, auricular mange	7
away from	ab-	ahb	abnormal, abductor muscles	5, 6
back or top	dors/o	**dohr**-sō	dorsal, dorsum	3
back surface of the forelimb distal to the carpus	palm/o	**pahl**-mō	palmar	3

Continued

Definition of Word Part	Word Part	Pronunciation	Example Word	Chapter
back surface of the forelimb distal to the carpus	palmar/o	pahl-**mahr**-ō	palmarodorsal	3
back surface of the rear limb distal to the tarsus	plant/o	**plahn**-tō	plantar	3
back surface of the rear limb distal to the tarsus	plantar/o	plahn-**tahr**-ō	plantarodorsal	3
bacteria	bacteri/o	bachk-**tehr**-ē-ō	bacterium	14
bad, defective, painful, or difficult	dys-	dihs	dysplasia	2
before (in time and place)	pre-	prē	prefix	10
before, anterior, in front of	pro-	prō	prognosis	2, 5
before, in front of, prior to	ante-	**ahn**-tē	antebrachium, anterior, antechamber	5, 8
belly	ventr/o	**vehn**-trō	dorsoventral	3
below, beneath	infra-	**ihn**-frah	infraspinous	3
below, decrease, under	sub-	suhb	subdorsal	3
between, among	inter-	**ihn**-tər	interchondral, intercostal, interphalangeal	3, 5
beyond, after, next	meta-	**meht**-ah	metastasis, metaplasm	3, 5
beyond, excess, on the other side of	ultra-	**uhl**-trah	ultrasound	3
bile, gall	chol/e	**kō**-lē	cholangitis	10
bilirubin	bilirubin/o	**bihl**-ē-**roo**-bihn-ō	bilirubinuria	14
black	melan/o	**mehl**-ah-nō	melanocyte, melanoma	4, 5
bladder, a sac containing fluid	cyst/o	**sihs**-tō	cystitis	14
bleeding	-staxis	**stahck**-sihs	epistaxis	9
blister, small sac	vesicul/o	veh-**sihk**-ū-lō	vesiculectomy	4
blood	sanguin/o	**sahng**-gwihn-ō	exsanguination	8
blood	hemat/o	hē-**mah**-tō	hematothorax, hematogenous, hematology	3, 5, 8
blood	hem/o	**hē**-mō	hemostasis, electrohemostasis	3, 8
blood condition (usually abnormal)	-emia	**ē**-mē-ah	hydremia, anemia	7, 8
blood vessel	vascul/o	**vahsk**-yoo-lō	cardiovascular	7
blue	cyan/o	**sī**-ahn-ō	hypercyanosis	5
body	corp/o	**kohr**-pō	corpus	11
body	somat/o	**sō**-mah-tō	somatology	2
bone	os	ohs	os penis, os cordis, os rostri	5
bone	osse/o	**ohs**-ē-ō	osseous tissues	5
bone	oss/o	**ohs**-sō	ossicle	12
bone	oste/o	**ohs**-tē-ō	osteochondritis, osteoliposarcoma, osteoarthritis	2, 3, 5
bone marrow	myel/o	mī-**eh**-lō	periosteomyelitis	5
bone marrow or spinal cord	myel/o	mī-**eh**-lō	myelitis, neuromyelitis	5, 11
both, on both sides	ambi-	**ahm**-bē	ambidextrous	5
both, on both sides	amphi-	**ahm**-fih	amphicranitis	5
brachium	brachi/o	**brā**-kē-ō	cervicobrachial	5
brain	cerebr/o	sehr-**ē**-brō	cerebroatrophy	11
brain	encephal/o	ehn-**sehf**-ah-lō	electroencephalograph	11

Definition of Word Part	Word Part	Pronunciation	Example Word	Chapter
break into pieces	-clast	klahst	osteoclast, chondroclast	5, 8
break into pieces	clast/o	**klahs**-tō	karyoclastic	8
break, rupture	-rrhexis	**rehx**-sihs	arteriorrhexis	7
breath or respiration	-pnea	pah-**nē**-ah	apnea	9
breath or respiration	pne/o	**nē**-ō *or* pah-**nē**-ō	pneopneic	9
breathing	hal/o	**hah**-lō	exhalation, inhalant	9
breathing	spirat/o	**spī**-rah-tō	inspiration	9
breathing or coil or spiral	spir/o	**spī**-rō	spirograph	9
bronchus	bronch/o	**brohng**-kō	bronchospasm	9
bud, germinal, seed, formative cell	-blast	blahst	osteoblast, hematoblast	5, 8
capable of, pertaining to	-ity	**ih**-tē	abnormality	12
capable of, pertaining to	-ile	īl	infantile	12
carbon dioxide	capn/o	**kahp**-nō	hypercapnia	9
carpus	carp/o	**karh**-pō	intercarpal	5
carry, produce	gest/o	**jehs**-tō	gestation	15
cartilage	chondr/o	**kohn**-drō	osteochondritis, chondrectomy	2, 3
cause	eti/o	**ē**-tē-ō	etiopathology	2
cecum	cec/o	**sē**-cō	cecorrhaphy	10
cell	cellul/o	**sehl**-yoo-lō	cellulitis	3
cell	-cyte	sīt	chondrocyte, osteocyte, plasmocyte	3, 5, 8
cell	cyt/o	**sī**-tō	chondrocytosis, polycythemia	3, 8
cheek	bucc/o	**būk**-ō	buccal	10
chemically basic	baso-	**bā**-sō	basophil	8
chest	steth/o	**stehth**-ō	stethoscope	7
chyle	chyl/o	**kī**-lō	chylorrhea	10
claw, nail	onych/o	**ohn**-ih-kō	onychectomy	4
clotting process	coagul/o	kō-**ahg**-ū-lō	coagulation	8
colon	col/o	**kō**-lō	colocentesis	10
colon	colon/o	**kō**-lohn-ō	colonoscopy	10
color	chrom/o	**krō**-mō	achromodermic	5
coming together; to fasten together; sexual intercourse	coit/o	**kō**-ih-tō	coitophobia	15
coming together; to fasten together; sexual intercourse	copul/o	**kohp**-ū-lō	copulation	15
common bile duct	choledoch/o	**kō**-lē-dō-kō	choledochohepatostomy	10
cornea	corne/o	**kohr**-nē-ō	corneitis	12
cornea or hard, horn-like tissue	kerat/o	**kehr**-ah-tō	keratitis	12
cough	tuss/o	**tuhs**-sō	tussiculation, antitussive	9
crown	coron/o	**kohr**-ō-nō	coronary	7
crushing, grinding	-tripsy	**trihp**-sē	lithotripsy	14
death	necr/o	**neh**-krō	necrobiosis, avascular necrosis	4, 7
destruction, dissolution, dissolving, breakage	-lytic	**liht**-ihck	cellulolytic	8
destruction, dissolution, dissolving, breakage	lys/o	**lī**-sō	rhabdomyolysis, hemolysis	6, 8

Continued

Definition of Word Part	Word Part	Pronunciation	Example Word	Chapter
different, other, unlike	heter/o	**heht**-tər-ō	heterophil	8
digestion	peps/o	**pehp**-sō	apepsia	10
digestion	pept/o	**pehp**-tō	bradypeptic	10
digit or toe or finger	digit/o	**dihg**-iht-ō	interdigital	5
digit or toe or finger	dactyl/o	**dahk**-tihl-ō	polydactyly	5
disease	-pathy	**pahth**-ē	arthropathy, myopathy	2, 6
disease	path/o	**pahth**-ō	chondropathology, myopathologist	2, 6
disease or abnormal condition; condition, process, or action	-osis	**ō**-sihs	osteochondrosis	2
diseased, bad, abnormal, defective	mal-	mahl	malformation, malodorous	5, 10
do, to cause, to act upon	-ate	āt	medicate	2
down, reverse, backward, degenerative	cata-	**kaht**-ah	catabiosis	6
downward placement, drooping	-ptosis	pah-**tō**-sihs	enteroptosis, nephroptosis	10, 14
dry	xer/o	**zē**-rō	xeroderma	4
duodenum	duoden/o	**doo**-ō-də-nō	esophagoduodenostomy	10
ear	ot/o	ō-**tō**	otorhinolaryngology	12
eardrum	myring/o	**mihr**-ihng-ō	myringectomy	12
eardrum	tympan/o	**tihm**-puh-nō	tympanocentesis	12
eat	phag/o	**fā**-gō	dysphagia, hyperphagia	8, 10
eat, devour, swallow	-vore	vohr	omnivore	10
eject, discharge, to throw out	ejacul/o	ē-**jahck**-yoo-lō	ejaculation	15
electricity	electr/o	ē-**lehck**-trō	electromyography, electrocardiograph	6, 7
embryo	embry/o	**ehm**-brē-ō	embryectomy	15
empty, emptiness	vacu/o	**vahck**-ū-ō	vacuole	8
engage in a specific activity, to become like, to treat	-ize	īz	crystallize	2
entrance, cavity, or channel that is an entrance to another cavity	vestibul/o	veh-**stihb**-ū-lō	vestibular	9
enzyme	-ase	ās	lipase	10
epididymis	epididym/o	ehp-ih-**dihd**-ih-mō	epididymoplasty	15
equal	is/o	**ī**-sō	anisocytosis	8
esophagus	esophag/o	ē-**sohf**-ah-gō	esophagoplegia	10
examine, view	scop/o	**skō**-pō	necroscopy	4
excessive flow	-rrhage	rihdj	hemorrhage	7
expansion, dilation, distention	-ectasis	**ehck**-tah-sihs	cardiectasis	9
eye	ocul/o	**ohk**-ū-lō	oculocutaneous	12
eye	ophthalm/o	**ohf**-thahl-mō	ophthalmologist	12
eye	opt/o	**ohp**-tō	optometrist	12
eyelid	blephar/o	**blehf**-ər-ō	blepharospasm	12
eyelid	palpebr/o	**pahl**-peh-brō	palpebration	12
false, deception	pseud/o	**soo**-dō	pseudoarthrosis, pseudoanorexia	13, 15
fast	tachy-	**tahck**-ē	tachyrhythmia	7
fat	adip/o	**ahd**-ih-pō	adipocyte, adipose	3, 4
fat	lip/o	**lī**-pō	lipectomy, lipoma, lipolysis	3, 4, 10

Definition of Word Part	Word Part	Pronunciation	Example Word	Chapter
fat	steat/o	stē-**aht**-ō	steatorrhea	10
feces	copr/o	**kohp**-rō	coprophagia	10
feeling, experience, sensation	-esthesia	ehs-**thē**-zē-ah	anesthesia	12
feeling, experience, sensation	esthesi/o	ehs-**thē**-zē-ō	esthesiogenesis	12
femur	femor/o	**fehm**-ohr-ō	pubofemoral	5
fiber	fibr/o	**fīb**-rō	myofibrosis, deacutaneous fibrolysis	6, 8
fibrin	fibrin/o	**fī**-brihn-ō	fibrinolysis	8
fibula	fibul/o	**fihb**-yoo-lō	tibiofibular	5
first	prim/i	**prī**-mah	primary	15
flank, loin	lapar/o	**lahp**-ah-rō	laparosplenotomy	10
flesh	sarc/o	**sahr**-kō	rhabdomyosarcoma	6
flesh, meat	carni-	**kahr**-nē	carnivore	10
flow, flowing	-rrhea	**rē**-ah	diarrhea	10
follicle	follicul/o	fohl-**lihck**-kuhl-ō	folliculitis	4
food	aliment/o	ahl-ih-**mehn**-tō	alimentary canal	10
foot	pod/o	**pō**-dō	pododerm	5
force, energy	dynam/o	**dī**-nah-mō	dynamoscope, dynamogenesis	6, 9
formation or beginning	-genesis	**jehn**-eh-sihs	pathogenesis	5
formation or beginning	gen/o	**jehn**-ō	pathogenic	2
formed material (as of a cell or tissue)	-plasm	plahzm	neoplasm, cytoplasm	2, 5, 8
four	quadri-	**kwohd**-rih	quadrilateral	6
four	tetra-	**teht**-rah	tetradactyly	6
freezing, icy-cold	cry/o	**krī**-ō	cryotherapy	6
front or before	anter/o	ahn-**tər**-ō	anterior	3
giving birth to a live fetus	para	**pehr**-ah	bipara	15
giving birth to a live fetus	parturi/o	**pahr**-tuhr-ē-ō	parturiometer	15
giving birth to a live fetus	partum	**pahr**-tuhm	postpartum	15
giving birth to a live fetus	par-	pehr	uniparous	15
gland	aden/o	**ahd**-ehn-ō	adenopathy	13
glottis	glott/o	**gloh**-tō	glottitis	9
glucose	gluc/o	**gloo**-cō	cytoglucopenia	10
glue, glial cells	gli/o	**glē**-ō	glioma	11
good, well, normal	eu-	ū	eupepsia	12
granule, small grain	granul/o	**grahn**-ū-lō	agranulocyte	8
gray	poli/o	**pohl**-ē-ō	poliomyelitis	11
green	chlor/o	**klohr**-ō	chlorosis	5
growth	-trophy	**trō**-phē	hypertrophy, amyotrophy	6, 13
growth, development, or formation	plas/o	**plā**-zō	hypoplasia, osteochondroplasia, erythroplasia, plasmodysplasia	2, 5, 6, 8
gums, gingiva	gingiv/o	**jihn**-jih-vō	gingivostomatitis	10
hair	trich/o	**trī**-kō	melanotrichia	4
hair	pil/o	**pī**-lō	piloerection	4
half, partial	hemi-	**hehm**-ih	hemialgia	6

Continued

Definition of Word Part	Word Part	Pronunciation	Example Word	Chapter
half, partial	semi-	**seh**-mē	semiconscious	6
hard	scler/o	**sklehr**-ō	arteriosclerosis	7
hard, horn-like tissue	kerat/o	**kehr**-ah-tō	keratodermia	4
head, origin of a muscle	cep	sehp	biceps	6
head, skull	cephal/o	**seh**-fahl-ō	cephalocaudal	6
head, skull	crani/o	**krā**-nē-ō	craniology, cranium, craniectomy, cranioplasty	3, 5
hearing, listening	acous/o	ah-**koo**-sō	acoustics	12
heart	cardi/o	**kahr**-dē-ō	cardiomyopathy, acardia	6, 7
heat	therm/o	**thər**-mō	catathermal	6
heat, high temperature	pyrex/o	pī-**rehx**-ō	pyrexia	6
heat, high temperature	pyr/o	**pī**-rō	pyrogen	6
height, altitude	hyps/o	**hihps**-ō	hypsography	10
hernia	herni/o	**hər**-nē-ō	herniorrhaphy	10
hidden	crypt/o	**krihp**-tō	cryptorchidism	15
hip	cox/o	**kohx**-ō	coxofemoral	5
horn or structure that looks like a horn	cornu/o	**kohr**-nū-ō	cornual nerve block	4
humerus	humer/o	**hū**-mər-ō	scapulohumeral	5
ileum	ile/o	**ihl**-ē-ō	ileostomy, ileopathy	5, 10
ilium	ili/o	**ihl**-ē-ō	iliocostal	5
immunity, immune	immun/o	ihm-**yoo**-nō	immunocyte	8
in, into, inward	em-	ehm	emphysema, embolus	11
in, into, inward	en-	ehn	enchrondroma	11
in, within, inward, into	in-	ihn	inside, inbreeding	3
incomplete, imperfect	atel/o	aht-**ehl**-ō	atelectasis	9
inflammation	-itis	**ī**-tihs	arthritis	2
injury, pain, harm	noci-	**nō**-sē	nociperception	12
instrument for examining or viewing	-scope	skōp	endoarthroscope	4
instrument used to write or record	-graph	grahf	myograph, polygraph	4, 6
intense or abnormal fear	-phobia	**fō**-bē-ah	hydrophobia, hippopotomonstroses-quipedaliophobia	7, 8
intestines in general	enter/o	**ehn**-tehr-ō	enterokinesia	10
iris	irid/o	ihr-ih-**dō**	iridocele	12
ischium	ischi/o	**ihs**-kē-ō	ischiococcygeal	5
jaw	gnath/o	**gnahth**-ō	prognathism	5
jejunum	jejun/o	jeh-**joo**-nō	esophagojejunoplasty	10
joint	arthr/o	**arth**-rō	arthropathy, arthrodysplasia	2, 5
joint	articul/o	ahr-**tihck**-yoo-lō	articular	5
ketone bodies	keton/o	**kē**-tōn-ō	ketonuria	14
ketone bodies	ket/o	**kē**-tō	ketosis	14
kidney	nephr/o	**nehf**-rō	nephroblastoma	14
kidney	ren/o	**rē**-nō	renogram	14
kidney pelvis	pyel/o	**pī**-eh-lō	pyeloplasty	14
knot	nod/o	**nohd**-ō	nodule	4

Definition of Word Part	Word Part	Pronunciation	Example Word	Chapter
knowledge	-gnosis	**nō**-sihs	diagnosis	2
lack, deficiency	-penia	**pē**-nē-ah	leukopenia	8
large or enlarged	megal/o	**mehg**-ah-lō	cardiomegaly	7
large or enlarged	mega-	**mehg**-ah	megagnathia	7
large, enlarged	macro-	**mahck**-rō	macrobiotic	8
larynx, voice box	laryng/o	lah-**rihng**-gō	laryngospasm	9
left	sinistr/o	sihn-**ihs**-trō	sinistrodextral	3
life	bi/o	**bī**-ō	endobiosis, biology	4, 6
lip	cheil/o	**kī**-lō	cheilophagia	10
lip	labi/o	**lā**-bē-ō	labionasal	10
little, few, small	olig/o	**ohl**-ih-gō	oligodendroglia	11
liver	hepat/o	heh-**paht**-ō	hepatocyte	10
loin	lumb/o	**luhm**-bō	lumbocostal	5
loving, or more than normal	phil/o	**fihl**-ō	ergophilous, hydrophilic	7, 8
loving, or more than normal	-philia	**fihl**-ē-ah	thermophilia, hematophilia	7, 8
lung	pneumon/o	**nū**-mohn-ō	pneumonoultramicroscopic-silicovolcanoconiosis	9
lung	pulmon/o	**puhl**-mohn-ō	pulmonologist	7
lymph	lymph/o	**lihm**-fō	lymphangitis	8
made up of, characterized by	-ose	ōs	cellulose	2
made up of, characterized by	-y	ē	fruity	2
make grow, to produce	physi/o	**fihz**-ē-ō	physiology	5
making, producing	-poiesis	poy-**ē**-sihs	hematopoiesis	8
male, masculine	andr/o	**ahn**-drō	androgen	13
malignant neoplasm arising in bone, cartilage, or striated muscle that spreads into neighboring tissue or by way of the bloodstream	-sarcoma	**sahr-kō**-mah	chondrosarcoma	2
mammary gland; breast	mamm/o	**mahm**-mō	mammogram	15
mammary gland; breast	mast/o	**mahs**-tō	mastopathy	15
mandible (lower jaw bone)	mandibul/o	mahn-**dihb**-ū-lō	mandibulectomy	5
maxilla (upper jaw of skull)	maxill/o	mahck-**sih**-lō	maxillotomy	5
meal	prandi/o	**prahn**-dē-ō	postprandial	10
measure	metr/o	**meh**-trō	metric system	6
measure, a device to measure	-meter	**mē**-tər	cytometer	6
mediastinum; space between the two lungs that contains all the thoracic viscera except the lungs	mediastin/o	mē-dē-ah-**stī**-nō	mediastinoscopy	9
meninges	mening/o	meh-**nihng**-ō	meningocele	11
metacarpal bones	meta- + carp/o	**meht**-ah-**kahr**-pō	metacarpectomy	5
metatarsal bones	meta- + tars/o	**meht**-ah-**tahr**-sō	metatarsophalangeal	5
method of recording	-graphy	**grahf**-ē	myography, autobiography	4, 6
middle	medi/o	**mē**-dē-ō	mediolateral	3

Continued

Definition of Word Part	Word Part	Pronunciation	Example Word	Chapter
middle	mesi/o	**mēs**-ē-ō	mesial	3
middle	mes/o	**mēs**-ō	mesoappendix	3
mouth	stom/o	**stō**-mō	anastomosis	10
mouth	or/o	**ohr**-ō	oral	10
mouth	stomat/o	stō-**mah**-tō	stomatomalacia	10
movement	kinesi/o	kih-**nē**-sē-ō	kinesiology	6
much or many	multi-	**muhl**-tī	multiarticular	6
much or many	poly-	**pohl**-ē	polyarthritis, polypathia	2, 6
mucus (noun) or mucous (adjective)	muc/o	**myoo**-kō	mucogenesis, mucous cell	9
muscle	muscul/o	**muhs**-kyoo-lō	cervicomuscular	6
muscle	my/o	**mī**-ō	myodysplasia, myopathology, cardiomyopathy	3, 6, 7
narrow	sten/o	**stehn**-ō	arteriostenosis	7
near, beside, abnormal, apart from	para-	**pahr**-ah	parabiosis, paranuclear	4, 6
nearest	proxim/o	**prohck**-sih-mō	proximal	3
neck; cervix (neck of the uterus)	cervic/o	**sihr**-vih-cō	cervicodorsal, cervicoplasty	5, 15
nerve, nervous system	neur/o	**nər**-ō	neuritis, neuropathy	3, 11
neutral	neutr/o	**nū**-trō	neutrophil	8
new	neo-	**nē**-ō	neogenic	2
nitrogen	azot/o	**āz**-oht-ō	azotemia	14
no color	albin/o	ahl-**bī**-nō	albinism	5
none, zero	nulli-	**nuhl**-lih	nulliparous	15
normal	norm/o	**nohr**-mō	normocytic	8
nose	nas/o	**nā**-zō	nasology	9
nose	rhin/o	**rī**-nō	rhinoplasty, rhinitis	9, 12
nose	rostr/o	**rohs**-trō	rostral	3
not	in-	ihn	inappropriate, inapt	3
nucleus	kary/o	**kehr**-ē-ō	karyogenic, karyorrhexis	3, 8
oil, sebum	sebac/o	seh-**bā**-shō	pilosebaceous	4
oil, sebum	seb/o	**seh**-bō *or* **sē**-bō	sebum	4
omasum	omas/o	ō-**mā**-sō	omasal stenosis	10
omentum	oment/o	ō-**mehn**-tō	omentopexy	10
on or upon	epi-	**ehp**-ih	epidermis, epibiosis	3, 5
one thousand	kilo-	**kihl**-ō	kilosecond	6
one-billionth or extremely small	nano-	**nah**-nō	nanosecond, nanocranous	6
one-hundredth, or one hundred	centi-	**sehnt**-ah	centimeter	6
one-millionth or small, very small	micro-	**mī**-krō	microcurie, microbiologist, microscope	6
one-tenth	deci-	**deh**-sih	decibel	6
one-thousandth	milli-	**mihl**-ih	milligram	6
one-trillionth	pico-	**pī**-cō	picoliter	6
one, single	mono-	**mohn**-ō	mononeuropathy	6
one, single	uni-	**ū**-nah	unicellular	6
orange-yellow	cirrh/o	**sihr**-ō	cirrhosis	5
order, coordinated movement	tax/o	**tahck**-sō	ataxia	11

Definition of Word Part	Word Part	Pronunciation	Example Word	Chapter
organ	organ/o	ohr-**gahn**-ō	organectomy	3
other than, abnormal	par-	pahr	paresthesia	6
out, outside, outer, away from	exo-	**ehcks**-ō	exogenous, exoskeleton	3, 5
out, outside, outer, away from	ex-	ehcks	exostosis, excise	3, 5
outside	extra-	**ehcks**-trah	extracellular	3
outside, external	ecto-	**ehct**-tō	ectodermatosis	3
outside, external	ect-	ehct	ectosteal	3
ovary	oophor/o	ō-**ohff**-ohr-ō	hysterosalpingo-oophorectomy, oophorrhagia	2, 15
ovary	ovari/o	ō-**vahr**-ē-ō	ovariohysterectomy, ovariectomy	2, 15
oviduct	salping/o	sahl-**ping**-ō	hysterosalpingo-oophorectomy	2
ovum, egg	o/o	**ō**-ō	oocyte	15
ovum, egg	ovul/o	**ōhv**-yoo-lō	ovulation	15
ovum, egg	ov/o	**ō**-vō	ovum	15
oxygen	ox/o	**ohck**-sō	hypoxia	9
pain	-algia	**ahl**-jē-ah	analgia	5
pain	-dynia	**dihn**-ē-ah	ischiodynia, craniodynia	5
palate, roof of mouth	palat/o	**pahl**-ah-tō	palatorrhaphy	10
pancreas	pancreat/o	**pahn**-krē-aht-ō	pancreatitis	10
pancreas	pancre/o	**pahn**-krē-ō	pancreopathy	10
paralysis	-plegia	**plē**-jē-ah	myoplegia	6
partial paralysis, weakness	-paresis	pah-**rē**-sihs	hemiparesis	6
patella	patell/o	pah-**tehl**-ō	patellectomy	5
pathological condition that results from	-iasis	**ī**-ah-sihs	lithiasis	10
pathological growth	-phyte	fīte	chondrophyte, dermatophyte	2, 4
pelvis	pelvi/o	**pehl**-vē-ō	pelvioplasty	5
pelvis	pelv/i	**pehl**-vī	pelviscope	5
penis	pen/i	**pē**-nih	penectomy	15
penis	priap/o	**prī**-ah-pō	priapitis	15
person or thing that does something specified	-or	ohr	injector	2
person or thing that does something specified	-ist	ihst	pathologist	2
person or thing that does something specified	-ant	ahnt	assistant	2
pertaining to	-(t)ic	tihck *or* ihck	asthmatic	2
pertaining to	-ar	ahr	binocular	2
pertaining to	-ide	īd	carbon dioxide	2
pertaining to	-ac	ahck	cardiac	2
pertaining to	-ous	uhs	enormous	2
pertaining to	-ia	**ē**-ah	hypothermia	2
pertaining to	-ory	**ohr**-ē	inflammatory	2
pertaining to	-ic	ihck	microscopic	2
pertaining to	-ive	ihv	positive	2
pertaining to	-al	ahl	thermal	2
phalanges	phalang/o	fah-**lahn**-jō	metacarpophalangeal	5

Continued

Definition of Word Part	Word Part	Pronunciation	Example Word	Chapter
pharynx, throat	pharyng/o	fah-**rihng**-gō	pharyngostomy	9
physician, medicine	iatr/o	**ī**-aht-rō	iatrogenic	9
pimple, solid lesion <1 cm	papul/o	**pahp**-yool-ō	papular	4
pipe	tub-	toob	tubule	14
plant, green crop	herbi-	**hərb**-ih	herbivore	10
plasma or related to plasma	plasm/o	**plahz**-mō	plasmocytoma, plasmodysplasia	8
pleura, thin membrane with two layers that lines the lungs and the chest cavity	pleur/o	**ploor**-ō	pleuritis, pleurisy	9
pore, small opening, or cavity	por/o	**pohr**-ō	osteoporous	5
potassium, kalium	kali/o	**kā**-lē-ō	kaliopenia	14
pregnancy	pregn/o	**prehg**-nō	pregnant	15
pregnancy	-cyesis	sī-**ē**-sihs	pseudocyesis	15
pregnant female	gravida	**grahv**-ihd-ah	primigravida	15
pressure, tension	ton/o	**tō**-nō	myotonia	6
process of an action	-esis	**ē**-sihs	morphogenesis	8
protrusion, hernia	-cele	sēl	tracheoaerocele	10
pubis	pub/o	**pehw**-bō	pubocaudal muscles	5
pupil of the eye or skin or heart	cor/o	**kohr**-ō	corectasis	12
purple	purpur/o	**pər**-pər-ō	purpura	4, 5
pus	py/o	**pī**-ō	pyoarthrosis, ureteropyosis	4, 14
pylorus	pylor/o	pī-**lohr**-ō	pyloric sphincter	10
radiation	radi/o	**rā**-dē-ō	radiodermatitis	5
radius	radi/o	**rā**-dē-ō	radiohumeral	5
rear, behind, after	poster/o	pō-**stēr**-ō	posterior	3
rectum	proct/o	**prohck**-tō	proctologist	10
rectum	rect/o	**rehck**-tō	rectalgia	10
red	eosin/o	ē-ō-**sihn**-ō	eosinophil	8
red	erythemat/o	ehr-ih-**thēm**-ah-tō	erythematous	8
red	erythr/o	eh-**rihth**-rō	erythrocyanosis, erythrocyte	5, 8
red	rubr/o	**rū**-brō	rubricity, rubric	5, 8
red	rubri-	**rū**-brih	rubricyte	8
remote, farther away from any point of reference	dist/o	**dihs**-tō	distal	3
removal, separation, reduction	de-	dē	deoxygenation	6
reproduction; sex organs	genit/o	**jehn**-eh-tō	genitalia	15
resembling	-oid	oyd	osteoid, myoid	2, 6
reticulum	reticul/o	reh-**tihck**-yoo-lō	reticulorumen	10
retina	retin/o	**reht**-ih-nō	neuroretinitis	12
returned sound	echo-	**ehck**-ō	echocardiogram	7
rhythm, regularly occurring motion	rhythm/o	**rihth**-mō	arrhythmia	7
ribs	cost/o	**kohs**-tō	costectomy, cervicocostal	2, 5
right or toward the right	dextr/o	**dehcks**-trō	dextroposition	3
rod, cylinder	rhabd/o	**rahb**-dō	rhabdomyoma	6
rounded projection, knob	tuber/o	**too**-bər-ō	tuberous	5

Definition of Word Part	Word Part	Pronunciation	Example Word	Chapter
rumen	rumen/o	**roo**-mehn-ō	rumenotomy	10
rumen	rumin/o	**roo**-mihn-ō	ruminant	10
sac containing fluid, a bladder	cyst/o	**sihs**-tō	pilocystic	4
sacrum	sacr/o	**sā**-krō	sacrocaudal	5
saliva, salivary gland	ptyal/o	**tī**-uh-lō	hypoptyalism	10
saliva, salivary gland	sial/o	sī-**ahl**-ō	sialectasis	10
salpinx; a trumpet-shaped tube, oviduct in the reproductive system	salping/o	sahl-**ping**-ō	salpingotomy, rhinosalpingitis	15
same, self	ipsi-	**ihp**-sē	ipsilateral	6
scanty, small	olig/o	**ohl**-ih-gō	oliguresis	14
scapula	scapul/o	**skahp**-yoo-lō	scapulopexy	5
secrete	crin/o	**krihn**-ō	endocrinology	13
self	aut/o	**ahw**-tō	autodermic	4
self, one's own	propri/o	**prō**-prē-ō	proprioception	12
serum	ser/o	**sehr**-ō	serosanguineous	8
several, more than one	plur/i	**ploor**-ē	pluripotent	8
short	brachy-	**brahk**-ē	brachydactyly	10
side	later/o	**laht**-ər-ō	lateral	3
similar	home/o	**hō**-mē-ō	homeostasis	9
skeleton	skelet/o	**skehl**-eh-tō	skeletal	5
skin	cor/o	**kohr**-ō	corium	4
skin	dermat/o	**dər**-mah-tō	dermatitis, dermatologist	3, 4
skin	derm/o	**dər**-mō	dermopathy, hypodermic	3, 4
skin	cutane/o	**kyoo-tā**-nē-ō	subcutaneous	4
slow	brady-	**brā**-dē	bradycardia	7
smell	osm/o	**ohz**-mō	aosmia	12
smell	odor/o	**ō**-dər-ō	malodorous	12
smell	olfact/o	ohl-**fahck**-tō	olfaction, olfactory nerve	9, 12
sodium	natr/o	**nā**-trō	hypernatremia	14
sodium	natr/i	**nā**-trē	natriuresis	14
soft, softening	malac/o	mah-**lā**-shō	osteomalacia	5
something small	-ule	ūhl	glandule	2
something small	-ole	ohl	ovariole	2
sound	audi/o	**ahw**-dē-ō	audiology	12
spasm (intermittent involuntary abnormal muscle contractions)	spasm/o	**spahz**-mō	myospasm	6
spermatozoa; male productive cell	spermat/o	**spər**-mah-tō	spermaturia	15
spermatozoa; male productive cell	sperm/o	**spər**-mō	spermous	15
spider, spider web	arachn/o	ah-**rahck**-nō	arachnoid	11
spinal cord or bone marrow	myel/o	mī-**eh**-lō	myelitis, neuromyelitis	5, 11
spine	spin/o	**spī**-nō	spinous	3
spitting	-ptysis	pah-**tuh**-sihs	hemoptysis	10
spleen	splen/o	**splehn**-ō	splenomyelomalacia	8

Continued

Definition of Word Part	Word Part	Pronunciation	Example Word	Chapter
star	astr/o	**ahs**-trō	astrocyte	11
starch	amyl/o	**ahm**-mehl-ō	amylodyspepsia	10
state, condition, action, process, or result	-tion	shuhn	absorption	2
state, condition, action, process, or result	-ism	ihsm	dwarfism	2
state, condition, action, process, or result	-sion	shuhn	exclusion	2
state, condition, action, process, or result	-ation	**ā**-shun	retardation	2
state, condition, action, process, or result	-sis	sihs	thesis	2
state, condition, action, process, or result	-ion	shun	vision	2
sternum, breastbone	stern/o	**stər**-nō	costosternoplasty	5
stiff, not movable, bent, crooked	ankyl/o	**ahng**-kih-lō	ankylosis	5
stomach in ruminants	abomas/o	ahb-ō-**mā**-sō	abomasopexy	10
stomach in simple-stomached animals	gastr/o	**gahs**-trō	gastropexy	10
stone	-lith	lihth	cholelith	10
stone	lith/o	**lihth**-ō	lithogenesis, nephrolithotomy	10, 14
stop, keep back, suppress	isch/o	**ihs**-kō	ischemia	7
stopping, slowing, or a stable state	-stasis	**stā**-sihs	diastasis, venostasis, arteriostasis	2, 7
straight, normal, correct	orth/o	**ohr**-thō	orthodigitia	5
structure, shape	morph/o	**mohr**-fō	morphology	8
structure, thing	-um	uhm	aquarium	2
structure, thing	-is	ihs	analysis	2
structure, thing	-a	ah	aquaria	2
structure, thing	-ium	**ē**-uhm	bacterium	2
study, or to have knowledge of	log/o	**lō**-gō	chondrology	2
study, or to have knowledge of	-logy	**lō**-jē	chondrology	2
sugar	glyc/o	**glī**-co	hypoglycemia	10
sugar	sacchar/o	**sahck**-ahr-ō	monosaccharide	10
surgical creation of a new permanent opening	-stomy	**stō**-mē	hysterosalpingostomy	4
surgical fixation, stabilization	-pexy	**pehck**-sē	hysteropexy	4
surgical incision	-tomy	**tō**-mē	craniotomy	4
surgical puncture	-centesis	sehn-**tē**-sihs	abdominocentesis, pericardiocentesis	4, 7
surgical removal	-ectomy	**ehck**-tō-mē	hysterectomy, onychectomy	2, 4
surgical repair	-plasty	**plahs**-tē	epidermatoplasty	4
suture	-rrhaphy	**rahf**-ē	dermorrhaphy	4
sweat	hidr/o	**hī**-drō	hidrosis	4
sweat	sudor/o	**soo**-dohr-ō	sudoral	4
swelling	edem/o	eh-**dē**-mō	dactyledema	7
system	system/o	sihs-**tehm**-ō	systemic	3
tail	caud/o	**kahw**-dō	caudal, caudectomy	3
tail	coccyg/o	kohck-**sihd**-jō	coccygectomy	5
tarsus	tars/o	**tahr**-sō	tibiotarsal	5
taste	gust/o	**guh**-stō	gustation	12
tears	dacry/o	**dahck**-rē-ō	dacryopyorrhea	12
tears	lacrim/o	**lahck**-rih-mō	nasolacrimal duct	12

Definition of Word Part	Word Part	Pronunciation	Example Word	Chapter
teeth	dent/o	**dehn**-tō	dentist	10
teeth	odont/o	ō-**dohn**-tō	odontopathy	10
teeth	dont/o	**dohn**-tō	orthodontic	10
tendon	tendin/o	**tehn**-dihn-ō	tendinitis, polytendinitis	3, 6
tendon	tendon/o	**tehn**-dohn-ō	tendonectomy, tendonitis	3, 6
tendon	tenont/o	**tehn**-ohnt-ō	tenontology, tenontomyoplasty	3, 6
tendon	ten/o	**tehn**-ō	tenophyte, tenotomy	3, 6
testicle	orch/o	**ohr**-kō	orchectomy	15
testicle	orchi/o	**ohr**-kē-ō	orchiectomy, orchialgia	15
testicle	orchid/o	**ohr**-kih-dō	orchidotomy	15
testicle	test/o	**tehs**-tō	testicular artery	15
thick	pachy-	**pahck**-ē	pachyderma, pachydermia	4, 5
thin, fine, slender, small	lept/o	**lehp**-tō	leptocephaly	11
thirst	dips/o	**dihp**-sō	polydipsia	10
thorax	thorac/o	**thōr**-ah-cō	thoracopathy, thoracoscopy	3, 5
three	tri-	trī	triphalangia	6
thrombus, clot	thromb/o	**throhm**-bō	thrombectomy	8
through, between, apart, across, complete	dia-	**dī**-ah	dialog, diagnosis, diadermal	2, 3
thyroid gland	thyr/o	**thī**-rō	thyroidectomy	13
tibia	tibi/o	**tihb**-ē-ō	femorotibial	5
tissue	histi/o	**hihs**-tē-ō	histiocytosis	3
tissue	hist/o	**hihs**-tō	histology	3
together, joined	syn-	sihn	synchondrosis, synergic muscles	5, 6
tongue	gloss/o	**glohs**-ō	glossopalatolabial	10
tongue	lingu/o	**lihng**-gwah-ō	lingual	10
touch	tact-	tahckt	tactile agnosis	12
toward	ad-	ahd	adneural, admaxillary, adductor muscles	5, 6
trachea, windpipe	trache/o	**trā**-kē-ō	tracheotomy, tracheostomy	9
tree, dendrite	dendr/o	**dehn**-drō	dendroid	11
tumor or abnormal new growth, a swelling	-oma	**ō**-mah	osteoma, multiple myeloma	2, 5
two	bi-	bī	bicycle, bicaudal	4, 6
two, twice, double	di-	dī	dichromic	6
ulna	uln/o	**uhl**-nō	ulnar	5
under, beneath, below	hypo-	**hī**-pō	hypodermic	3
ureter	ureter/o	ū-**rē**-tər-ō	ureteralgia	14
urethra	urethr/o	ū-**rē**-thrō	urethroscope, urethrocele	14, 15
urine	-uria	**uhr**-rē-ah	dysuria	14
urine	ur/o	**ū**-rō	uremia	14
uterus	hyster/o	**hihs**-tehr-ō	hysterosalpingo-oophorectomy, hysterectomy	2, 15
uterus	metr/o	**meh**-trō	metrorrhagia	15
uterus	uter/o	**ū**–tər-ō	uterocystostomy	15

Continued

Definition of Word Part	Word Part	Pronunciation	Example Word	Chapter
vagina	colp/o	**kohl**-pō	colpocentesis	15
vagina	vagin/o	vah-**jī**-nō	vaginodynia	15
valve	valvul/o	**vahl**-vū-lō	valvulosis	7
vein	ven/o	**vĕ**-nō	intravenous	7
vein	phleb/o	**flĕ**-bō	phlebotomy	7
ventricle (lower chamber of the heart)	ventricul/o	vehn-**trih**-kū-lō	atrioventricular	7
vertebra	vertebr/o	vehr-**tĕ**-brō	intervertebral	5
vertebral column, spine	spondyl/o	spohn-**dih**-lō	spondylosis	5
vessel (for blood or other fluids)	vas/o	**vahs**-ō	vasodilation	7
vessel, often a blood vessel	angi/o	**ahn**-jē-ō	hemangioma	7
vessel, often a blood vessel	ang/o	**ahn**-jō	periangitis	7
viscera (internal organs)	viscer/o	**vihs**-ər-ō	viscerate	3
vulva	episi/o	uh-**pē-zē**-ō	episiorrhaphy	15
vulva	vulv/o	**vuhl**-vō	vulvitis	15
water	hydr/o	**hī**-drō	hydrant, hydruria	4, 14
water, watery solution	aqua-	**ah**-kwah	aquatic	12
water, watery solution	aque/o	**ah**-kwē-ō	aqueous	12
white	leuc/o	**loo**-kō	leucocytometer	8
white	leuk/o	**loo**-kō	melanoleukoderma, leukocyte	5, 8
within	intra-	**ihn**-trah	intracellular	3
within, inner	endo-	**ehn**-dō	endoarthritis, endopelvic	3, 5
within, inner	end-	ehnd	endosteitis, endosteoma	3, 5
within, inside	intra-	**ihn**-trah	intracranial	5
without, no, not	a-	ah *or* ā	amyoplasia, acellular	4, 6
without, no, not	an-	ahn	anhidrosis, anerythroplasia	4, 6
work	erg/o	**ər**-gō	ergometer	6
written record produced, something recorded or written	-gram	grahm	myogram, arthrogram	4, 6
yellow	xanth/o	**zahn**-thō	xanthoma	5

Abbreviations

Abbreviation	Definition	Chapter
<	less than	10
>	greater than	10
µg	microgram	6
ad lib	as much as needed	6
Afib	atrial fibrillation	7
AI	artificial insemination	15
ASAP	as soon as possible	10
BAR	bright, alert, responsive	4
BD/LD	big dog/little dog	4
bid	twice a day	6
BM	bowel movement	10
bpm	beats (or breaths) per minute	7
BUN	blood urea nitrogen	14
BW	body weight	4
bx	biopsy	4
C	castrated	2
c or $\bar{c}$	with	7
cap	capsule	6
cath	catheter, catheterization	14
CBC	complete blood count	8
CC	chief complaint	4
cc	cubic centimeter	6
CCL	cranial cruciate ligament	5
CHF	congestive heart failure	7
cm	centimeter	6
CNS	central nervous system	11
CO_2	carbon dioxide	9
CPR	cardiopulmonary resuscitation	9
C-section	Cesarean section	15
CSF	cerebrospinal fluid	11
CVP	central venous pressure	7
cysto	cystocentesis or cystoscopic examination	14
DA	displaced abomasum	10

Abbreviation	Definition	Chapter
DDN	dull, depressed, nonresponsive	4
ddx	differential diagnosis	4
diff	differential white blood cell count	8
dL or dl	deciliter	6
DLH	domestic longhair (cat)	2
DNA	deoxyribonucleic acid	15
DOA	dead on arrival	4
DSH	domestic shorthair (cat)	2
dx	diagnosis	4
ECG	electrocardiogram	7
EDTA	ethylenediaminetetraacetic acid	8
EMG	electromyography	6
ETT	endotracheal tube	9
F	female, Fahrenheit	2
FLUTD	feline lower urinary tract disease	14
FUO	fever of unknown origin	4
fx	fracture	5
g	gram	6
GFR	glomerular filtration rate	14
GI	gastrointestinal	10
GSW	gunshot wound	4
Hb	hemoglobin	8
HBC	hit by car	4
Hct	hematocrit	8
Hgb	hemoglobin	8
HR	heart rate	7
hx	history	4
IA	intra-arterial	6
ICU	intensive care unit	10
ID	intradermal	6
IM	intramuscular	6
IP	intraperitoneal	6
IV	intravenous	6
K^+	potassium	14

Continued

Abbreviation	Definition	Chapter
K-9	canine (dog)	2
kg	kilogram	6
Ⓛ	left	4
L or l	liter	6
LA	large animal	2
lac	laceration	4
LDA	left displaced abomasum	10
LRI	lower respiratory infection	9
M	male	2
m	meter	6
mcg	microgram	6
med	medication	6
mg	milligram	6
mL or ml	milliliter	6
MM	mucous membrane, muscles	10
mm	millimeter	6
mm	mucous membrane, muscles, millimeter	10
N	neutered	2
NA or N/A	not applicable	10
Na$^+$	sodium	14
NPO	nothing by mouth	6
O$_2$	oxygen	9
oid	once a day	6
PCV	packed cell volume	8
PD	polydipsia	10
PE	physical exam	4
pH	potential hydrogen; scale to indicate degree of acidity or alkalinity	14
PLR	pupillary light reflex	12
PMN	polymorphonuclear	8
PO	by mouth, orally	6
PRN	as often as necessary, as needed	10
pt	patient	4
PU/PD	polyuria/polydipsia	14
q24h	once a day	6
qh	every hour	6

Abbreviation	Definition	Chapter
qid	4 times a day	6
QNS	quantity not sufficient	9
qxh	every x number of hours	6
Ⓡ	right	4
R/O	rule out	4
RAO	recurrent airway obstruction	9
RBC	red blood cell	8
RDA	right displaced abomasum	10
Rx	prescription	6
S	spayed	2
s or s̄	without	7
SA	small animal	2
SC	subcutaneous	6
SG	specific gravity	14
sid	once a day	6
sp gr	specific gravity	14
SQ	subcutaneous	6
Stat	immediately	4
subcu	subcutaneous	6
subq	subcutaneous	6
sx	surgery	5
tab	tablet	6
tid	3 times a day	6
TNTC	too numerous to count	8
TP	total protein	8
TPN	total parenteral nutrition	10
TPR	temperature, pulse, respiration	4
tx	treatment	6
UA	urinalysis	14
URI	upper respiratory infection	9
UTI	urinary tract infection	14
Vfib	ventricular fibrillation	7
WBC	white blood cell	8
wt	weight	4
xs	excessive	9
YOB	year of birth	4

Terms That Defy Word Analysis

Term	Definition	Chapter
aberrant	abnormal; deviating from the usual or ordinary	11
abortion	removal of an embryo or fetus from the uterus to end a pregnancy; a miscarriage is a spontaneous abortion	15
abrasion	a skin scrape	4
abscess	a localized collection of pus	4
acidic	pH less than 7.0 (neutral)	8
acute	sudden onset; having a short duration	2
afferent	to carry to or bring toward a place	11
agonal breathing	pertains to the last breaths taken near or at death, or after cardiac arrest; breathing is gasping and labored	9
alkaline	pH greater than 7.0 (neutral)	8
allodynia	a painful response to a normally nonpainful stimulus	12
alopecia	loss of hair, wool, or feathers	4
amplify	increase in size, effect, volume, extent, or amount	12
amplitude	the loudness of a sound	12
anomaly	a deviation from the average or norm	11
antagonistic	acting in opposition	13
antrum	cavity within a structure	10
aorta	large artery that directly leaves the heart to deliver blood to the body; largest artery in the body	7
aponeurosis	sheet-like dense fibrous collagenous connective tissue that binds muscles together or connects muscle to bone; the linea alba is an aponeurosis	6
artificial insemination (AI)	injecting semen into the vagina or uterus by use of a special syringe rather than by natural copulation	15
ascites	accumulation of fluid in the abdominal cavity; also known as *dropsy*	7
asthma	a chronic disease that often causes bronchoconstriction, making breathing difficult; sometimes caused by an allergic response	9
auscultate	to evaluate by listening, usually with the aid of a stethoscope	7
avulsion	an acute tendon injury in which the tendon is forcibly torn away from its attachment site on the bone	6
axon	the long branch off a nerve cell (neuron) that carries impulses away from the cell	11
benign	does not recur and has a favorable outlook for recovery	2
blood–brain barrier	the separation of brain nervous tissue (which is bathed in a clear cerebrospinal fluid) from capillaries within the brain tissue	11
borborygmus	a rumbling noise that gas makes as it moves through the stomach and intestines	10
bowel	another name for the intestines	10
cachexia	generalized wasting of the body as a result of disease	10
calculus	a stone	14

Continued

	Definition	Chapter
callus	a bridge that forms as part of the healing process across the two halves of a bone fracture; composed of cartilage that becomes ossified over time	5
cannon bone	the lay term for the third metacarpal or metatarsal bone in four-legged mammals such as cattle and horses; located between the hock and fetlock joints	5
canthus	the corner of each eye formed by the junction of the upper and lower eyelids; there is a lateral and a medial canthus for each eye	12
carbuncle	a group of furuncles in adjacent hairs	4
catheter	tube for injecting or removing fluids	14
cerebellum	"little brain"; the second-largest portion of the brain	11
cerebrum	the largest portion of the brain	11
Cesarean section	C-section; surgical delivery of a fetus through an incision in the dam's abdominal wall	15
chronic	slow onset; an abnormal condition that lasts a long time	2
chyme	a semifluid mass of partially digested food that enters the small intestine from the stomach	10
cicatrix	(*plural* = cicatrices)—a scar	4
cilia	(*singular* = cilium)—small, hair-like structures on the surface of the epithelium that beat rhythmically; originates from the Latin word for "eyelash"	9
circadian rhythm	biological cycles that occur at approximately 24-hour intervals	13
clitoris	a sensitive female external organ homologous to the penis; an erectile body	15
clonic spasm	alternating spasm and muscle relaxation	6
cochlea	snail shell—spiral organ in the inner ear that turns sound waves into sensory impulses	12
concretion	a solid or calcified mass formed by disease and found in a body cavity or tissue	14
condyle	smooth end of a bone that forms part of a joint	5
congenital	pertaining to a condition existing at birth or dating from birth	15
conjunctiva	the mucous membrane that lines the exposed portion of the eyeball and the inner surface of the eyelids	12
constipation	bowel movements that are infrequent or hard to pass	10
cornus	horn	15
corpus	body	15
corpus callosum	"tough body"; the bundle of nerve fibers that connect the right and left hemispheres of the cerebrum	11
cortex	"outer shell"; the outer layer of nervous tissue in the brain	11
cough	reflex stimulated by irritation or foreign matter in the trachea or bronchi	9
creatinine	the end-product of muscle metabolism; waste product excreted in urine	14
crest	a raised ridge along the surface of a bone	5
cud	the portion of partially digested food that a ruminant returns to the mouth for further mastication before sending it to the omasum	10
cull	take out an animal (especially an inferior one) from a herd; or reduce the size of a herd or flock by removing a proportion of its members	5
deciduous	temporary teeth; also known as milk teeth or baby teeth	10
denude	loss of epidermis, caused by exposure to urine, feces, body fluids, wound drainage, or friction; not associated with necrosis of the tissue	14
diaphragm	a thin, dome-shaped sheet of muscle that separates the thorax from the abdomen	9
diestrous animals	species that have two estrous cycles per year; dogs	15
displacement	movement of one segment of the digestive tract to an abnormal location	10
distention	abnormal enlargement of a part of the digestive tract	10

Term	Definition	Chapter
DNA	deoxyribonucleic acid—the molecule that carries the genetic information (genetic code) that is the basis of heredity	15
dura mater	"tough mother"; the thick, fibrous outer membrane covering the brain	11
dystocia	abnormally slow, difficult birth	15
ecchymosis	blood leaking from a ruptured blood vessel into subcutaneous tissue; a bruise	4
ectopic pregnancy	abnormal development of an embryo occurring somewhere other than inside the lumen of the uterus, usually in the oviduct; also known as *eccyesis*	15
edema	excess fluid accumulation around the cells of connective tissue	7
efferent	to carry out or take away from a place	11
electrolyte	chemical element (e.g., potassium, sodium) that carries an electrical charge when dissolved in water; proper balance in blood is maintained by the kidneys	14
embolism	abnormal material circulating in blood that could become lodged in a vessel and block blood flow; could be composed of a blood clot, parasites, fat, gas bubbles, or clumps of bacteria	8
emesis	vomiting of food from the stomach	10
emetic	a substance that causes vomiting	10
emphysema	overexpansion of alveolar walls causing the walls to break down and block other airways, resulting in less oxygen/carbon dioxide exchange in the lungs	9
endorphin	a compound produced in the brain and in other body tissues that reduces the sensation of pain; the body's natural painkiller	13
enema	injection of a fluid into the rectum to stimulate a bowel movement	10
enzootic	a disease found in nearly every animal of a species within a limited geographical area; a disease embedded in an area that will occur naturally in unprotected animals	2
enzyme	protein produced by living cells that initiates a chemical reaction (e.g., digestion) but is not affected by the reaction	10
epidemic	the equivalent of an epizootic in human medicine	2
epithelium	the cells that cover the internal and external body surfaces and also form many glands	4
epizootic	a disease that appears suddenly and spreads rapidly over a large geographical area like a state, province, or country	2
eructation	burp; the method by which ruminants continually get rid of fermentation gases	10
eschar	dried serum, blood, pus; a scab; the charred surface of a burn	4
estrous	an adjective used to describe events associated with the breeding cycle	15
estrus	a noun; the period when the female accepts the male	15
eustachian tube	also known as the *auditory canal;* a canal that runs from the middle ear to the pharynx	12
exacerbation	worsening severity of a disease	2, 5
excoriate	scratch the skin	4
fatigue	muscle contractions get feebler under repeated stimulation until they stop altogether	6
fecund	fertile; capable of producing offspring	15
fetus	an animal in later stages of development within the womb	15
fibrillation	rapid, irregular myocardial contractions resulting in loss of a simultaneous heartbeat and pulse	7
filtration	process in the kidney whereby blood pressure forces materials through a filter (the glomerulus)	14
fimbria	a fringe-like structure, found in the infundibulum of the oviduct	15
fissure	a crack-like lesion in the skin	4
flatus	intestinal gas produced by the action of bacteria	10
follicle	a small cavity or sac	15
foramen	small opening or perforation	5

Continued

Term	Definition	Chapter
fossa	a depression, trench, or hollow area	5
fracture	a break or rupture	5
frequency	the pitch of a sound	12
friable	crumbly, easily crumbled	9
furcation	divided, branched	9
furuncle	a boil or skin abscess, usually around follicles	4
gamete	a mature sexual reproduction cell; a sperm or an ovum	15
ganglia	(*singular* = ganglion)—cell bodies in the peripheral nervous system that cluster together in groups	11
gavage	tube-feeding through a stomach tube	10
geriatric	pertaining to old age or the aging process	11
gland	a group of specialized cells in the body that produce and secrete a specific substance, such as a hormone	13
globin	protein; the protein portion of hemoglobin and myoglobin	8
globulin	a class of simple proteins that are insoluble in water	8
granulation tissue	new tissue that grows to fill in a wound defect	4
gyrus	(*plural* = gyri)—a convolution or raised area between grooves	11
head	rounded proximal end of a bone (e.g., femur); also the end of a muscle nearest the origin	5
heat	a common name for estrus	15
heatstroke	a considerable elevation in body temperature (hyperthermia)	12
hermaphroditism	a condition whereby an animal has both male and female reproductive organs	15
hiccups	spasms of the diaphragm accompanied by sudden closing of the glottis; may be caused by nerve irritation, indigestion, or central nervous system damage; most often temporary and harmless	9
hook bones	in cattle, the two prominent raised areas on either side of the tailhead and backbone; the caudal raised area is the pin bone, and the cranial raised area is the hook bone	5
hormone	a substance produced by one tissue or by one group of cells that is carried by the bloodstream to another tissue or organ to affect its physiological functions such as metabolism or growth	13
humor	an antiquated word meaning any one of the four cardinal fluids in the body: blood, phlegm, yellow bile, and black bile	12
hyperesthesia	an increased response to a painful stimulus	12
hypothalamus	the part of the brain that links the endocrine system to the nervous system	11
idiopathic	a disease of unknown origin	2
ileus	lack of neuromuscular control of the intestines, which prevents ingesta from moving through the intestines at a normal rate	10
impaction	physical blockage of one part of the digestive tract by abnormal amounts of material	10
impulse	an electrical signal that travels along an axon	11
in vitro	within a glass, test tube, or other container outside the body	2
in vivo	within a living body	2
induced ovulator	species that must be bred before they ovulate; cats	15
infarct	a localized area of tissue that is dying or dead because of lack of blood supply	7
infection	invasion and multiplication of a disease-causing organism in a body tissue	2
inflammation	tissue response to injury or destruction, with signs of pain and swelling, redness, and a feeling of warmth; inflammation does not necessarily mean that an infection is involved—only that tissue is injured	2
infundibulum	the flared end of a funnel-shaped duct or passageway such as the oviduct	15
ingest	to take into the body (e.g., food, liquids)	10
ingesta	ingested material, especially food taken into the body via the mouth	10

Term	Definition	Chapter
intussusception	slipping or telescoping of one part of a tubular organ into a lower portion, causing obstruction; seen especially in the intestines	10
keloid	an overgrowth of scar tissue at the site of injury	4
kyphosis	abnormal convex curvature of the spine	11
laceration	a rough or jagged skin tear	4
lavage	washing out a hollow organ by rinsing with fluid that is introduced into the organ and suctioned out	7
laxative	a substance that induces bowel movements or loosens the stool; most often taken to relieve constipation	10
lesion	localized pathological change in an organ or tissue; a wound or injury	10
lethargic	drowsy, dull, listless, unenergetic	8
luxation	a joint dislocation where the joint is displaced or goes out of alignment	5
malignant	becoming progressively worse, recurring, leading to death	2
matrix	a surrounding-substance in which something else is contained	12
melena	passing dark, tarry feces containing blood that has been acted upon by bacteria in the intestines	10
micturition	urination; also called *voiding*	14
miosis (myosis)	prolonged constriction of the pupil of the eye	12
modulate	change, regulate, adjust	12
monestrous animals	animals that cycle only one time per year; wolves, foxes, bears	15
morbidity	the number of animals in a population that become sick expressed as a percent of the entire population; also known as the *morbidity rate*	2
mortality	the number of animals in a population that die from a disease expressed as a percent of the entire population; also known as the *mortality rate*	2
murmur	an atypical heart sound associated with a functional or structural valve abnormality	7
mutant	the result of altered DNA; a genetic abnormality	15
mydriasis	prolonged dilation of the pupil of the eye	12
myelin	a fatty, white substance that surrounds some axons and is produced by special cells in the central nervous system	11
natal	birth	15
neural transmission	passage of a nerve impulse across a synapse	12
neutral	pH = 7.0, neither acidic or alkaline	8
nocturnal	active at night	12
nosocomial	hospital-acquired	10
occlude	to close off or shut	8
occlusion	the way the upper and lower teeth line up against each other	10
olecranon	large process on the proximal end of the ulna that forms the point of the elbow; literally means "the head of the elbow"	5
oosik	the os penis of a walrus	5
palliative	treating the symptoms, but not curing the cause	4
papilla	(*plural* = papillae)—a small, round, or cone-shaped projection or peg on the top of the tongue that may contain taste buds	12
papule	a small, solid, usually somewhat pointed elevation of the skin; does not contain pus but is inflamed	4
paralumbar fossa	the dorsal area of the flank; the dorsal, soft, triangular portion of the flank	10

Continued

Term	Definition	Chapter
paranasal sinus	a hollow cavity in the skull connected to the nasal passages; usually just called a *sinus*	9
parenchyma	the functional tissue of an organ, as opposed to supporting tissue	14
perception	conscious interpretation of sensory information	12
perineum	the region between the scrotum and the anus in males; also the region between the vulva and the anus in females	15
peristalsis	a progressive wave of contraction and relaxation of the smooth muscles in the wall of the digestive tract that moves food through the digestive tract	10
petechia	(*plural* = petechiae)—tiny ecchymosis within the dermal layer	4
pH	potential hydrogen; a scale from 0 to 14 that measures the acidity or alkalinity of a substance	8
pheromone	a liquid substance released in very small quantities by an animal that causes a specific response if it is detected by another animal of the same species	12
pia mater	"delicate, soft mother"; the thin, innermost membrane covering the brain	11
pin bones	in cattle, the two prominent raised areas on either side of the tailhead and backbone; the caudal raised area is the pin bone, and the cranial raised area is the hook bone	5
pinna	ear flap	12
pituitary	the master endocrine gland that affects nearly all hormonal activity in the body	11
placenta	a vascular, membranous organ between a mother and her offspring in the womb, formed by membranes from the mother and the embryo, providing nourishment to and taking waste products away from the embryo/fetus during the entire pregnancy	15
plaque	a raised, flat papule greater than 1 cm	4
polyestrous animals	species that have estrous cycles throughout the year; humans, cattle, pigs	15
potential space	the space or cavity that can exist between two adjacent body parts that are not tightly adjoined; does not appear during normal functioning	11
presentation	the orientation of the fetus when parturition begins	15
process	a natural outgrowth or projection	5
proud flesh	overgrowth of granulation tissue at the site of injury; also known as *exuberant granulation tissue* (horses)	4
pruritus	itching	4
pseudocyesis	false pregnancy; the physical symptoms of pregnancy develop without conception	15
purulent	containing or consisting of pus	4
pyometra	an accumulation of pus in the uterus; the cervix can be open (open pyometra) or closed (closed pyometra)	15
receptor	a protein molecule on a cell wall with a unique shape that will allow only one type of molecule, such as a hormone, to attach to it	13
reflex	automatic, unthinking reaction or behavior	10
regurgitation	bringing back to the mouth food that has not yet reached the stomach	10
relapse	to fall back into a disease state after an apparent recovery	10
remission	improvement in or absence of signs of disease	2
retained placenta	all or part of the placenta is left in the uterus after the third stage of labor	15
retch	involuntary spasms of ineffective vomiting; dry heaves	10
retrograde	inverted, reversed, backward, recede, deteriorate	10
rigor mortis	temporary muscular stiffening that follows death, resulting from lack of energy to allow muscle fibers to relax	6
ruminal tympany	overdistention of the reticulorumen as a result of rumen gas being trapped in the rumen when the ruminant is unable to eructate; also known as *bloat* or *hoven*	10
rumination	bringing ingesta from the reticulorumen back to the mouth, followed by remastication and reswallowing	10

Term	Definition	Chapter
seasonally polyestrous animals	species that have more than one estrous cycle per year, but only during certain times of the year (e.g., spring, fall); cats, horses, sheep, goats, hamsters	15
sedative	a drug that depresses (makes it quieter) an animal and slows down body functions; no painkilling action	12
sensation	awareness of stimuli from the environment	12
sensory receptor	a nerve ending that responds to a stimulus, found in the internal or external environment of an animal; sends an impulse to the brain	12
sensory transduction	conversion of a signal from one form (e.g., light) to another (e.g., electrical impulse)	12
sepsis	the systemic inflammatory response induced by invasion and multiplication of a disease-causing organism	4
shivers	rapid involuntary muscle contractions that release waste heat, which will warm the animal's body; seen in response to a cold environment	6
sigh	a deep breath through the nose that usually is taken in response to a slightly low blood oxygen level or a slightly high blood carbon dioxide level	9
signalment	a detailed description, including distinctive features, of an animal	4
signs	the objective evidence of disease; observable indicators like body temperature and bleeding	2
sinus	a cavity, recess, or passage in any organ or tissue	9
slough	a mass or layer of necrotic tissue that separates from the underlying healthy tissue	14
sneeze	similar to a cough, but the irritation is in the nasal passages	9
solute	a substance dissolved in a solution (e.g., glucose in blood)	14
spasm	an acute involuntary muscle contraction	6
sphincter	a circular band of voluntary or involuntary muscle that encircles an opening of the body or one of its hollow organs	10
spine	a hard, pointed process that runs the length of the lateral surface of the scapula	5
sprain	the result of stretching or tearing a ligament, which connects bone/cartilage to bone/cartilage	5
sterile	not able to produce offspring; can affect both males and females	15
stillborn	born dead	15
strain	the result of stretching or tearing a ligament, which connects bone/cartilage to bone/cartilage	5
stranguria	painful urination due to muscle spasms in the urinary bladder and urethra	14
subluxation	a partial dislocation of a joint	5
sulcus	a groove	11
suppurate	to produce or discharge pus	4
suture	the line of junction of two bones forming an immovable joint	5
symptoms	the subjective evidence of disease as reported by the patient; what the patient tells you is wrong	2
synapse	the junction across which a nerve impulse passes from an axon to another neuron, a muscle cell, or a gland cell	11
synchronized estrus	the use of hormones to create a group of females that will come into estrus at the same time; used with artificial insemination	15
syrinx	a pathological tube-shaped lesion in the brain or spinal cord	11
target cells	cells that have appropriate receptors on their cell walls to allow attachment of a specific molecule	13
teat	nipple of the breast or mammary gland	15
tetanus	painful, sustained muscle contractions caused by toxins released from the *Clostridium tetani* bacteria	6
tetany	intermittent, painful, sustained muscle contractions related to defective calcium metabolism	6
thalamus	the part of the brain that relays sensory impulses to the cerebral cortex	11
thrombus	a blood clot that forms and adheres to the wall of a blood vessel at its site of formation (it becomes an embolus when it breaks away from the endothelium and circulates in blood)	8

Continued

Term	Definition	Chapter
tonic spasm	a continuous spasm	6
topical	applied to, designed for, or an action on the surface of the body	4
torsion	twisting or rotating on a long axis	10
tranquilizer	a drug that makes the animal less anxious; no painkilling action	12
trochanter	two knobs at the proximal end of the femur where muscles of the thigh and pelvis attach	5
tuberosity	a rough projection on a bone; usually an area of muscle attachment	5
tumor	any mass or swelling; a nodule greater than 2 cm	4
turbinate	scroll-shaped bone on the wall of a nasal passage; also known as a *nasal concha* (shell-shaped)	9
ulcer	a circumscribed crater-like lesion of the skin or mucous membrane; a depressed lesion on the skin or mucous membrane accompanied by inflammation, pus formation, and necrosis	4, 10
urea	a water-soluble, nitrogen-based compound that is the waste material of protein metabolism by the body's cells; a major component of mammalian urine	14
ventilate	breathing in and out	9
ventilator	a machine that artificially moves air into and out of the lungs	9
viable	capable of living, workable, capable of being done	10
vitreous	resembling glass	12
volvulus	abnormal twisting of the intestines, causing an obstruction	10
wheal	(hives, urticaria)—a circumscribed, elevated papule (pimple) caused by localized edema (collection of fluid between cells)	4
wings	transverse processes on the first cervical vertebra (atlas) so named because they give the appearance of wings on the bone	5
yawn	a slow, deep breath taken through the wide open mouth; can be caused by mildly low blood oxygen levels, fatigue, boredom, or drowsiness	9
zoology	the study of animal life	2
zoonosis	a disease transmitted from animals to humans (noun)	2
zoonotic	a disease transmitted from animals to humans (adjective)	2
zygote	a cell produced by the union of two gametes	15

Note: Page numbers followed by f indicate figures; t, tables; and b, boxes.